Backpacking **Idaho**

From the book . . .

SNAKE RIVER TRAIL (TRIP 5)

Your efforts are rewarded by the superb scenery, which features a continuous series of amazing views of the raging river, the ruggedly contorted canyon walls, and even occasional glimpses of the high Summit Ridge in Oregon.

CHAMBERLAIN BASIN LOOP (TRIP 8)

Try to picture what the American mountain west looked like 200 years ago. . . . One of those scenes sometimes pictured in Western movies showing vast forests, an endless series of lonesome ridges and peaks, pristine lakes, and lots of wildlife. Now . . . head for the Frank Church–River of No Return Wilderness . . . perhaps the last place where you can still hike for days, weeks, or even months, and never even come close to a road.

MIDDLE FORK SALMON RIVER (TRIP 11)

Like all of the hot springs in this canyon, this is a great place to spend some time soaking sore muscles and enjoying the scenery.

PETTIT LAKE: HELL ROARING LOOP (TRIP 15)

Lake Lucille is surely one of the most spectacular lakes in the Sawtooth Mountains. It is backed on three sides by tall spires and reddish-colored cliffs and is one of those spots that really has to be seen to be appreciated.

BIG BOULDER LAKES (TRIP 17)

Every one of these bodies of water is tucked amid rocky shores, flower fields, and shimmering mountains of incredible beauty. The larger lakes even have fish. For added scenic interest, as if any were needed, the stream connecting the larger lakes tumbles over lovely little cascades and small waterfalls, and pink and white heather scattered all around provide color.

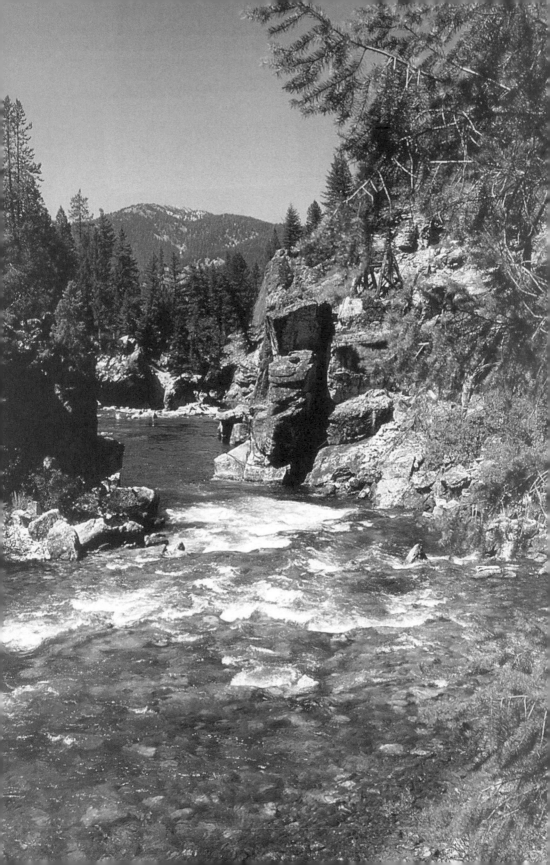

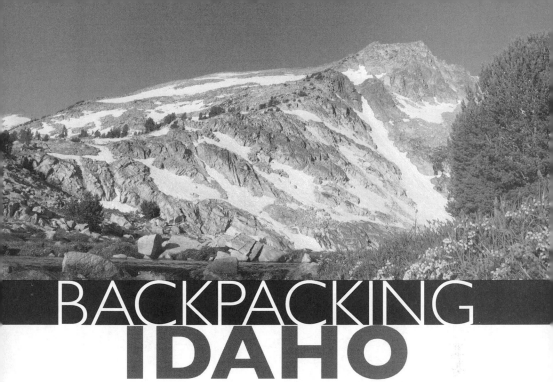

BACKPACKING
IDAHO

From Alpine Peaks to Desert Canyons

DOUGLAS LORAIN

 WILDERNESS PRESS . . . **on the trail since 1967**

Backpacking Idaho: From Alpine Peaks to Desert Canyons
2nd Edition 2015, third printing 2022

Library of Congress Cataloging-in-Publication Data

Lorain, Douglas, 1962-
  Backpacking Idaho / Doug Lorain. — Second edition.
     pages cm
  "Distributed by Publishers Group West"—T.p. verso.
  Includes index.
  ISBN 978-0-89997-773-7 (pbk.) — ISBN 0-89997-773-1 — ISBN 978-0-89997-774-4 (ebook)
     1. Backpacking—Idaho—Guidebooks. 2. Idaho—Guidebooks. I. Title.
  GV199.44.I24L67 2015
  796.5109796—dc23
                                    2014047531

Manufactured in the United States of America

Published by: **WILDERNESS PRESS**
             An imprint of AdventureKEEN
             2204 First Avenue South, Suite 102
             Birmingham, AL 35233
             800-678-7006; fax 877-374-9016
             info@wildernesspress.com
             wildernesspress.com

Visit our website for a complete listing of our books and for ordering information.

Distributed by Publishers Group West

Front cover photos (clockwise from top): Emerald Lake in the Four Lakes Basin (Trip 16), an outlet creek from Sapphire Lake (Trip 17), a meadow below Lake 10,148 (Trip 18), and a section of the remote East Fork Owyhee River Canyon (Trip 25).

Back cover photo: White Cloud Peaks from Ants Basin (Trip 16).

Frontispiece: Dagger Falls (Trip 10)

SAFETY NOTICE: Although Wilderness Press and the author have made every attempt to ensure that the information in this book is accurate at press time, they are not responsible for any loss, damage, injury, or inconvenience that may occur to anyone while using this book. You are responsible for your own safety and health while in the wilderness. The fact that a trail is described in this book does not mean that it will be safe for you. Be aware that trail conditions can change from day to day. Always check local conditions and know your own limitations.

CONTENTS

FEATURED TRIPS

OTHER BACKPACKING TRIPS

Map Legend

─────────	Paved road
─────────	Gravel road
─────────	Dirt road
= = = = = = = = = =	Primitive road (may require four-wheel drive)
▬ ▬ ▬ ▬ ▬ ▬	Featured trail
- - - - - - - - - - - - - - -	Other trail
• • • • • • • • • • • • • • •	Cross-country route
⬭	Lake
∿∿∿	Stream/falls/major rapids
∿∿∿	Intermittent creek
♂	Spring
⤬	Pass
▲ *6844′*	Mountain (with elevation)
🔭	Fire lookout
🅰	Car campground
🅰	Backcountry campsite
🅣	Featured trailhead (with parking)
🅿	Parking
(12)	US highway
(75)	State highway
281	Forest Service road
✈	Airport/landing strip
■	Point of interest/building

ACKNOWLEDGMENTS

The help of many people made this book possible. First of all, I would like to thank the many wilderness rangers and fellow hikers who provided trip companionship, reviewed some of the material, and offered recommendations.

SPECIAL THANKS GO TO THE FOLLOWING PEOPLE:

My occasional hiking partner—Dave Elsbernd.

My friends—Bob, Barbara, and Natalie Fink, who graciously provided this dirty, bedraggled author with a place to shower, do laundry, and resupply on one of my long trips while doing research for this book.

As usual, my sister, Christine Ebrahimi, was invaluable in providing answers for all questions botanical.

The leaders and friendly young men of Boy Scout Troop 152 in Rigby, Idaho, who kindly provided this tired hiker with much needed transport that saved me many miles of arduous road walking during a spell of record 100°F weather.

Most of all, for her continuing love, support, and willingness to take care of house and home while her husband is off exploring new trails, I thank my wife, Becky Lovejoy.

While the contributions and assistance of the persons listed above were invaluable, all of the text, maps, and photos herein are my own work and sole responsibility. Any and all omissions, errors, and just plain stupid mistakes are strictly mine.

FEATURED TRIPS SUMMARY CHART

RATINGS (1–10)			LENGTH		ELEVATION GAIN
SCENERY	SOLITUDE	DIFFICULTY	DAYS	MILES	
10	6	6	4–7	54	5,300'
9	10	8	2–4	19	3,400'
7	5	5	4–6	50	4,200'
8	9	8	4–6	45	10,300'
10	9	8	4–5	38	11,200'
8	6	5	2–4	33	5,850'
9	7	6	3–4	30	5,800'
8	7	5	3–4	25	2,800'
5	7	7	4–7	50	10,300'
7	6	7	3–5	40	7,500'
9	4	6	3–6	46	9,000'
7	6	6	3–4	37	8,200'
9	7	5	3–4	37	8,100'
9	8	9	3	18	4,200'
9	3	6	6–10	65	12,700'
8	8	7	3–4	27	6,100'
7	7	6	3–5	27	5,450'
9	3	5	3–4	30	6,000'
10	5	8	3–5	31	6,850'
10	3	6	3–5	19	4,050'
7	3	3	3–5	41	1,700'
7	5	9	3–5	41	11,350'
7	8	10	5–8	68	12,150'
7	6	6	6–8	67	4,200'
8	6	8	3–6	45	9,800'

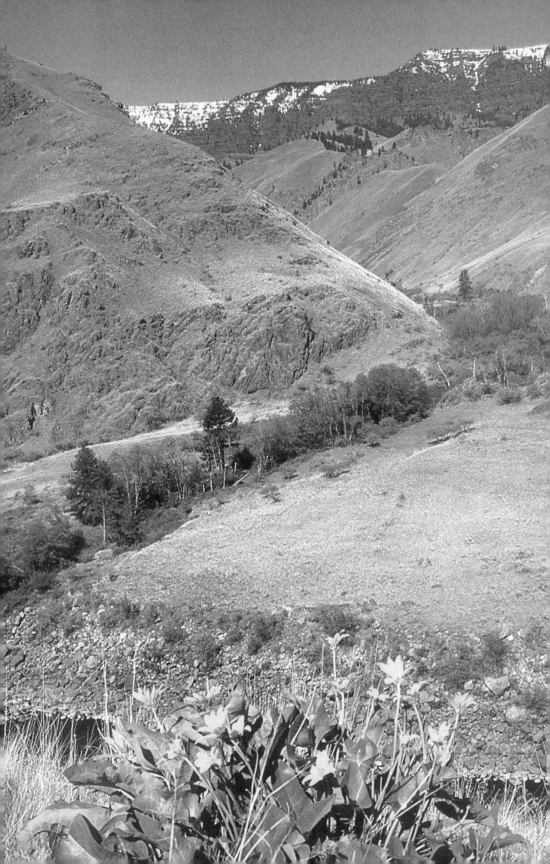

INTRODUCTION

I daho is a virtually undiscovered backpacker's paradise. Though the state has millions of acres of wilderness, it has no national parks and few well-known destinations to draw the crowds. As a result, Idaho remains a great place to "get away from it all."

What all those crowds heading for more famous hiking areas don't realize is that Idaho hides some of North America's most beautiful scenery. The mountains of Idaho are at least as scenic as anything found elsewhere in the American West and, in fact, they are far better than most. The canyon country is great too and is, if possible, even more spectacular than the mountains. These great gashes in the earth are incomparable in their depth, their scenic grandeur, and the abundance of their wildlife.

Idaho's nearly ideal climate helps to make exploring the state's natural wonders a joy. The weather here is consistently better than in bordering geographic regions, with fewer thunderstorms than in the Rocky Mountain states to the south and east, and much less rain than in soggy Oregon and Washington to the west. So Idaho boasts the ideal combination of solitude, outstanding scenery, and good weather—in other words, Shangri-la for backpackers.

There are many ways to see and appreciate the beauty of Idaho. Many parts of the state can be seen just as easily on day hikes, rafting trips, bicycle tours, or even from your car. The focus of *this* book, however, is on the best ways for *backpackers* to see the state. Most of Idaho's best scenery is far from roads and can be truly appreciated only by those willing to hit the trails. After many years and thousands of trail miles, I have selected what I believe to be Idaho's very best backpacking trips. The focus is on longer trips—from three days to two weeks. These go beyond a simple weekend outing, but they make terrific vacations, and give you enough time to fully appreciate the scenery. Best of all, you'll have the chance to really get to know and love the state.

Opposite: Scenery above Rush Creek Rapids (Trip 5)

1

A WORD ABOUT THE SECOND EDITION

Thanks to the consistent support of backpackers from every corner of Idaho and beyond, *Backpacking Idaho* now proudly goes into its second edition, bigger and better than ever. Readers familiar with the first edition will recognize the user-friendly format as well as most of the trips, but they will also find four exceptional, all-new outings to explore.

A few of the trips from the first edition have been taken out, mostly to make room for the new trips that offer even better scenery and are more enjoyable overall to hike. I have also made major revisions to five of the trips that were retained from the first edition, adding excellent new side trips, changing the recommended ending points to remove poor road access or add new areas of great scenery, or removing areas where trails have now been destroyed or abandoned. One of the trips (Trip 18 in the Pioneer Mountains) has been changed so much that it is effectively a new trip as well.

Though these old trips have been, I believe, significantly improved, most readers will probably be more excited about the new trips. Most of these great new adventures are in parts of the state unfamiliar to many Idaho outdoor lovers, and some have never been fully described in any guidebook before. A wildlife-rich corner of the Selway-Bitterroot Wilderness, a spectacular string of alpine lakes tucked away in the virtually unknown Italian Peaks region, some of the best alpine scenery in North America (no exaggeration) in the trailless upper basin of the Big Boulder Lakes, and amazing views into the dramatic depths of one of the most impressive but almost-never-visited system of desert canyons in the United States—all await your discovery on these hikes.

In addition to the new trips and major changes to some of the old ones, all of the original hikes have been carefully updated, new and improved maps are included for all trips, and a wealth of new photos is to be found throughout this edition for you to really see the beauties of the backcountry of Idaho. Also, nearly every trip now includes a section at the end that describes the best way for readers to at least get a sampling of the beauties of the described area in day hikes or shorter backpacking trips.

Finally, in line with suggestions from readers of the first edition, I have made an effort in this edition to include a few more somewhat-shorter trips for those with less time for a backcountry vacation, and trips that are best suited for those who prefer to hike into a base camp and then explore from there. On the other end of the spectrum, a few readers have asked for suggestions on trips that include some challenging off-trail sections, so I have included a couple of those as well.

I invite all readers, whether you're new to hiking and this book or already wearing boots worn ragged from years of backpacking, to use this second edition as a guide to many years of great adventures in the wildlands of Idaho. I hope you enjoy touring these trails as much as I did.

HOW TO USE THIS GUIDE

Each featured trip begins with an information box that provides a quick overview of the hike's vital statistics and important features. This lets you rapidly narrow down your options based on your preferences, your abilities, how many days you have available, and the time of year.

Scenery: This is a subjective opinion of the trip's overall scenic quality, on a 1-to-10 scale, with 1 being an eyesore and 10 being absolutely gorgeous. This rating reflects my personal biases in favor of flowers, photogenic views, and clear streams. If your tastes run more toward lush forests or rolling grasslands, then your own rating may be quite different. Also keep in mind that the rating is relative. All the featured trips are beautiful, and if they were located almost anywhere else in North America, they would justifiably draw crowds of admirers.

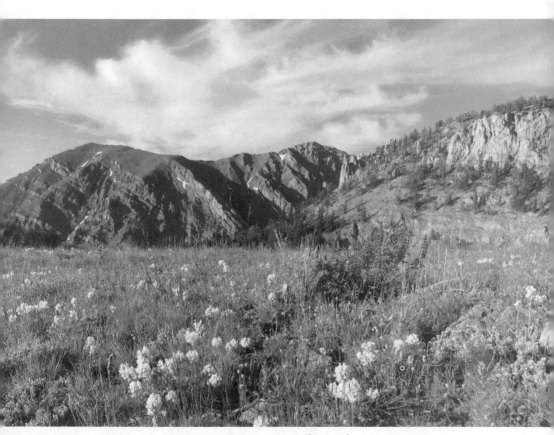

Looking south from the ridge above Webber Creek (Trip 21)

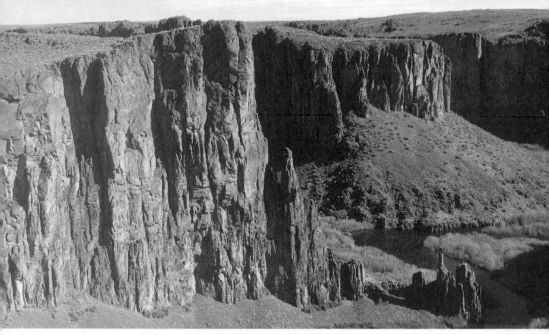

Rock pinnacles beside Owyhee River at The Tules (Trip 25)

Solitude: Because solitude is one of the things that backpackers are seeking, it helps to know roughly how much company you can expect. This rating is also on a 1-to-10 scale, with 1 meaning you'll need stilts to see over the crowds, and 10 meaning it will be just you and the mountain goats. It is worth noting, however, that by comparison to almost any other state, the Idaho backcountry is remarkably free of crowds. With few exceptions, it is rare to see more than one or two other parties during a full day of hiking. In the years of research for this book, I spent hundreds of memorable nights camped near scenic lakes, fish-filled streams, and other idyllic locations throughout Idaho, and more than 75% of the time I had these choice spots all to myself. Hikers who are accustomed to the relatively crowded trails of other states should, therefore, take this rating with a grain of salt.

Difficulty: This is yet another subjective judgment. The rating is intended to deter you from the most difficult outings if you're not in shape to try them. The scale is relative only to other backpacking trips. Many Americans would find even the easiest backpacking trip to be a very strenuous undertaking. So this 1-to-10 scale is only for people already accustomed to backpacking, and 1 means you're practically still on the La-Z-Boy, while 10 means you may as well be doing the Ironman Triathlon.

Mileage: This is the total mileage of the recommended trip in its most basic form, including only those side trips that are integral to the basic itinerary. I have never, however, seen the point of a bare-bones, Point-A-to-Point-B kind of trip. After all, if you're going to go, you may as well explore a bit. Thus, for many trips, there is a second mileage number (in parentheses) that includes distances for additional recommended side trips. These side trips are also shown on the maps and included in the "Possible Itinerary" section.

I have made every reasonable effort (and some unreasonable ones) to ensure that the mileages shown are accurate. However, users should not assume that the numbers are exact. Idaho hiking guidebooks are notoriously lax about including mileages. Wilderness maps for the state rarely, if ever, include mileages. Even the distances indicated on trail signs (when they are given at all) are often contradictory and usually unreliable.

The overall trip mileages for this book are shown to the nearest 1 mile (0.5 mile for short distances) and are based on a combination of map extrapolation and my own pedometer readings. These numbers can be considered accurate to within a margin of error of perhaps +/- 10%. To attempt to give mileages with any more precision would give the reader a false sense of accuracy. Hikers accustomed to tracking their progress with a higher degree of precision will need to adjust their mindset. Such exactness is not possible when traveling in the vast backcountry of Idaho.

Elevation Gain: For many hikers, how far up they go is even more important than the distance. This box shows all of the trip's ups and downs in a total elevation gain, not merely the net gain. As with the mileage section, a second number (in parentheses) includes the elevation gain in recommended side trips.

Days: This is a rough figure for how long it will take the average backpacker to do the trip. In general, it is based on my preference for traveling about 10 miles per day. Also considered were the spacing of available campsites and the trip's difficulty. Hardcore hikers may cover as many as 25 miles a day, while others saunter along at 4 or 5 miles per day, a good pace for hikers with children. Most trips can be done in more or fewer days, depending on your preferences and abilities.

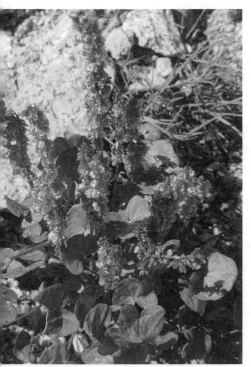

Mountain sorrel in the Pioneer Mountains (Trip 18)

Shuttle Mileage: This is the shortest driving distance between the beginning and the ending trailheads. Because most trips in this book are loop trips, a shuttle mileage is usually not applicable.

Map(s): Every trip includes a map that is as up-to-date and accurate as possible. These maps use bold lines to indicate the main route and all recommended side trips, so you can get an instant overview of the hike. As every hiker knows, however, you'll also need a good contour map of the area. This entry identifies the best available map(s) for the described trip.

Season: There are two seasonal entries shown for each trip. The first tells you when a trip is usually snow-free enough for hiking (which can vary considerably from year to year). The second lists the particular time(s) of year when the trip is at its very best—when the flowers peak, or the fall colors are at their best, or the mosquitoes have died down, and so on.

Permits and Rules: Compared to more crowded states in the American West, Idaho has very few restrictions on backcountry visitors. Except for Yellowstone National Park, most of which is in Wyoming, there are no trail quotas anywhere in the state, and hikers don't need to worry about making reservations. Very few areas even require that you fill out a free permit. Some places do have regulations that restrict the use of fires or the number of people in each party. These and other rules are noted in this section.

Contact: This is the telephone number for the local land agency responsible for the area. You can contact it to check on road and trail conditions before your trip.

Unfortunately, you should not expect to get much useful or reliable information from these local land managers. In researching this book, I asked dozens of U.S. Forest Service personnel hundreds of questions about trail lengths, when trail maintenance was last done (which can range from last week to not since the trail was built more than 50 years ago), if a trail was snow-free enough for travel, and if a trail shown on the map even exists (they often don't). The answer was almost always, "I don't know. We don't keep track of that information." Only once did I receive accurate and reliable information. Similarly, the websites of these agencies don't usually include updated information about current conditions, so that won't help you either.

Special Attractions: This section focuses on attributes of a particular trip that are rare or outstanding. For example, almost every trip has views, but some have views that are especially noteworthy. The same is true of areas where you have a better than average chance of seeing wildlife, excellent fall colors, and so on.

Challenges: This is the flip side to the "Special Attractions" section. It lists the trip's special or especially troublesome problems. Expect to read warnings about areas with particularly abundant mosquitoes, poor road access, grizzly bears, or limited water.

Tips and Warnings: Throughout the text are numerous helpful hints and ideas that come from my personal experience. Hopefully, these prominently labeled "Tips" and "Warnings" will make your trips safer and more enjoyable.

Possible Itinerary: This is given at the end of each trip. To be used as a planning tool, it includes daily mileages and total elevation gains, as well as recommended side trips. Though I have hiked every mile of every trip, many were not done exactly as written here. If I were to re-hike a trip, I would follow the improved itinerary shown here.

Best Shorter Alternative: Because many readers no longer have the time or desire to tackle a longer backpacking trip, nearly every featured trip now includes a section at the end that details the best way to get a sampling of the area with day hikes or shorter backpacking adventures. These options usually miss some of the better areas that are farther from the roads, but this will at least give today's time-strapped hikers the opportunity to see some of the wonders that each described area has to offer.

Opposite: Snag along Mosquito Ridge (Trip 8)

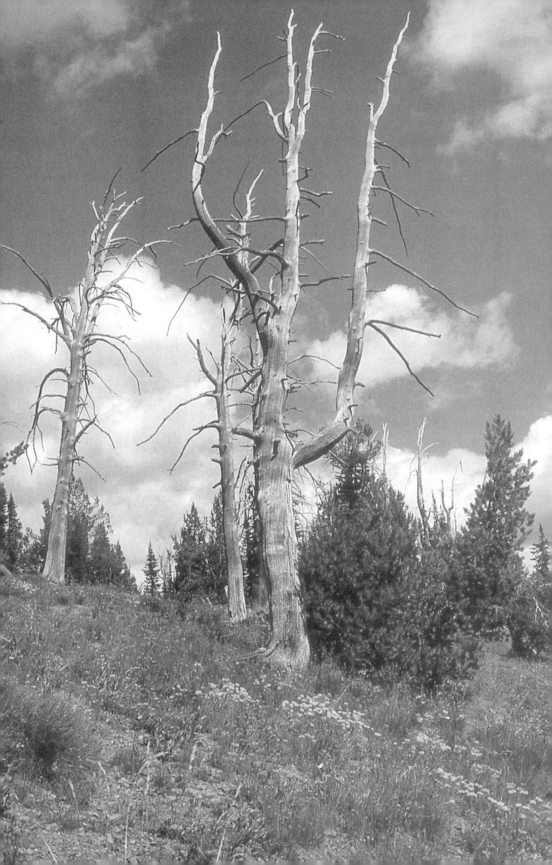

BACKPACKING IN IDAHO

Authors of hiking guidebooks face a paradox. Without dedicated supporters, the wilderness would never be protected in the first place. The best and most enthusiastic advocates are those who have actually visited the land, often with the help of a guidebook. On the other hand, too many boots can also be destructive. It is the responsibility of every visitor to tread lightly on the land and to speak out strongly for its preservation.

Though Idaho has more than 4 million acres of officially designated wilderness, the job of protecting Idaho's precious wildlands is far from complete. You are strongly encouraged to join in the efforts to set aside more of the state's millions of acres of unprotected roadless terrain. But even land that is officially protected as wilderness needs continued citizen involvement. Issues such as use restrictions, grazing rights, mining claims, all-terrain vehicle damage, and entry fees all continue to present challenges. Remember: You own this land. Treat it with respect and get involved in its management.

To their credit, almost every agency official who reviewed this material stressed the need for hikers to leave no trace of their visit. But the time has come for us to go beyond the well-known Leave No Trace principles and leave behind a landscape that not only shows no trace of our presence, but is also in *better* shape than before we visited it.

GENERAL BACKPACKING GUIDELINES

This book is not a how-to guide for backpackers. Anyone contemplating an extended backpacking vacation will (or at least *should*) already know about equipment, the Leave No Trace ethic, conditioning, how to select a campsite, food, first aid, and all the other aspects of this sport. Many excellent books cover these subjects. It is appropriate, however, to review a few general backpacking guidelines and discuss some tips and ideas that are specific to Idaho:

- **Obviously, be sure not to leave litter of your own.** Even better, remove any litter left by others (blessedly little these days).

- **Do some minor trail maintenance as you hike.** Kick rocks off the trail, remove limbs and debris, and drain water from the path to reduce mud and erosion. Report major trail-maintenance problems, such as large blowdowns or washouts, to the land managers, so they can concentrate their limited dollars where those are most needed.

  If you are a plant expert, **remove any introduced noxious weeds that you see.** Musk thistle, spotted knapweed, leafy spurge, and purple loosestrife are just some of the invasive species that land managers need help in eliminating.

  Always camp in a place that either is compacted from years of previous use or can easily accommodate a tent without being damaged—sand, rocks, or a densely wooded area is best.

- **Never camp on fragile meadow vegetation or immediately beside a lake or stream.** If you see a campsite "growing" in an inappropriate place, be proactive: Place a few limbs or rocks over the area to discourage further use, scatter horse apples, and remove fire-scarred rocks. Report those who ignore the rules to rangers (or offer to help the offenders move to a better location).

- **Never feed wildlife,** and encourage others to refrain.

- **Do not build campfires.** I have backpacked tens of thousands of miles in the last 25 years and built just one fire (and that was only in an emergency). While there are still places in the forests of Idaho where you may be able to build a small campfire with a clear conscience, you simply don't need a fire to have a good time, and it damages the land. When you discover a fire ring in an otherwise pristine area, scatter the rocks and cover the fire pit to discourage its further use.

- **Leave all of the following at home:** soap, as even biodegradable soap pollutes; pets, because even well-mannered pets are instinctively seen as predators by wildlife; anything loud; and any outdated attitudes you may have about going out to "conquer" the wilderness.

IDAHO-SPECIFIC GUIDELINES

The winter's snowpack has a significant effect not only on when a trail opens, but also on peak wildflower times, stream flows, and how long seasonal water sources will be available. The best plan is to check the snowpack on about April 1, and make a note of how it compares

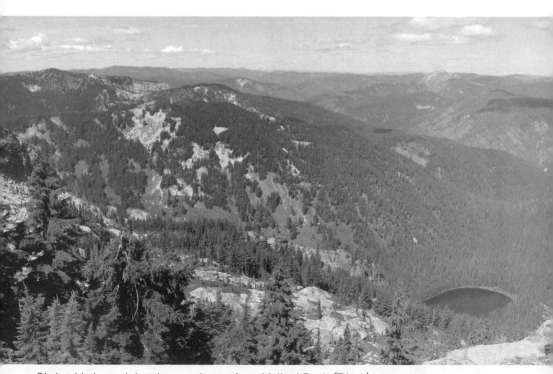

Skyland Lake and the view northwest from Mallard Peak (Trip 2)

to normal. This information is available through the local media or by checking the snow survey website at **nrcs.usda.gov/wps/portal/nrcs/main/id/snow.** If the snowpack is significantly above or below average, then adjust a trip's seasonal recommendation accordingly.

Except on popular trails in places like the Sawtooth Mountains, trail maintenance in Idaho is not as regular as in most other western states. Most trails are cleared only once every few years, and many trails get no maintenance at all. You should expect to encounter downed logs or other obstacles as you hike. You should also expect that many minor trail junctions will not be signed, so watch the map and the surrounding terrain closely to locate obscure junctions.

A bit of advice for urbanites visiting the Idaho backcountry: In rural Idaho (and, for that matter, in much of the rural American West) the correct pronunciation of the word *creek* is "crik," with a short "i" sound rather than a long "e" sound. Keep this in mind so you don't end up sounding like "ignorant city folk." Also, when you are passing an oncoming car on rarely used rural roads, it is considered good etiquette to acknowledge the other driver with a small wave, whether you know the person or not. Failing to do so identifies you as a rude city visitor.

When driving on rural roads, beware of free-ranging livestock, which typically show little fear of cars and have a habit of loitering in the middle of the road. It may take considerable patience, honking, and/or swearing to get the animals to move off the road. Calves are particularly notorious for darting in front of cars when you least expect them to. In addition, ranchers regularly use the roadways to push their herds of sheep and cattle between pastures. Be prepared to occasionally get stuck behind (or in the middle of) slow-moving masses of smelly livestock.

General deer-hunting season in Idaho runs from early October to sometime in November. For safety, anyone traveling in the forest during this period (particularly those doing any cross-country travel) should carry and wear a bright red or orange cap, vest, pack, or other conspicuous article of clothing.

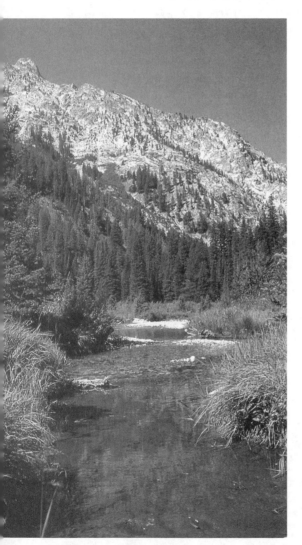

Grandjean Peak over Baron Creek (Trip 13)

For most of Idaho, the general elk-hunting season begins in early to mid-October and runs to mid-November, but in many backcountry game units the season begins on September 15. The exact season varies in different parts of the state. The seasons for hunting moose, mountain goats, bighorn sheep, and black bears usually do not attract enough hunters to cause a problem for backpackers.

Though Idaho's black bears are generally quite shy, they are common throughout the state's mountains and forests. You should hang all food and garbage at least 10 feet off the ground and 4 feet from the nearest tree trunk, so the bruins cannot reach it. This will also protect your food supply from an even more common and destructive group of thieves—chipmunks.

Grizzly bears are a subject of interest (and sometimes nightmares) for many hikers. In Idaho, there is a reasonable chance of encountering these impressive, but potentially dangerous, animals only in the mountains of the northern panhandle (Trip 1) and in or near Yellowstone National Park (Trip 22). When hiking in these areas, the following precautions are in order: Never hike alone or at night, avoid areas with recent signs of bears, take special care to avoid spilling food or garbage near your camp, make plenty of noise while you hike, and hang all food and garbage at least 15 feet from the ground and 500 feet away from your camp. Because most of the trees along the ridgetops are rather small, it is sometimes difficult to properly hang your food. You may want to bring a bear canister instead. Finally, remember that bears and dogs do not get along. Accordingly, the National Park Service prohibits dogs, and the U.S. Forest Service strongly discourages bringing your dog. If you must bring your pet, be sure that the animal is on leash at all times. If you see a grizzly bear, consider yourself fortunate that you saw one of these rare and magnificent creatures in the wild, and report the sighting to the land managers—they like to keep track of such things.

Hikers frequently have to ford streams (large and small) on the trips described in this book and in Idaho in general. Early in the season, rivers and creeks run high with meltwater, which makes fording them a cold and potentially dangerous undertaking. The typical depth of the stream for the recommended season of the hike is noted in the text, but this can vary considerably from year to year. If a ford looks too deep, swift, or dangerous when you get there, don't risk it! Turn around and head back the way you came. The best and safest way to make a ford is to wear lightweight wading shoes or sandals, which will give you better traction, protect your feet from cuts and scrapes, and allow you to keep your boots and socks dry. Trekking poles to provide a third and fourth leg of support are also highly recommended.

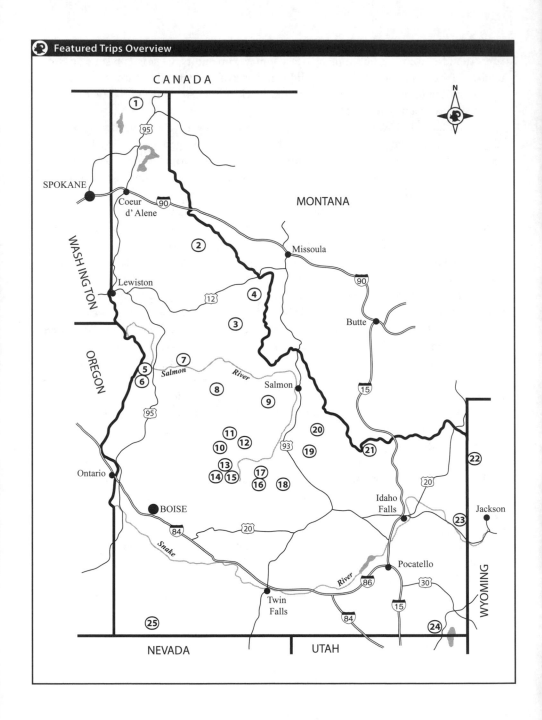

CANADA

SPOKANE

Coeur
d' Alene

MONTANA

Missoula

WASHINGTON

Lewiston

Butte

OREGON

Salmon River

Salmon

Ontario

BOISE

Idaho
Falls

Jackson

Snake

Pocatello

WYOMING

Twin
Falls

NEVADA

UTAH

Opposite: Near North Indian Creek Pass (Trip 23)

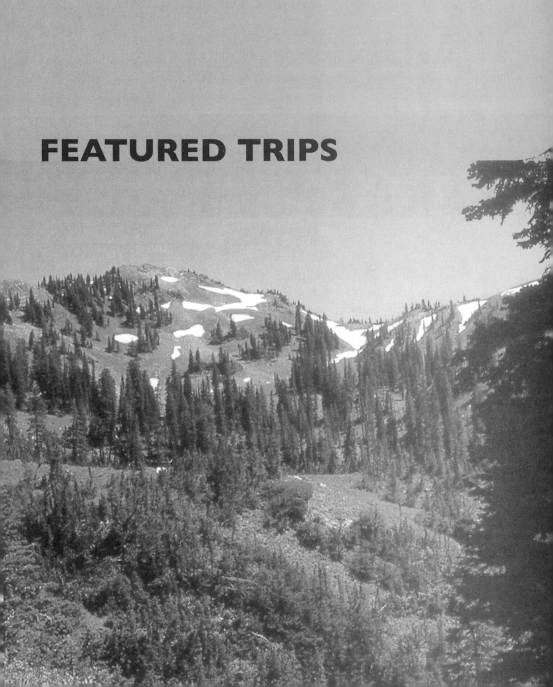

FEATURED TRIPS

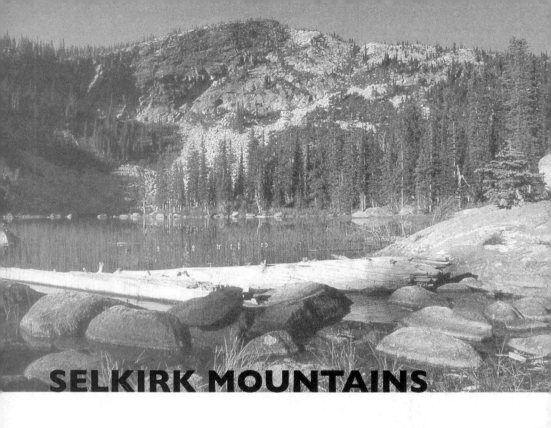

SELKIRK MOUNTAINS

T ucked in the far northern panhandle of Idaho, the craggy Selkirk Mountains are a long way from the state's main population centers. From Boise, for example, it's a nine-hour drive to the nearest Selkirk trailheads. As a result, most visitors to these mountains come from the much nearer metropolis of Spokane, Washington, to the west.

Pacific storms, also coming from the west, dump a lot more snow and rain in the Selkirk Mountains than they do in mountains to the south, making this the wettest part of Idaho. All this precipitation, along with the more northerly latitude, results in a relatively low timberline, so even though the peaks here are all below 8,000 feet, there is plenty of alpine scenery to enjoy.

The precipitation also leads to incredibly lush forests, featuring species like western hemlock and western red cedar, which are rare or absent from the rest of the state. These dense forests have suffered from two recurring catastrophes over the last 125 years: first, the insatiable desire of human beings for big trees to cut down; and second, a series of enormous fires that have repeatedly blackened the area. The rampant logging has left behind a landscape riddled with clear-cuts that despoil most distant views. Evidence of the fires comes in the form of silvery snags along the ridgetops.

Above: Pyramid Lake on Long Canyon Loop (Trip 1)

These mountains are the southern tip of a 250-mile-long range of peaks that stretch down from the interior of British Columbia, Canada. As a result, this range hosts an unusual assortment of northern animals not found in other parts of the state. Hikers may be fortunate enough to see mountain caribou—the most endangered large mammal in the United States—moose, lynxes, gray wolves, or grizzly bears. Even though they are rarely seen, just knowing that these impressive animals inhabit the Selkirk Mountains adds a thrilling sense of possibility to your adventure.

These mountains provide many joys in addition to the wildlife. The biggest attraction is impressive scenery, mostly in the form of lovely cirque lakes and jagged granite peaks. A less obvious advantage this area has over the mountains in southern Idaho is that the lower elevations here don't require extra time for lowlanders to get accustomed to thin air.

One of the few disadvantages of hiking in the Selkirk Mountains is that this area has a higher percentage of cloudy and rainy days than the rest of the state (though it's still nowhere near as soggy as the mountains of Oregon and Washington to the west). Another disadvantage is the thick undergrowth, which makes cross-country travel much more difficult than in drier ranges to the south. But even with these problems, it is the rare pedestrian who, after a hike in these mountains, doesn't believe that the Selkirks' scenery, solitude, and wildlife far outweigh any downsides of the trip.

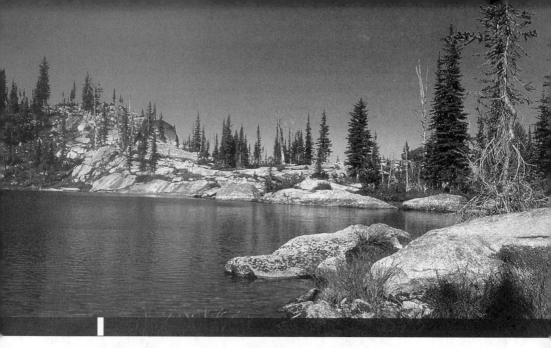

LONG CANYON LOOP

RATINGS: Scenery 7   Solitude 6   Difficulty 6
MILES: 37 (52) (These numbers exclude the road walk back to the Canyon Creek trailhead.)
SHUTTLE MILEAGE: 4
ELEVATION GAIN: 8,200' (13,000')
DAYS: 3–4
MAP(S): USGS *Pyramid Peak,* USGS *Smith Falls,* USGS *Smith Peak*
USUALLY OPEN: Mid-July–early October
BEST: Late July–September
PERMITS: None
RULES: Maximum group size of 12 people, unless you specifically notify the Bonners Ferry Ranger District; fires are strongly discouraged; staying more than three nights at any given campsite is prohibited.
CONTACT: Bonners Ferry Ranger District, 208-267-5561

SPECIAL ATTRACTIONS

Unusual wildlife; lush rain forests

CHALLENGES

Grizzly bears; relatively wet weather; limited water and few campsites along Parker Ridge

Above: Long Mountain Lake

HOW TO GET THERE •

From the junction of US 2 and US 95 about 2 miles north of Bonners Ferry, drive 12.6 miles north on US 95 to a junction. Go straight on ID 1 for 1.1 miles, and then turn left (west) on a county road, following signs to Copeland Bridge and Westside Road. Stay on this paved road for 3.5 miles, taking a bridge over the Kootenai River, and come to a T-junction. Turn right on the paved Westside Road and drive 3.5 miles to the Parker Creek trailhead, which has room for only one or two cars to park. If you have two cars, leave one here.

To reach the recommended starting point, continue another 3.5 miles on Westside Road, and then turn left (uphill) at a signed junction with a narrow, gravel, dead-end road that goes 0.1 mile to the small parking lot for the Canyon Creek trailhead. *Note:* This trailhead is on private land. The public is allowed to park but not camp here.

INTRODUCTION •

As the wettest range in the state of Idaho, the Selkirk Mountains support forests that are so lush they resemble the rain forests of the Pacific Northwest coast. The trees include such relatively unusual Idaho species as western red cedar, western hemlock, western yew, and Pacific dogwood, while the undergrowth is a mass of ferns, mosses, and lichens that assail the hiker with a stunning display of greenery. In a grand sampling of this wet environment, the first half of this hike takes you up Long Canyon, the last major unlogged valley in the Selkirk Mountains, where a magnificent shady forest provides a hiking experience unlike anything else in the state.

But there is more to admire here than dense forests. Along the ridges are jagged peaks; hidden cirques filled with small, scenic lakes; and expansive views of the deep, green valleys below. In addition, wildflowers bloom in profusion, especially along the open ridgetops, where the forests have yet to recover from a series of large forest fires. This superior hike is the finest backpacking adventure in the Selkirk Mountains because it includes the best of the area's low-elevation forests as well as some of the range's most beautiful lakes and ridgetop views.

> **WARNING:** This is grizzly bear country. Please heed the guidelines given on page 11. Remember that bears and dogs do not get along. Accordingly, the U.S. Forest Service strongly discourages bringing your dog. If you *must* bring your pet, be sure that the animal is on leash at all times.

DESCRIPTION •

The trail, which has been significantly rerouted from what is shown on the U.S. Geological Survey (USGS) maps, follows an overgrown road the first 200 yards, and then narrows to a foot trail and wanders gradually uphill through a nicely varied forest. The mix of evergreen trees here is more diverse than just about anywhere else in the state. Douglas-firs and western red cedars are the most common species, but there are also western larches and grand firs, as well as ponderosa pines, western white pines, and western hemlocks. The ground cover is kept in check by the deep shade of the canopy, but in places you will find pipsissewa, Oregon grape, lady fern, and thimbleberry, among other species.

RECOMMENDED LONG CANYON SIDE TRIPS

To do the shorter side trip, turn sharply right and wander down a few gentle switchbacks to a junction beside a visitor registration box. You turn right and make a circuitous, 0.5-mile ascent to the irregularly shaped Pyramid Lake, a shallow pool with good campsites near its outlet and a superb view of an unnamed, craggy peak to the southwest. For more scenery and exercise, continue on the trail to the equally scenic Ball Lakes. To reach them, turn sharply left at the outlet of Pyramid Lake and climb a boulder-strewn slope on seven moderately steep switchbacks to the top of a ridge. You then wander up and down through lovely subalpine fir forests for 0.5 mile to a signed fork. The trail to the left descends several hundred yards to Lower Ball Lake, while the path to the right goes just 50 yards to the slightly larger Upper Ball Lake. Both lakes are set in very scenic granite basins and have good campsites.

The well-maintained trail climbs seven moderately long but well-graded switchbacks, and then cuts through a woodsy gap in the ridge and emerges high on the slopes of Long Canyon. The trail then curves to the right and makes a rather steep and rocky uphill traverse well above cascading Long Canyon Creek, which can be heard, but not seen, deep in the canyon on your left. Though this traverse stays above the best forests, it has the advantage of going past some excellent viewpoints of Long Canyon and densely forested Parker Ridge to the south.

The trail levels briefly, and then goes downhill at an irregular grade to a nice campsite beside rollicking Long Canyon Creek. Above this campsite, you travel across a forested hillside a little above the stream, maintaining a steady uphill grade that keeps pace with the cascading creek. About 3 miles from where it first met the creek, the trail drops to a pair of good campsites on either side of where you cross the stream on a log.

You make two quick switchbacks away from the creek and walk upstream for 1.5 miles through some of this area's best forests to a second creek crossing, which requires a knee-deep ford in early summer or a slippery rock-hop in late summer. A fair campsite can be found immediately after the crossing hidden in the creek's dense riparian undergrowth of devil's club, lady fern, horsetail, and Douglas maple. For the next few miles you make several steep little ups and downs through a dense forest that has no views, but which provides plenty of up-close green scenery. Though the trail generally stays well away from Long Canyon Creek, finding water is never a problem because you hop over numerous tiny side creeks along the way. In fact, if anything, there is *too much* water, as frequent rains leave behind lots of mud and wet vegetation that overhangs the trail and soaks passing hikers. Fortunately, several wooden boardwalks have been installed over the muddiest places to help keep you clean and dry.

About 2.5 miles from the second creek crossing, you pass a good campsite just before a rock-hop crossing of a fairly large, unnamed creek that flows down from Smith Lake. From there, it's another 0.5

mile to the third and final crossing of Long Canyon Creek, which is usually an easy ford, though by late summer it is possible to cross on slippery rocks. About 200 yards later, you pass a decent campsite beside a small tributary creek, and then walk a little less than 1 mile to a signed junction. The unmaintained trail straight ahead goes a short distance to a good creek-side campsite.

You turn left at the junction and begin the long, steady climb out of Long Canyon. The 2,200-foot ascent starts with 30 mostly short and always gently graded switchbacks, followed by a 0.5-mile-long traverse. Though there isn't much in the way of views, it's interesting to observe the changes in vegetation as you climb. The cedars and Douglas-firs in the lower canyon slowly give way to lodgepole pines, Engelmann spruces, and western white pines, while the understory makes a transition to huckleberries, alders, and bear grass. Once the traverse ends, 20 more switchbacks take you up to a nice viewpoint and a junction.

The return route of your loop goes sharply left on Parker Ridge Trail #221, but first you'll want to spend a day or two on a pair of extended side trips to the high lakes and scenic terrain at the head of Trout Creek Canyon. To do so, go straight and wind gradually uphill past the base of the aptly named Pyramid Peak to the narrow, viewless defile of Pyramid Pass. The trail then descends several switchbacks on a hillside covered with huckleberries to a junction beside a small wooden bridge. Here you have a choice of side trips, both of which are highly recommended.

To finish the loop trail, go back over Pyramid Pass and return to the junction with the Parker Ridge Trail. Go north (uphill) and steeply climb through an area that was swept by fire several decades ago and still hides some silvery snags amid the new forest. After a little more than 0.5 mile of steep uphill, you reach the ridgecrest at a rocky saddle, where you'll have exceptional views west to Smith Peak, north down Long Canyon, and northeast down the wooded canyon of Parker Creek and up to Fisher Peak. The trail then turns to follow the ridgecrest and slowly climbs for 400 yards to a junction with

To do the longer side trip, return to the junction below Pyramid Pass and go northeast, following signs to Trout and Big Fisher Lakes. This trail goes gradually uphill across the partly forested southeast side of Fisher Ridge, where you'll have fine views ahead of Trout Creek Canyon and back to the peaks around Pyramid Lake. After about 1 mile the trail levels off, contours around a high point in the ridge, and then descends 250 feet to Trout Lake. This gorgeous lake sits beneath a high granite mountain and has a couple of very good campsites above its east shore. Beyond Trout Lake the trail makes a moderately steep, 1-mile climb to the top of Fisher Ridge, and then ascends the ridgeline to a 7,400-foot pass with fine views down to Big Fisher Lake. From here, you steeply descend to the shores of this very scenic lake, where the trail ends. The best campsites are on the lake's southwest shore, but the best views are from the east shore back up to the high ridgeline you just descended.

Long Canyon Loop

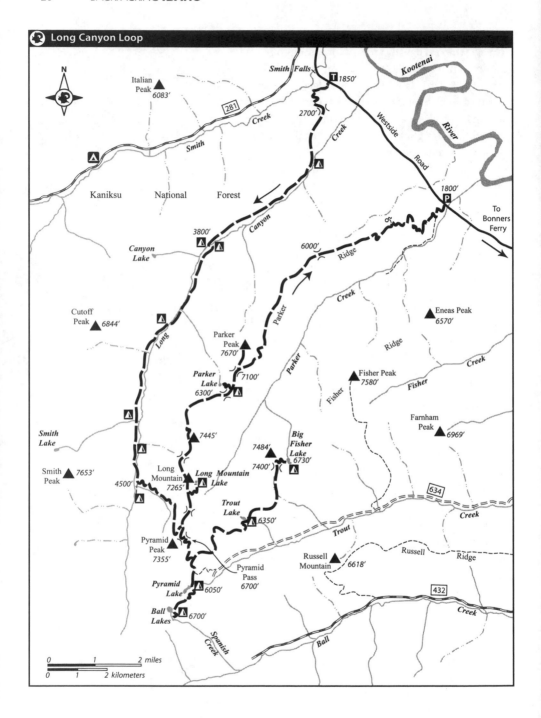

N

Italian
Peak
6083'

Smith Falls

Kootenai

T 1850'

281

Creek

2700'

Creek

Westside
Road

River

1800'
P

To
Bonners
Ferry

Kaniksu   National   Forest

Smith

Canyon

3800'

*Canyon
Lake*

6000'

Ridge

Creek

Eneas Peak
6570'

Cutoff
Peak   6844'

Long

*Parker
Peak
7670'*

Parker

Ridge

Fisher Peak
7580'

Fisher

Creek

*Parker
Lake
6300'*

7100'

Parker

Fisher

Farnham
Peak
6969'

*Smith
Lake*

7445'

7484'

*Big
Fisher
Lake
6730'*

7400'

634

Smith   7653'
Peak

4500'

Long
Mountain
7265'

*Long Mountain
Lake*

Creek

Pyramid
Peak
7355'

*Trout
Lake*

6350'

Trout

Russell
Mountain   6618'

Russell   Ridge

*Pyramid
Lake*   6050'

Pyramid
Pass
6700'

432

*Ball
Lakes*   6700'

*Spanish
Creek*

Ball

Creek

0   1   2 miles

0   1   2 kilometers

the 0.5-mile spur trail that switchbacks down to Long Mountain Lake. This side trip would be worthwhile if only to appreciate this small, deep lake's lovely setting surrounded by heather and perky subalpine firs in a basin of white granite rocks. But the best reasons to make the side trip are that this lake is one of the few permanent water sources on Parker Ridge and it has an excellent campsite.

The main trail continues straight from the Long Mountain Lake junction and ascends Parker Ridge to a point just below the rolling summit of the 7,265-foot Long Mountain. High-elevation wildflowers are abundant on this open ridge, especially pussytoes, lousewort, and white heather. Views are similarly grand, featuring outstanding vistas up and down the spine of the Selkirk Mountains, into the green depths of Long Canyon, and north to the vastness of Canada.

From Long Mountain, you go down to a saddle, and then climb partway up a tall, rocky, pyramid-shaped summit. Before reaching the top, the trail cuts to the left, makes an up-and-down traverse across the west side of this peak, and then drops again in steep switchbacks and follows the undulating ridgecrest as it curves east. Plenty of possible campsites are along this scenic ridge, but the only water is from snowfields that may, if you are lucky, linger into early August. At a saddle about 3.5 miles from Long Mountain is the junction with the 0.7-mile side trail to Parker Lake. This lake has excellent fishing, but it isn't as spectacular as most of the other lakes in this range, and camping near the shore is limited by brush and steep slopes. You'll still want to visit this lake, however, because it's the last reliable source of water until a small spring about 6 miles ahead. If you choose to camp here, the best sites are on the ridge near the main trail, though they force you to walk a long way to get water.

The main trail bears right at the Parker Lake junction and climbs fairly steeply to a long, ridgetop saddle and another junction. The trail that goes straight makes a steep, 0.5-mile climb to the former lookout site atop the prominent Parker Peak, where you can take in many of the same views you had along the ridge, but from a higher and better grandstand. The Parker Ridge Trail bears right at the junction, goes steadily downhill across the rocky east face of Parker Peak, and then regains about 250 feet and returns to the wide and heavily forested ridgetop.

It's all downhill from here, most of the time traveling in dense woods, where you will notice a reversal of the pattern of change in the tree species that you noted on the way up. The descent starts quite gently as it goes through a long, woodsy saddle, and then makes a series of well-graded switchbacks. At the third switchback turn, a trail goes straight about 10 yards to a small spring with welcome water. Unfortunately, there is no flat ground nearby to accommodate a tent. The last part of the descent takes you across large, grassy areas with good views of the farmland and meandering river in the Kootenai River Valley. At the 43rd switchback, a little before the bottom of the long downhill, you meet Parker Creek Trail #14. Here you turn left and go down nine short switchbacks to the Parker Creek trailhead on Westside Road.

POSSIBLE ITINERARY

	CAMP	MILES	ELEVATION GAIN
Day 1	First crossing of Long Canyon Creek	8.0	2,300'
Day 2	Pyramid Lake	11.0	3,200'
Day 3	Pyramid Lake (day hike to Ball Lakes and Big Fisher Lake)	13.0	3,700'
Day 4	Ridge above Parker Lake	7.0	2,200'
	Side trip to Long Mountain Lake	1.0	500'
Day 5	Out	11.0*	500'*
	Side trip to Parker Peak	1.0	600'

* These numbers exclude the road walk back to the Canyon Creek trailhead.

BEST SHORTER ALTERNATIVE ●

To focus exclusively on this trip's best viewpoints and alpine lakes, drive Road 634 (it's rough) up Trout Creek to the trailhead just before the end of the road (see map). From there, make a day hike up to Pyramid and Ball Lakes, a day hike to Long Mountain and Long Mountain Lake, and either a long day hike or a short backpacking trip to Trout and Big Fisher Lakes.

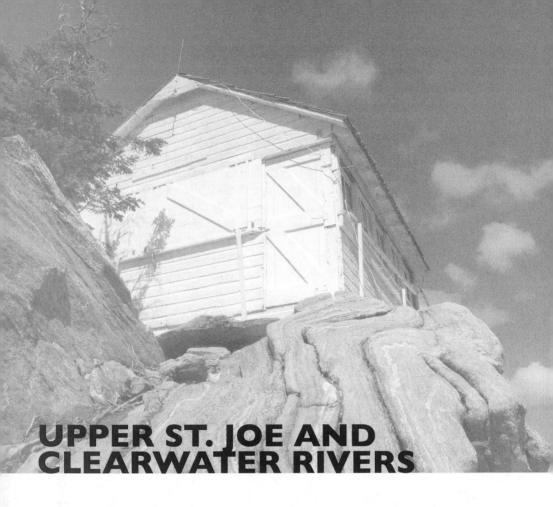

UPPER ST. JOE AND
CLEARWATER RIVERS

M ost of Idaho's mountains feature skyscraping peaks and towering cliffs that can accurately be described as spectacular. That word, however, would *not* be appropriate for the millions of acres of rolling, forested hills of north-central Idaho. The relatively gentle and picturesque hills and valleys of this region probably won't take a visitor's breath away, but that is only by comparison to other mountains in this scenery-rich state. Were these mountains located in almost any other state, they would be visited by thousands of hikers every year. In Idaho, however, this area is generally over-looked, except by anglers who enjoy the region's excellent fishing streams.

For decades, loggers and miners have eaten away at the wild character of this region, so there are few areas left where backpackers can get a meaningful distance from the nearest road. The wildest country, and the best scenery, is in the south near the watershed divide between the St. Joe and Clearwater Rivers. Hikers here can enjoy some fine mountain scenery, lots of wildlife (especially elk and mountain goats), and hundreds of miles of pleasant trails. These trails typically either follow the area's famous streams or climb to small lakes and huckleberry-covered ridges.

Above: Mallard Peak Fire Lookout (Trip 2)

This entire region was at the center of one of the largest forest fires in recorded history. In August 1910, a fire of almost unbelievable size and ferocity swept across northern Idaho, northwest Montana, and parts of northeast Washington. In the process it killed at least 85 people, most of them firefighters, and burned approximately 3 million acres. Incredibly, the firestorm consumed most of that vast acreage in just two horrific days! This catastrophe was the catalyst for an aggressive fire-suppression policy by the U.S. Forest Service, which continued until recent times, when foresters realized that periodic natural fires are needed for forest health. In response to the 1910 disaster, the U.S. Forest Service built numerous fire lookouts and an extensive system of trails to service these remote facilities. Most of the lookouts are gone now, made obsolete by modern fire-detection techniques, but those that remain are among the area's most popular hiking destinations. This is understandable, because the lookouts provide not only a colorful history but also great views, which is, after all, why these locations were selected in the first place.

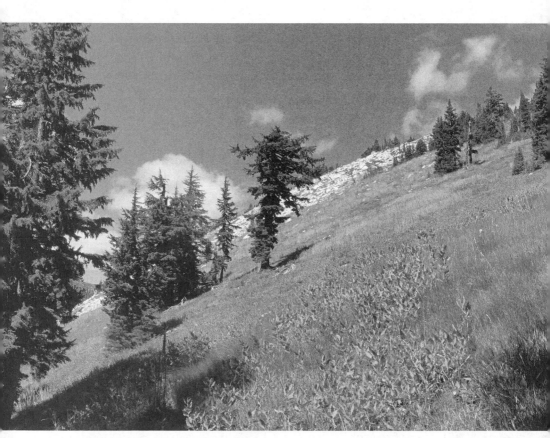

A sloping meadow west of Mallard Peak

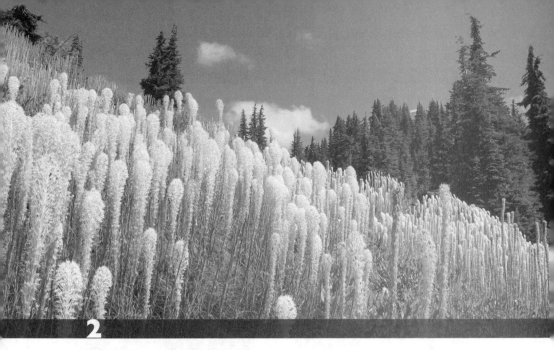

2

SNOW PEAK: MALLARD-LARKINS LOOP

RATINGS: Scenery 7   Solitude 5   Difficulty 9
MILES: 41 (44.5)
ELEVATION GAIN: 11,350' (12,600')
DAYS: 3–5 (4–6)
MAP(S): USGS *Bathtub Mountain,* USGS *Buzzard Roost,* USGS *Mallard Peak,* USGS *Montana Peak*
USUALLY OPEN: July–early October
BEST: Mid-July (for flowers) or August–early September (for huckleberries)
PERMITS: None
RULES: The usual Leave No Trace principles apply.
CONTACT: St. Joe Ranger District, Avery Office, 208-245-4517

SPECIAL ATTRACTIONS ·

Huckleberries; wildlife; great views from two fire lookouts; lovely mountain lakes

CHALLENGES ·

Long road access; rough, obscure, and very brushy trail from Snow Peak down to the Little North Fork Clearwater River

Above: Bear grass on Mallard Peak

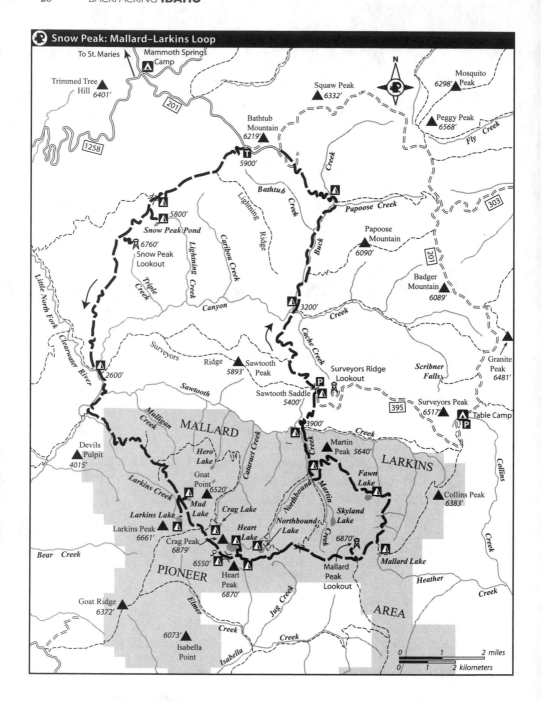

Snow Peak: Mallard–Larkins Loop

To St. Maries
Mammoth Springs Camp

Trimmed Tree Hill 6401'

Mosquito Peak 6298'

Squaw Peak 6332'

Peggy Peak 6568'

201

1258

Bathtub Mountain 6219'

T 5900'

Papoose Creek

303

Fly Creek

5800'

Bathtub Creek

Lightning Creek

Buck Creek

Papoose Mountain 6090'

Snow Peak Pond 6760'
Snow Peak Lookout

Caribou Creek

Lightning Ridge

201

Badger Mountain 6089'

Little North Fork

Triple Creek

Canyon

3200'

Cache Creek

Granite Peak 6481'

Surveyors Ridge

Sawtooth Peak 5893'

Surveyors Ridge Lookout

Scribner Falls

Clearwater River

2600'

Sawtooth

P

Sawtooth Saddle 5400'

395

Surveyors Peak 6517'

Table Camp

Mulligan Creek

MALLARD

Cataract Creek

3900'

Creek

Creek

Martin Peak 5640'

LARKINS

Collins

Devils Pulpit 4015'

Hero Lake

Gnat Point 6520'

Larkins Creek

Mud Lake

Crag Lake

Northbound Creek

Fawn Lake

Martin Creek

Collins Peak 6383'

Larkins Lake

Larkins Peak 6661'

Crag Peak 6879'

Heart Lake

Northbound Lake

Skyland Lake

6870'

Creek

Bear Creek

6550'

PIONEER

Heart Peak 6870'

Elmer

Jug Creek

Mallard Peak Lookout

Mallard Lake

Heather

Creek

AREA

Goat Ridge 6372'

Creek

Isabella

Creek

6073'
Isabella Point

0   1   2 miles

0   1   2 kilometers

HOW TO GET THERE ● ● ● ● ● ● ● ● ● ● ● ● ● ● ●

From the small town of St. Maries, go 1 mile north on ID 3; then turn right (northeast) onto St. Joe River Road, following signs to Calder and Avery. Stay on this paved road, which eventually becomes Forest Service Road 50, for 69 miles to a junction with Bluff Creek Road (FS 509). Turn right, immediately cross a bridge over the St. Joe River, and climb 8.1 miles on this narrow gravel road to a fork. Bear left onto FS 1250, following signs to Pineapple Saddle, and drive 3.4 miles to a four-way junction. Turn left onto FS 201, following signs to Beaver Creek, and proceed 3.9 miles to the Snow Peak trailhead in a saddle below the rounded summit of Bathtub Mountain. The trailhead comes complete with an outhouse, a horse feeding station, and a primitive car campground near a small spring just west of, and below, the parking lot.

INTRODUCTION

This ruggedly difficult loop takes you into the heart of the very scenic Mallard-Larkins Pioneer Area. A pioneer area does not offer the same permanent protection as official wilderness status does, but it is managed the same as wilderness areas in that it is both roadless and machine-free. Regardless of what you call it, this lovely region features plenty of crowd-pleasing attributes, including very scenic lakes, good fishing, and great views.

A special feature of this area is its unusual abundance of wildlife. Elk seem to be everywhere, and moose can sometimes be seen near the rivers and lakes. Mountain goats are found on all of the area's craggy mountains, and a particularly well-known herd lives on the cliffs of Snow Peak. In addition, black bears are common enough that hikers should hang their food to keep it safe from marauding bruins.

All this wildlife attracts hunters during the elk season in October. If you visit then, make yourself conspicuous by wearing bright red or orange clothing.

Larkin was the name of an early homesteader in this area, but the origin of the name Mallard is unknown, though it probably does not refer to the duck because the only waterfowl found on the area's high lakes are a few goldeneyes.

TIP: Do not do this loop clockwise. Going *up* the exposed, hard-to-find, and mostly dry trail between the Little North Clearwater River and Snow Peak would be no fun at all.

DESCRIPTION

Snow Peak Trail #55, which is closed to motor vehicles to reduce the impact of noise for the mountain goats, begins in a dense ridgetop forest of firs and mountain hemlocks. Beneath these lichen-draped trees, the forest floor is covered with huckleberries, bear grass, and grouse whortleberries. The wide and well-maintained trail immediately gets your thigh muscles warmed up with a 450-foot ascent on a wide ridge. This climb is the first of many ups and downs along this rolling ridge, none of which is overly steep, but when taken together add up to a significant amount of elevation gain. At the 1-mile point you bear right at the junction with the Lightning Ridge Trail, and then spend the next 2 miles going down, up, then down again to a saddle and a junction with the Spotted Louis Trail #104.

You bear slightly left at the junction and, 30 yards later, come to a pleasant campsite with water from a tiny spring to the east. Though there are no views here, at night you will be rewarded with the sounds of an unusually high concentration of owls, which hoot for hours from their perches in the trees. Expert birders will recognize the calls of great horned, barred, and screech owls, and they may pick up the distant sound of a great gray or a pygmy owl as well.

A relatively short but steady uphill from this campsite takes you to an unsigned junction at a forest opening with a first-rate view of the rugged Snow Peak. The 0.5-mile dead-end trail to the left winds downhill to the shallow Snow Peak Pond, where an excellent campsite awaits with a terrific view up to the nearby cliffs of Snow Peak. This pond is also a fine spot to watch mountain goats leap from ledge to ledge in a display that would make a prima ballerina look clumsy.

The main trail goes straight at the unsigned junction and climbs around the back side of a rocky ridgeline to an unsigned fork. The trail to the left (uphill) is the not-to-be-missed side trip to the top of Snow Peak. This short, scenic path steeply ascends through open forests and sloping meadows with nice displays of colorful arnica, yarrow, paint-brush, lousewort, pink heather, and other wildflowers. From the wooden lookout building atop the rocky pinnacle of Snow Peak, the views are breathtaking. No single landmark dominates the scene, but the view over a seemingly endless sea of wooded peaks, ridges, and river canyons is inspiring. In addition to the views, you stand a good chance of seeing mountain goats on the crags near the lookout. A sign tells the history of the prolific Snow Peak herd, which has been used since 1960 as a "mother herd" for transplanted goats throughout the American West.

Back on the main trail, you go south, make a gentle descent across a partly forested hillside, and then contour around a sloping basin and go gradually down the spine of a ridge on the southwest side of Snow Peak. After this deceptively gentle start, you plunge very steeply downhill on a rarely, if ever, maintained trail that includes a fair amount of deadfall and is overgrown with miles of miserable brush. The builders of this trail were of the old-school, shortest-distance-between-two-points mentality, so there are few switchbacks to ease the grade. The brush combines with numerous elk paths to make things very confusing. The proper trail generally stays close to the top of the ridge, though you need to watch carefully because several confusing detours go down the hillside on your left. If you get lost (and you almost certainly will) just persevere in struggling along the ridgetop until you relocate the trail and, when you get back to civilization, write a letter to the U.S. Forest Service asking them to send a trail crew to maintain this important connecting trail at least once every 10 or 15 years. After descending 3,700 feet, the seemingly endless downhill finally concludes at an unsigned junction just above the confluence of Canyon Creek and the Little North Fork Clearwater River.

TIP: A considerably longer but better maintained alternate route to reach this point follows the Spotted Louis Trail from the junction northeast of Snow Peak to Little North Fork Clearwater River. From there, you turn left and hike Trail #50 to Canyon Creek.

Delighted to have that rough and miserable section completed, you turn left (downstream) on well-maintained Trail #50 and make a knee-deep ford of clear Canyon Creek. Immediately on the south side of the creek is a broken-down building called Trappers Cabin and a very good campsite, or rather it *would* be good if not for the almost constant presence of large horse parties that make the spot very aromatic and home to thousands of horseflies. Atop a little spur ridge just past this camp is a junction with the Surveyors Ridge Trail, where you go straight, sticking with the Little North Fork Clearwater River Trail. Less than 0.5 mile later, you make an easy ford of Sawtooth Creek, and then gradually climb a heavily forested hillside to a junction just after you begin to switchback down the south side of a spur ridge.

You bear left (uphill), following signs to Larkins Lake, and start a long ascent of the steep-sided canyon that holds the cascading Larkins Creek. The climb has an irregular grade, but it is often very steep as it works its way up the southwest-facing slope of the canyon. The first mile goes across mostly open, sun-exposed slopes; then the canyon walls become increasingly wooded, so the remainder of the climb is in the shade. The trail eventually pulls away from the creek, climbs six moderately steep switchbacks, and then turns southeast and steadily climbs a wide, wooded ridge to an unsigned and unmapped junction with an outfitter's trail that goes sharply left.

You go straight and keep slowly plugging away uphill, often under the shade of huge, old-growth western red cedars, to a signed junction with the rough Hero Lake Trail. Bear right and soon you will reach a confusing junction with a very good outfitter's horse trail that is not shown on any map. Your trail turns left (uphill) and ascends through a series of small, brushy meadows filled with aster, coneflower, groundsel, pearly everlasting, paintbrush, and other tall wildflowers. Eventually, the trail leaves these lush meadows and crosses an open, view-packed hillside carpeted with huckleberries. Partway up this hillside is a signed junction with the 0.5-mile side trail, right, to Larkins Lake. Set directly beneath the cliffs of Larkins Peak, this scenic lake has plenty of fish and some good campsites. Just 10 yards beyond the Larkins Lake turnoff is an unsigned junction with the 150-yard side trail that goes left and uphill to Mud Lake. This beautiful, misnamed lake has an excellent campsite of its own and a fine view of the long ridge of Gnat Point.

The main trail goes straight at both of these junctions and keeps climbing the open hillside for 0.5 mile to the top of the ridgeline east of Larkins Peak. The trail then curves left and traverses the south side of a knoll to an unsigned junction with Trail #240, which angles in from the right. Go straight and, just 200 yards later, reach a junction with the irregularly maintained Cataract Creek Trail.

TIP: For a nice side trip, turn left and go 1 mile down this trail to scenic Crag Lake, which has a couple of nice, secluded campsites.

Your route, now called Heart Pass Trail, goes straight and makes a gradual uphill traverse around the south side of Crag Peak. After a little more than 0.5 mile, you pass a view-packed campsite beside a (really) tiny spring, and then reach a high saddle between Crag Peak and Heart Peak. Just north of this saddle is sparkling Heart Lake, the largest and arguably the most scenic lake in the Mallard-Larkins area.

From the saddle, the trail goes downhill across the steep, rocky north face of Heart Peak to an unsigned but obvious junction. The rocky trail to the left drops very steeply for 0.3 mile to the shores of the large, deep, and gorgeous Heart Lake, which is well worth a visit. If you want to spend the night at this deep lake, you'll find a couple of excellent but popular campsites above the northeast shore. Here you can happily while away several hours fishing, swimming, or watching mountain goats on the sheer cliffs that drop into three sides of the lake.

WARNING: Treacherous snowfields often remain on the north-facing slope of Heart Peak until late July or early August.

After returning to the main trail, you hike 0.2 mile to a little meadow with a trickle of water and a fine campsite, and then cross a north-facing slope and descend through forest to the junction with Northbound Creek Trail #111, a little more than 1 mile east of the Heart Lake junction. This trail provides a somewhat shorter alternate route back toward your starting point, but going that way misses some of this area's most attractive scenery at Mallard Peak and Fawn Lake.

If you have the time, it is much better to go straight at this junction, staying on Heart Pass Trail #65. This path contours across mostly forested slopes for 0.5 mile to a second junction, this time with Martin Creek Trail #479, which goes left and is closed to horses. Go straight again and make a moderately long climb before leveling off and walking across a delightful landscape of meadows and partial forest to a four-way junction atop the northern spur ridge coming off of the tall Mallard Peak.

> **WARNING:** If you leave your heavy packs at this junction to make the side trip to Mallard Peak, you may want to either hang them from a tree limb or leave a member of your party behind as a guard. A small herd of mountain goats is often found near this junction and has been known to chew on sweaty pack straps and hip belts for the salt.

The main trail goes straight at the Mallard Peak junction, soon turns to the left (north) and begins descending the mostly open east face of Mallard Peak. There are fine views here, especially down to the meadow holding the small but pretty Mallard Lake. This circuitous route descends the partly forested slope for about 0.8 mile to reach a junction.

If you need water or a campsite, consider the short side trip from here to Mallard Lake. To reach it, you turn sharply right (downhill) and descend through forest at a moderate grade for about 0.3 mile to the short side trail that goes right to Mallard Lake. There are good campsites here, and the shallow lake is in a very attractive setting in a meadow with fine views back up to Mallard Peak.

To continue the recommended loop trip, go north from the junction above Mallard Lake, following signs to Fawn Lake. This trail takes you through a series of small ups and downs as it traverses a partly forested hillside. You also cross a couple of small creeks and several seasonal trickles as you make your way across this east-facing slope. After topping a small ridge, the trail cuts to the left (southwest) and descends to a superb campsite next to Fawn Lake. This deep, fish-filled lake is outstandingly scenic, surpassed in this area only by Heart Lake, and even that is a close call. The entire south side of the lake is rimmed by cliffs, making it very photogenic and a choice spot to spend the night in the wilderness.

From Fawn Lake the loop trail climbs briefly to a forested ridgetop, and then follows the top of this ridge to the northwest for the next mile. The route then begins a series of 10 often-long switchbacks that take you down the mostly forested west side of a ridge to a junction with the Martin Creek Trail. Go right at this junction and soon come to a second junction, this time with Northbound Creek Trail #111, the upper end of which you passed not far from Heart Lake.

You go straight (downstream) at this junction and, in the next mile, make two rock-hop crossings of Northbound Creek to a good campsite just before the shallow ford of Sawtooth Creek. By late summer the water is low enough to reveal a string of conveniently placed stepping-stones, which will get you across with dry feet. Rest and fill your water bottles here, because you now face a long, tough uphill. It begins with three short switchbacks that take you to a junction with the Sawtooth Creek Trail. Go straight on the dusty and more heavily used trail; then climb at a relentless, moderately steep grade for nearly 2 miles on an open, south-facing slope that can be oppressively hot in midsummer. Eleven switchbacks keep the grade from becoming excessively steep, but it's still a tiring climb. At the top of Surveyors Ridge, you intersect a primitive road, where you turn left and walk 50 yards to the road-end trailhead at Sawtooth Saddle. This is an alternate starting point for this trip if you are willing to make the long, bumpy drive to this remote location.

To continue the loop, take Surveyors Ridge Trail #40, which angles down from the north side of the trailhead parking area. This gently graded trail slowly loses elevation for 1 mile on the heavily forested north side of Surveyors Ridge to a junction with Buck Creek Trail #100. You turn right (downhill) and steadily lose 1,600 feet in a little less than 2 miles to a calf-deep ford of Canyon Creek. About 50 yards up the opposite bank is a junction with Upper Canyon Creek Trail #99.

You bear left, staying on the Buck Creek Trail, and, 100 yards later, come to a nice campsite beside Buck Creek. A short distance past the camp, the trail appears to cross the creek, but the correct route stays above the east bank and heads upstream through lush woods. Frequent crisscrossing elk paths and several muddy spots confuse backpackers in this area, but numerous blazes make the proper route obvious. A little more than 0.5 mile from Canyon Creek, you ford Buck Creek, and then, just 100 yards later, get wet again as you recross the flow at a calf-deep ford.

A bit less than 0.5 mile past these two crossings, you hop over a tiny side creek, and then make a short, steep climb to a junction with Papoose Mountain Trail #101. You go straight and descend to a third crossing of Buck Creek, this time on a log.

WARNING: The section of trail above this crossing is rarely maintained, so you are forced to struggle through dense riparian vegetation and to make frequent, frustrating detours around some huge blowdown. Fortunately, you will endure only about 0.5 mile of this tough hiking before the trail heads up onto the hillsides above the water, where the route is in much better shape.

MALLARD PEAK FIRE LOOKOUT

Take some time here for the scenic side trip to the historic fire lookout atop Mallard Peak. To reach it, you turn left at the four-way junction and climb steeply for a little more than 0.5 mile to the rocky, cliff-edged mountaintop. The wooden lookout building here was built in 1929 and is now on the National Register of Historic Places. It was restored in the 1980s through the volunteer efforts of Ray Kresek, an avid lookout buff from Spokane, Washington. From this site, you can enjoy views north and west over most of the area covered by this hike, as well as south to the rugged Clearwater River country

Not quite 1 mile from the Papoose Mountain junction is the first of five more creek crossings, none of which is very deep, but nearly all of which require that you get your feet wet. Immediately after the fourth crossing, this time over Papoose Creek, you come to a junction with Papoose Creek Trail #627. Turn left and soon come to a nice campsite just before you cross Buck Creek for the last time.

The trail is now well maintained as it makes a long, 2,000-foot climb through forests back up to Bathtub Mountain. The climb begins with a dozen moderately graded switchbacks to the top of a ridgeline, and then the trail turns northwest and ascends along the top of the ridge. After 1.5 miles, you climb several short switchbacks, and then come to a junction with an abandoned road. The trail resumes on the other side of the overgrown road, and then goes uphill at a gentle grade, makes one switchback, and meets the road for a second time. This time you follow the road for 30 yards, and then angle to the right on a foot trail that travels through open woods to a signed trailhead on a good gravel road. To return to your car, turn left and follow this gently ascending road for 1 mile back to the Snow Peak trailhead.

POSSIBLE ITINERARY

	CAMP	MILES	ELEVATION GAIN
Day 1	Snow Peak Pond	4.0	1,000'
Day 2	Mud Lake	11.0	4,050'
	Side trip to Snow Peak	1.0	350'
Day 3	Fawn Lake	9.0	1,800'
	Side trip to Larkins Lake	1.0	100'
	Side trip to Heart Lake	0.5	350'
	Side trip to Mallard Peak	1.0	450'
Day 4	Lower Buck Creek	9.5	1,700'
Day 5	Out	7.5	2,800'

BEST SHORTER ALTERNATIVE

For a day hike from the starting trailhead, be sure to make the walk up to Snow Peak (with a side trip to Snow Peak Pond). To avoid the poorly maintained trail down from Snow Peak, but still see the impressive lakes and peaks of the Mallard-Larkins area, continue driving on the bumpy Road 201 to the trailhead just beyond Table Camp (see map). From there, hike into Mallard Lake and past Mallard Peak to a camp at Heart Lake. Return either along the same scenic trail or, for a partial loop, drop down past Northbound Lake and then hike back along the trail past Fawn Lake.

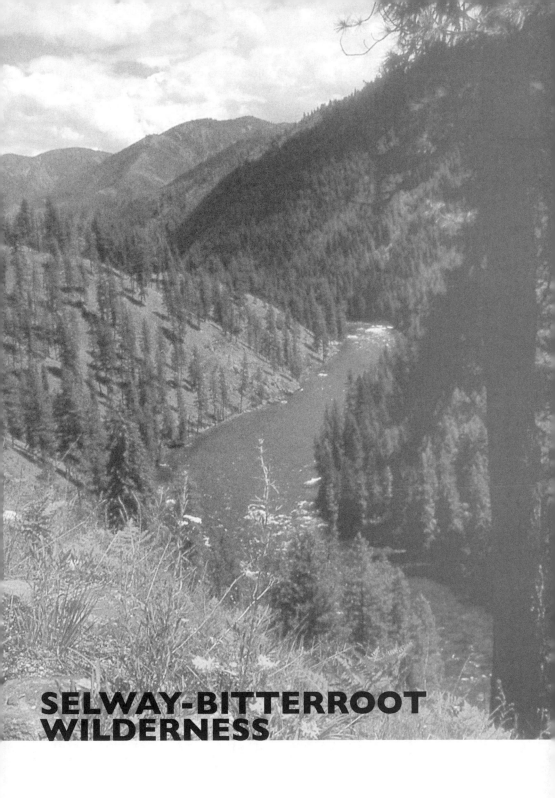

SELWAY-BITTERROOT WILDERNESS

Selway River Canyon near Dry Bar (Trip 3)

Were it not for the even larger, and adjoining, Frank Church–River of No Return Wilderness, Selway-Bitterroot Wilderness would be the largest wilderness area in the state. At approximately 1.8 million acres, it certainly covers a lot of territory. In fact, the mind-boggling size of this wilderness is one of its main attractions, because visitors here have the opportunity to find the kind of complete solitude that is rarely possible in other wild areas of the United States.

Most of the wilderness's vast acreage is a seemingly endless sea of forested ridges, stream canyons, and relatively low peaks. Only a few places feature truly dramatic scenery with high, jagged peaks and cirque lakes. The most impressive of these areas are the relatively small Selway Crags, in the west-central part of the wilderness, and the Bitterroot Divide along the border with Montana. These are the only places in the wilderness where the dense forest cover is broken by exposed portions of the Idaho Batholith, the huge, uplifted dome of granite that underlies almost all the mountains of central Idaho.

Cutting through the heart of the wilderness is the scenic canyon of the Selway River, a beautiful stream that runs clear and cold, due in no small part to the roadless nature of its watershed. Wilderness rafters and kayakers vie for coveted limited-use permits to run this river, but hikers can backpack along the trail that parallels this scenic stream without any restrictions.

The wilderness's size makes it ideal habitat for wildlife that requires large territories to survive. Though you might not see them, the wilderness is home to wolverines, black bears, gray wolves, and mountain lions. It has even been proposed that grizzly bears be reintroduced to the wilderness, and there is some anecdotal evidence that at least a few bears are recolonizing the area on their own. This unusual wildlife adds an extra level of excitement to a trip in the Selway-Bitterroot Wilderness.

The greatest problems of hiking in this wilderness are the difficulty of walking such long distances and the poor road access to some trailheads.

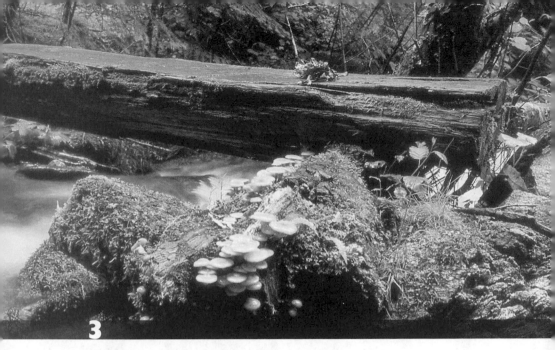

3

SELWAY RIVER TRAIL

RATINGS: Scenery 7   Solitude 5   Difficulty 5
MILES: 50
SHUTTLE MILEAGE: 252
ELEVATION GAIN: 4,200'
DAYS: 4–6
MAP(S): USFS *Selway-Bitterroot Wilderness: North Half,*
  USFS *Selway-Bitterroot Wilderness: South Half*
USUALLY OPEN: May–early November
BEST: July–October (for fishing)
PERMITS: None
RULES: Maximum group size of 20 people and 20 stock animals
CONTACT: Moose Creek Ranger District, 208-926-4258

SPECIAL ATTRACTIONS ·

Good stream fishing; whitewater rafters to watch; canyon scenery

CHALLENGES ·

Very long car shuttle; rattlesnakes

Above: Log bridge along the lower Selway River Trail

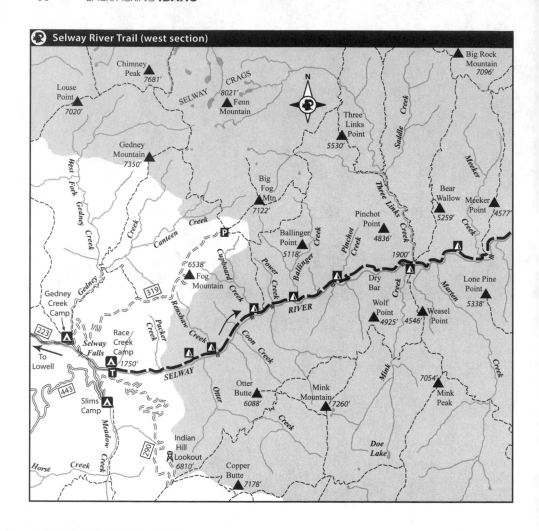

Selway River Trail (west section)

HOW TO GET THERE •

To reach the recommended starting point at the lower trailhead at Race Creek, drive 22 miles east from Kooskia on US 12 to a junction at the tiny resort town of Lowell. Turn right (southeast) onto the Selway River Road, following signs to the Selway Wild and Scenic River, and immediately cross a bridge over the Lochsa River. Drive 18.8 miles on this winding road, which turns from pavement to pothole-filled dirt and gravel after 6.8 miles, to a junction just past the Selway Falls Guard Station. Go straight and drive a final 1.1 miles to the signed trailhead at Race Creek Campground. The trail leaves from the east end of the large parking area.

To reach the upper Selway River trailhead, return to US 12, turn east, and drive 113 miles on this scenic road over Lolo Pass and into Montana, to a junction with US 93 at Lolo. Turn right (south) on US 93 and drive 58 miles to a junction just before a bridge over the Bitterroot River. Turn right (southwest) on ID 473 (also called West Fork Road), following signs to Trapper Creek Jobs Corps Center, and proceed 14.4 miles to a junction 0.5 mile past the West Fork Ranger Station and immediately before a bridge over West Fork Bitterroot River.

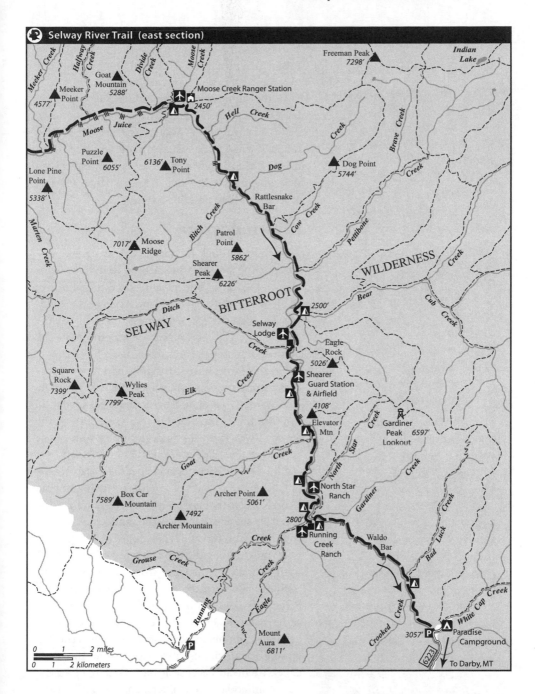

Selway River Trail (east section)

Bear right on Nez Perce Road and drive 16.5 miles on this alternating paved and gravel road to Nez Perce Pass, where you reenter Idaho. The pavement continues for another 8.4 miles as the road winds downhill beside the rushing waters of Deep Creek. Once the pavement ends, you follow a bumpy, gravel road for 10.5 miles to a junction with the Magruder Road to Elk City. Go straight, following signs to Paradise Campground, and drive 11.4 miles on

CAMP CRITTERS

The popularity of the riverside camps with both boaters and hikers has attracted a few animal pests. The most common thieves are black bears and chipmunks, which are easily foiled by hanging your food. You might also see a porcupine, which gives you the chance to get a good look at one of these common, slow-footed forest residents. On close inspection you soon realize that despite their prickly appearance, porcupines might even be described as cute, if not exactly cuddly. On the other hand, though porcupines are generally inoffensive, they have a destructive habit of chewing on sweaty pack straps, boots, and fly rod handles for the salt. So you'll need to hang these items with the food to keep them safe from the quilled pests. A final noteworthy resident of this area is the spotted sandpiper, which often flies up and down the shore here, piping out its distinctive alarm calls whenever a hiker temporarily intrudes on its territory.

the narrow and bumpy Forest Service Road 6223 to a bridge over White Cap Creek and the well-signed Selway River trailhead on the left. It takes a full day to complete this very long car shuttle.

In the summer months you may be tempted to try a shorter car shuttle that follows the very rough dirt road through the Magruder Corridor. Unfortunately, this route usually requires four-wheel drive, especially when the road is wet, and it is so slow it actually takes longer to drive than the recommended road described above.

INTRODUCTION • • • • • • • • • • • • •

Snaking through the heart of its namesake wilderness, the swift-flowing Selway River is a recreational mecca for rafters and kayakers who love challenging whitewater and pristine canyon scenery. To preserve the wilderness character of the canyon, the U.S. Forest Service strictly limits the number of rafting permits to one launch per day—a policy that forces floaters to apply for one of the coveted permits months in advance and makes this one of the country's toughest rivers to get permission to run. But hikers can enjoy the same scenery on the Selway River Trail without a permit or restrictions on the number of pedestrians.

The Selway River is managed as a catch-and-release fishery, with the season running late May–November; barbless hooks are required. On tributary streams you can catch and keep two fish, and the season runs July–November.

If you are doing the trip as a one-way hike, you'll want to walk downstream from the Selway River trailhead. But because the access road over Nez Perce Pass does not open until sometime in June, early-season hikers must use the Race Creek trailhead. In addition, hikers who want to do a shorter, up-and-back trip usually begin from the Race Creek trailhead because it has easier road access. To accommodate these hikers, I have described this trip from the Race Creek trailhead.

WARNING: Rattlesnakes are common along this trail, so watch your step and check the area carefully before you sit down to rest.

DESCRIPTION •

The first thing you notice as you start hiking upstream from Race Creek Campground is that in this relatively wet part of Idaho the vegetation is unusually lush. Droopy western red cedars hang over the riverbank, while grand firs, Douglas-firs, and ponderosa pines dominate elsewhere. Typical species in the thick undergrowth include thimbleberry, bracken fern, sword fern, wild rose, and honeysuckle, which blooms in showy clusters of orange, tubular-shaped flowers in June.

> **WARNING:** Much of this thick vegetation hangs over the trail, so after it rains you will get soaked if you're not wearing gaiters and rain pants.

For variety, the trail also passes through a few open, rocky areas with lots of May and June wildflowers like harebells, clarkia, yarrow, stonecrop, and skyrocket gilia.

The trail's early miles are easy because there are almost no noticeable ups and downs, and you stay under the shady canopy of large trees. You also never stray far from the lovely, green-tinted river, which has frequent gravel bars and sandy beaches that are great for lazy rest stops beside the water. After about 1.5 miles, you take a log across small Packer Creek and pass a sign marking where you enter the Selway-Bitterroot Wilderness. The first good riverside campsite comes a mile later where the river bends around a large gravel bar, but if this doesn't suit you, even better camps are at Renshaw Creek just 0.5 mile farther. Shortly after Renshaw Creek, the trail leaves the big trees and crosses a relatively open, brushy slope, where a few blackened snags suggest that this is an old burn area. The sun can beat down rather mercilessly on this south-facing hillside, but the grade remains gentle, so the hiking is still comfortable.

Not quite 6 miles from the trailhead is a very good campsite just before you cross the bridge over the rushing Cupboard Creek. A few feet past the bridge is a junction with the Cupboard Creek Trail, which appears to be well used even though the sign indicates that the trail is not maintained.

> **TIP:** The next 2 miles of the canyon are a good area to watch for ospreys, large hawks that build bulky, treetop nests and dive for fish in the river. Ospreys compete with river otters, belted kingfishers, and human anglers for their share of the Selway's famous trout.

From Cupboard Creek it's 0.5 mile to Power Creek, whose title greatly overstates both the stream's size and its significance, and then another mile across view-packed slopes to the sturdy bridge over Ballinger Creek, where a grassy, river-level flat provides a choice of excellent campsites.

A short distance past Ballinger Creek the trail crosses the trickling flow of Cascade Creek, which would hardly be worth mentioning except that its water drops over a scenic, wispy waterfall just above the trail. You then hike across grassy, wildflower-filled slopes with good views of a series of noisy river rapids, to a sandy beach with a good boater's campsite. Just past this campsite you take a log across the clear flow of Pinchot Creek, and then gradually pull away from the water in two lazy switchbacks, followed by an extended uphill traverse. For the next 1.5 miles the trail goes up and down across a steep, grassy slope dotted with picturesque ponderosa pines, where the views 200 feet down to the river's rapids and across to the forest-covered walls on the opposite side of the canyon are excellent. The trail then gradually works its way downhill across the slopes of Pinchot Point, returns to the river near Dry Bar, and continues another mile to a wooden bridge over the loudly cascading Three Links Creek.

About 100 feet past this bridge is a major trail junction. Though the signs here are small and hard to find, it would be impossible to miss this junction, because the Mink Peak Trail that goes to the south (right) immediately crosses an elaborately large cable suspension bridge over the rampaging Selway River.

> **TIP:** If you want to camp in this area, the best sites are on the south side of the river. To find them, cross the bridge; then bear right on an unsigned boot path. This route takes a log over Mink Creek and, 100 yards later, dead-ends at a nice campsite.

Two other important trails converge at the junction on the north side of the river. The Three Links Trail goes sharply left (north) to follow the creek of the same name, and an unsigned path angles slightly left (northeast) on its way up to Sixty-Two Ridge and Big Rock Mountain.

Your trail goes straight and closely follows the north bank of the Selway River. The canyon scenery here is always pleasant and often spectacular, as the river alternates between loud rapids and quiet riffles, while the mostly forested canyon walls stretch skyward thousands of feet on either side. The river's many twists and turns give you the chance to enjoy this scenery from different angles.

About 1.5 miles from Three Links Creek, you pass an inviting riverside campsite and, 100 yards later, splash across the tiny Tango Creek, whose meager flow is just enough to provide water if you camp nearby. Another 1.5 miles takes you through a small burn area and across partly forested canyon slopes to the bridge over fairly large Meeker Creek, after which you make a quick, 150-foot ascent to a junction with the Meeker Ridge Trail. You go straight and for the next mile make a series of gentle ups and downs through a fairly large burn area. The fire that left behind this charred landscape must have been quite intense, because fire scars on the other side of the canyon indicate that the flames managed to jump the river. As often happens in a wildfire, many of the trees survived the blaze, giving the forest a patchwork appearance. The undergrowth was burned as well, leaving the ground crowded with bracken ferns, which thrive in the open sunlight.

You reenter the shady forest canopy shortly before a grove of impressive western red cedars, where you might camp, though the trickle of water here dries up by midsummer. From here, it's another 0.5 mile to the bridge over the clear-flowing Halfway Creek and a junction with the Halfway Creek Trail. The sign says that this trail is not maintained, which may explain why it is so overgrown and appears to be virtually unused.

You go straight and for the next 3.5 miles hike through a narrow section of the canyon where the river dances along in what is essentially one continuous, churning rapid. Rafters refer to this exciting section below Moose Creek as the "Moose Juice," and it's a good place to watch for boaters. You may even see one or two boats flip over in the maelstrom of Class IV whitewater.

> **TIP:** If you're a photographer, it's a good idea to have your camera immediately available to catch action shots of the boaters.

The trail makes its way through this ruggedly scenic section via a series of little ups and downs that take you over the top of several small cliffs and rock outcrops. In general, you never get very far from the river, though at one point you climb to an overlook that is 200 feet above the water. Eventually, you pass a signed junction with the unmaintained Goat Mountain Trail, and then cross the small Divide Creek on a log and come to a junction with the Big Rock Trail. You turn right and immediately cross a long suspension bridge over the boisterous flow of Moose Creek, which almost anywhere else would deserve to be called a river.

Once across the bridge, the trail ascends two short switchbacks to another junction, this time with the Moose Ridge Trail, which drops to some excellent, but very popular, boater's camps on either side of a prominent bridge over the Selway River. The main trail bears left and climbs the spine of a minor ridge to the large flat that holds the Moose Creek Airfield. This remote airfield gets a surprising amount of use and has two long runways that cross in the middle of the field.

You bear right at a signed junction with a spur trail to the airfield and loop around and below the south end of the two landing strips. The trail then curves to the left and makes its way through woods to a junction about 200 yards from the Moose Creek Ranger Station. Though the Selway River Trail turns sharply to the right here, it's worth your time to first go left and make a short side trip to visit the historic log buildings at the ranger station. It's particularly interesting because this facility is a throwback to the early twentieth century, when most ranger stations were so isolated they had no road access and were staffed by just one or two hardy rangers who rarely saw many visitors.

TIP: The station has piped water, which gives you the chance to refill your water bottles.

The main Selway River Trail follows the canyon in a prominent turn to the southeast, making a long, sun-exposed traverse on the canyon walls several hundred feet above the river. The trail stays high for about 1 mile, crossing several small gullies and side ridges along the way, and then gradually descends to a crossing of Hell Creek, a pretty little stream whose uninviting name is difficult to explain. The trail then remains above the river for another mile before it finally returns to the water's edge not far from a good boater's campsite.

For the rest of the trip the Selway River Trail rarely rises more than 100 feet above the water, and even though there are many ups and downs along the way, none of them is sustained for very long, so the hiking is relatively gentle and easy. In addition, the scenery remains excellent throughout and helps to pull you along as the trail goes through open forests and across dry slopes of rocks, grasses, and shrubs, where you can enjoy frequent views up and down the canyon.

The next major tributary stream is the clear-flowing Dog Creek, which you cross on a bridge. You then walk about 1 mile to Rattlesnake Bar, whose name serves as a useful reminder that these reptiles are common in the Selway River canyon. Still staying fairly close to the beautiful river, you travel upstream to a junction, where you go straight and almost immediately cross a bridge over the narrow gorge that holds swift-flowing Pettibone Creek.

Your trail keeps going south, following the twisting river through two short but particularly attractive sections where the Selway flows in deep, green pools through narrow chasms below the trail. You then make a short, woodsy climb over a small side ridge and descend through open, parklike stands of ponderosa pines to a junction with Bear Creek Trail. At the edge of a small, grassy flat near this junction is a good campsite.

You veer right, almost immediately cross a bridge over the wide Bear Creek, one of the Selway River's largest tributaries, and then walk 1 mile through the lush understory of a shady forest to a junction just before a bridge over the river. Turn right and cross the bridge to reach the private and cozy Selway Lodge, which has several scattered buildings and a dirt airstrip.

The public trail curves to the left past the main lodge buildings, and then goes through a gate and ascends a bit to the south end of the landing strip. You go through another gate and almost immediately reach a junction with the Ditch Creek Trail. Here you go straight and walk past a wooden storage building to a bridge over the rushing Ditch Creek. Now the wide trail climbs a bit through relatively dense forests to a fork. To visit the Shearer Guard Station and Airfield, bear left and soon walk past the station's two log cabins to the airfield's grassy landing strip. This public landing strip is often used as an access for backcountry fishing and hunting trips.

The main trail goes right at the fork, takes a log over Elk Creek, and then comes to a junction with the Goat Ridge Trail. You go straight and skirt the west side of the Shearer Airfield to the south end of the landing strip and a reunion with the trail that went past the guard station. About 0.5 mile beyond the airfield, you pass just above a superb campsite on a sandy, riverside beach beneath a grove of towering, old-growth pines, firs, and cedars. From here, it's an easy 2-mile walk past the impressive ramparts of Elevator Mountain to a sturdy wooden bridge over large Goat Creek. Some nice campsites are below the bridge just before you cross the creek.

Immediately after the Goat Creek bridge is an unsigned junction with a trail that angles right. You go straight, hike through some brushy areas near the river, and then break out onto relatively barren canyon slopes and come to a good (but heavily horse-impacted) campsite directly below some impressive rock pinnacles. On the other side of the river you can see the scattered buildings and private airstrip of the isolated North Star Ranch. About 1 mile south of this campsite you'll pass above two even better ones—before and after where the trail has been blasted into the rock about 30 feet above the water.

Soon after these campsites, the trail crosses a bridge over the wide and shallow Running Creek and comes to a junction. The Selway River Trail goes left, follows the fence around the private and comfortable-looking Running Creek Ranch, and comes to the last of the large, curving, wood-and-cable bridges over the Selway River. Some good campsites are in a sandy area on the right just before you cross the bridge.

Immediately on the other side of the bridge is a junction, where you turn right and soon cross the small Gardiner Creek on stepping-stones.

TIP: Fill your water bottles here, because this is the last reliable and easily accessible source for about 5 miles.

South of Gardiner Creek the trail goes up and down across open slopes that support lots of bracken fern and, in early summer, a colorful assortment of wildflowers. Unfortunately, by August the only thing still blooming is spotted knapweed, a noxious, introduced species that has become the bane of the northern Rocky Mountains.

About 2 miles past Gardiner Creek you come to a good viewpoint above Waldo Bar; hike another 3 miles over generally open and rather barren terrain to a rock-hop crossing of the small Bad Luck Creek. On the left just beyond the creek crossing is a fair campsite. About 400 yards after this campsite is an unsigned junction with a trail that goes sharply left on its way up the canyon of Bad Luck Creek. You go straight and complete the last 2 miles of the hike in a relatively dense forest of mixed ponderosa pines, Douglas-firs, and grand firs, with lots of western red cedars on the riverbanks. The lush understory is filled with elderberry, sword fern, Oregon grape, twisted stalk, Douglas maple, and mountain ash, all of which are rare or absent from the drier slopes to the north. The trail ends at the small parking lot for the upstream trailhead.

VARIATIONS

If you are hiking from mid-July through early October, when the surrounding high country is free of snow, you can make a long, rugged semiloop out of this trip by returning along high, ridgetop trails south and west of the Selway River corridor. One particularly scenic route goes west from Shearer Guard Station, climbs Goat Ridge, and then passes Grave Meadow Peak on its way to Indian Hill Lookout, which is just a short car shuttle from the Race Creek trailhead.

POSSIBLE ITINERARY

	CAMP	MILES	ELEVATION GAIN
Day 1	Ballinger Creek	7.5	300'
Day 2	Moose Creek	14.0	1,200'
Day 3	Bear Creek	11.0	1,500'
Day 4	Running Creek	9.5	600'
Day 5	Out	8.0	600'

BEST SHORTER ALTERNATIVE

The lower canyon is marginally more impressive than the upper, so if you only have three or four days (or you have just one car), then start from Race Creek, hike into a base camp near Mink Creek, and then make a day hike up to Moose Creek before returning to your car.

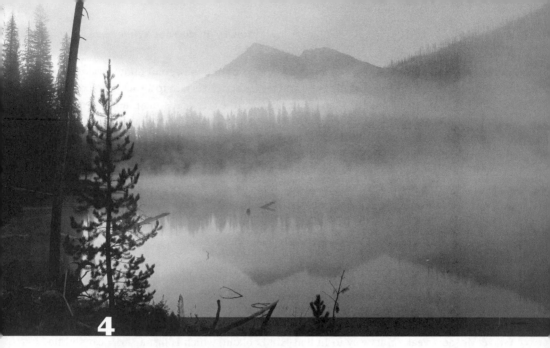

4

BIG SAND LAKE: HIDDEN CREEK LOOP

RATINGS: Scenery 7   Solitude 7   Difficulty 6
MILES: 27 (44.5)
ELEVATION GAIN: 5,450' (8,950')
DAYS: 3–5
MAP(S): USFS *Selway-Bitterroot Wilderness: North Half*
USUALLY OPEN: July–October
BEST: Any time it's open
PERMITS: None, just sign the trail register.
RULES: Maximum group size of 20 people and 20 stock animals
CONTACT: Powell Ranger District, 208-942-3113

SPECIAL ATTRACTIONS ·

Plenty of solitude in a remote region; abundant huckleberries in season; chance to see moose

CHALLENGES ·

Brushy trails; some large burn areas. Some route-finding skills are helpful.

Above: Morning fog at Big Sand Lake

HOW TO GET THERE •

Drive US 12 along the Lochsa River to a junction about 2 miles east of the Powell Ranger Station at milepost 163.4. Turn south here onto Elk Summit Road (also known as Forest Service Road 111) and follow the gravel, washboard road for 5.4 miles to a major fork. Turn right onto Road 360, and drive this narrow gravel road 3 miles to the heavily forested Savage Pass, where the road turns to dirt, but remains OK for passenger cars. Three miles later you go straight at a junction with Road 359, still following signs to Elk Summit, and proceed another 4.3 miles to a second junction, this time with Road 358. Go left here, still on Road 360 toward Elk Summit, and drive 3.8 miles to the turnoff for Big Sand Trail #4 and Elk Summit Campground. Go left, and drive about 100 yards to the trailhead parking area. The trailhead amenities include stock-loading facilities and a restroom.

INTRODUCTION •

Tucked away in the northeast corner of the Selway-Bitterroot Wilderness, this rugged and fun loop trip provides hikers with a fine sampling of the varied attractions of this huge preserve. The hike offers excellent wildlife-watching opportunities, especially for moose and a variety of birds. There are superb views from high ridges along the main trail and two lookouts that can be reached by relatively short side trips. You will go through many miles of old burn areas, which aren't particularly scenic, but which are common in this wilderness and offer a good study in how nature recovers from fire. One of the trip's main focal points, Big Sand Lake, offers both excellent scenery and fine camping. A long day hike can be made from here to the alpine glories around Blodgett Pass on the crest of the rugged Bitterroot Divide.

DESCRIPTION •

The trail begins along the campground loop road beside a signboard about 80 yards east of the parking area. The wide and rather dusty trail goes east through partly burned, open forests of Engelmann spruces, lodgepole pines, and subalpine firs, soon arriving at a trail register box and a junction with a trail that angles sharply in from the right.

You keep straight on the main trail and work your way up a gradual incline not far from small Horse Creek on your right. Eventually the bear grass–lined route works its way through forest on the outer edge of the expansive Horse Heaven Meadows, over which rises the scenic, rough outline of Diablo Mountain. At about 2.2 miles you reach a relatively low and partly burned-over high point with a signed trail junction.

The main loop trail goes straight, but for an excellent side trip, you'll first want to take the Diablo Mountain Lookout Trail that goes to the right. This path climbs rather gradually through a partial burn zone to the relatively open, higher elevations of a tall ridge. Here you'll be rewarded with great views to the west of the upper part of Horse Heaven Meadows and Grave Peak in the distance. Eventually the trail curves to the left (east) along the ridge, which now offers vistas to the south of a vast complex of forested peaks and ridges and the long drainage of Moose Creek. A half dozen switchbacks finally take you to the summit and its historic lookout building. The structure is maintained by volunteers, who also staff the facility throughout the summer—a nonpaying job but one with a benefits package that includes views that extend for miles.

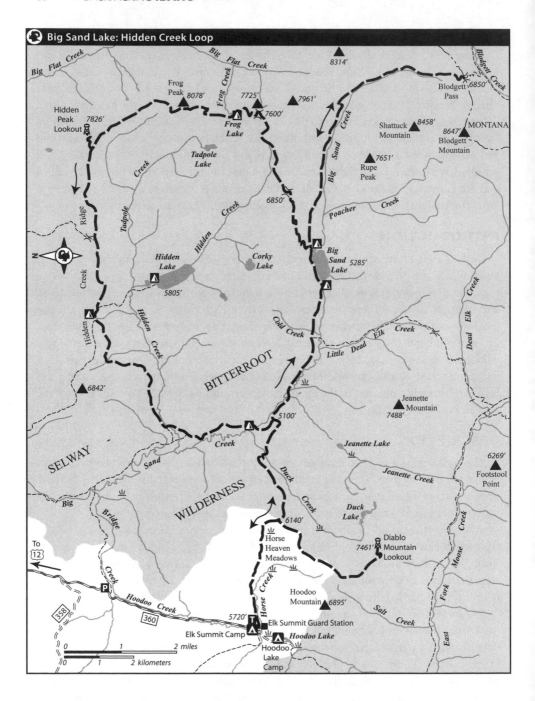

Back on the main trail, you go straight at the Diablo Mountain junction, almost immediately enter the Selway-Bitterroot Wilderness, and then make a long downhill traverse of
a rather brushy hillside. After a few lazy switchbacks you come to a crossing of the clear
and sliding Duck Creek. By midsummer this is an easy rock-hop. From here, a bit more

downhill, now in a small area of unburned forest, takes you to the bottom of the descent where you curve to the east up the wide canyon of Big Sand Creek.

Near 4.5 miles (excluding the Diablo Mountain side trip) is a junction with Big Sand Creek Trail #4. The return route of the recommended loop goes left here. For now, you go right and about 0.25 mile later come to a crossing of Big Sand Creek. For most of the summer this gently flowing stream requires a calf-deep ford to reach the other side, though by very late summer you can usually keep your feet dry with an easy rock-hop.

The trail now gradually ascends the valley of Big Sand Creek as you hike through the charred remains of a lodgepole pine forest. Shade is at a premium here, so it can get pretty uncomfortable on a hot afternoon. Enjoy the inviting rest stop along this section at a deep swimming hole on the creek, where a family of mergansers (a type of fish-eating duck) is often present.

Go straight at the signed junction with Little Dead Elk Trail #5, which goes right, and then hop over Cold Creek before arriving at the larger Big Sand Lake. This scenic, shallow lake has excellent views of a tall, open ridge to the east-northeast, and good fishing. A short spur trail leads to a fine and very scenic campsite on the lake's west end. Another good campsite is found near the inlet at the east end. Watch for moose feeding in the lake's shallow waters in the mornings and evenings. In fact, it is often possible to get quite close to these large and rather ungainly creatures.

At the northeast end of Big Sand Lake, which stretches for a half mile, is a spur trail to a campsite, and immediately thereafter is a signed junction. The recommended loop trail, signed as Frog Peak Trail #906, goes left. For an excellent day trip from Big Sand Lake, however, go right, still on Big Sand Creek Trail. This woodsy path is often quite brushy, but it is regularly maintained and the grade is very gentle, so the miles go by quickly. Starting at about 1.7 miles from the lake, you break out of the solid forest cover and begin passing through increasingly large meadows and rocky areas with good views of the nearby ridges and peaks. The trail is mostly gentle uphill, but the frustrating brush continues all the way to the Montana border at Blodgett Pass, not quite 5.8 miles from Big Sand Lake. Here you have superb views of Blodgett Mountain's tall pinnacle to the west, and on the other side of the pass you can see up and down the very deep defile of Montana's Blodgett Canyon.

Back at Big Sand Lake, complete the loop by turning left at the junction on the northeast side of the lake. The trail is somewhat bushy and overgrown but still easy to follow. The route generally goes northeast but has several irregularly spaced switchbacks as it works its way up a steep, badly burned slope. The lack of tree cover means no shade but allows for continuous views down to Big Sand Lake and of the numerous tall peaks all around. At the top of this 1,600-foot ascent you reach the ridgetop divide between the drainages of Big Sand and Hidden Creeks.

From this pass, you descend the mostly unburned north side of the divide, losing about 350 feet before reaching the bottom of a little basin and then turning uphill. The shady trail ascends beside the trickling headwaters of Hidden Creek before coming back to burned forests as you approach the top of an open ridge. The trail is faint in places, but if you have average route-finding skills, you should have no problem. Good views from this ridgetop look east to the Big Flat Creek Valley and the rugged Bitterroot Divide, as well as northeast to a nearby jagged, unnamed rocky peak.

The trail turns left at this ridgetop, following the ridge uphill through open, view-packed terrain. You top out 0.4 mile later at a 7,600-foot pass right beside the jagged peak you saw from the ridgetop earlier. There are excellent views from this pass to the north of island-dotted Frog Lake and the tall, rocky pyramid of Frog Peak. The trail descends steeply from this pass, negotiating a dozen or so switchbacks before reaching a camp next to the shallow waters of Frog Lake. Even though most of the shoreline and surrounding area is burned, the lake is still a pretty, isolated place to spend a night in the wilderness.

The trail soon pulls away from Frog Lake, going uphill and heading generally north along the west side of the ridge that climbs toward Frog Peak. The trail is obscure at times, but if you keep heading toward the top of Frog Peak and watch for old, cut logs amid the sea of picturesquely burned snags, you should be OK. You make a switchback to the right and then climb a talus slope on the east side of the ridge. At the top of this climb the route crosses back over the divide and traverses the west side of Frog Peak, only about 150 feet below the summit. There are terrific views from here to the west of the mostly burned Hidden Creek drainage and the rugged summits surrounding Grave Peak.

As you descend the north side of Frog Peak, where snow patches linger for most of the summer, there are nice views to the north-northwest of Hidden Peak, with its lookout building on top. Watch for cairns in this section as the tread can disappear in places. At one potentially confusing spot in a little meadow not far below the summit of Frog Peak, the trail makes a sharp turn to the right, away from a direct course toward Hidden Peak. After this detour, the route curves back to the left and makes a gradual but irregular descent through an attractive, unburned, high-elevation forest. You go in and out of burn areas and then complete an uphill traverse of the south side of Hidden Peak to a signed junction with Hidden Peak Lookout Trail #10.

To make the short and highly rewarding side trip to the lookout, turn sharply right at the junction and climb the steep and rocky trail up the west ridge of Hidden Peak. After a little less than 0.5 mile you reach the top with its outstanding views of the rugged Bitterroot Mountains. The old lookout building is no longer staffed and is starting to fall apart with age (aren't we all?); its ladder is collapsed and the wood is beginning to rot. But it's still a grand spot with world-class views and is well worth a visit.

Back on the main loop trail, you go west along Hidden Creek Ridge, traveling mostly downhill through partially burned forest. There is no water here, nor is there any dramatic scenery, but the hiking is pleasant and easy. In a woodsy saddle about 1.5 miles from the Hidden Peak Lookout turnoff is a signed junction with Big Flat–Hidden Ridge Trail #71.

You go straight, still on Hidden Peak Trail #10, and continue along the waterless and mostly downhill ridge walk. Through the blackened snags of this severely burned section, you can see the large Hidden Lake in the badly burned basin below you on the left. At a signed junction about 1.4 miles from the last junction, Hidden Lake Trail #9 goes sharply left. In 1.4 miles this side path drops to a simple ford of Hidden Creek, and then ascends past a smaller lake before reaching campsites next to Hidden Lake. This used to be a must-do side trip, but since a devastating wildfire in 2007, the scenery around this lake is no longer very attractive, so you might consider skipping it altogether.

The main trail goes straight at the Hidden Lake junction, and in a bit more than 0.1 mile reaches a comfortable campsite, used by a hunting outfitter in the fall, next to a bridge over a very small but reliable creek. Immediately on the other side of the bridge is a signed junction with Swamp Ridge Trail #22. *Note:* This junction is located about 0.5 mile before where the U.S. Forest Service wilderness map indicates it should be.

Go left at the junction and contour through partially burned terrain. After crossing several seasonal creeks, you begin a lengthy descent, which in a little less than 2 miles leads to an unmarked junction just above cascading Hidden Creek. Go left and immediately make a calf-deep ford of Hidden Creek. Even in late summer you should expect to have to ford this creek's chilly waters.

The trail soon curves away from Hidden Creek and takes you to a signed junction with a trail to Bridge Creek. You keep left, following signs to Elk Summit, and gradually make your way up the wide valley of Big Sand Creek. This area, like so much of the Selway-Bitterroot Wilderness, was burned many years ago and is now regrowing with thick stands of perky, little lodgepole pines. The slow-moving creek meanders through grassy meadows on your right. Watch for moose along the creek, especially on quiet mornings. Jeanette Mountain looms ahead and is easily viewed through the skinny snags of the old burn. After a quick 1.5 miles you come to a nice campsite beside the crystalline stream. Right next to the camp the trail goes down to the creek, taking you to a knee-deep ford of the sluggish waters. About 0.2 mile later you'll find yourself back at the signed junction at the close of the loop. Turn right and retrace your steps for 4.5 miles past Duck Creek and Horse Heaven Meadows, heading back to the Elk Summit Trailhead.

POSSIBLE ITINERARY

	CAMP	MILES	ELEVATION GAIN
Day 1	Big Sand Lake	7.5	550'
	Side trip to Diablo Mountain Lookout	5.0	1,400'
Day 2	Big Sand Lake	11.5	1,700'
	(day hike to Blodgett Pass)		
Day 3	Hidden Creek Ridge	10.0	3,700'
	Side trip to Hidden Peak Lookout	1.0	400'
Day 4	Out	9.5	1,200'

BEST SHORTER ALTERNATIVE •

Diablo Mountain Lookout makes an excellent day hike for a quick overview of this area. Strong hikers can also do Big Sand Lake as a long day hike, though it is much better as an overnight trip.

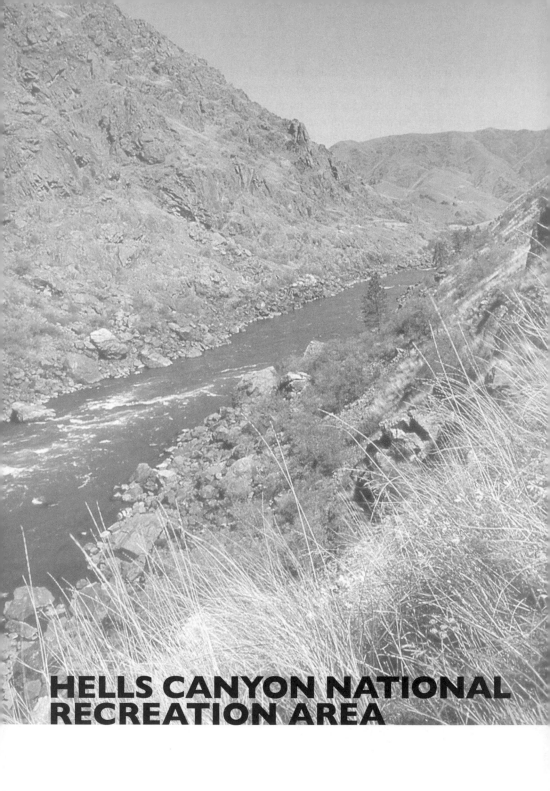

HELLS CANYON NATIONAL RECREATION AREA

Waterspout Rapids along the Snake River Trail (Trip 5)

From the lofty, 9,393-foot summit of He Devil, the highest point in the Seven Devils Mountains, you can see all the way down to the Snake River at the bottom of Hells Canyon, fully 8,000 feet below. All that elevation change leads to a great variety of life zones. In just 4 or 5 miles as the golden eagle flies, the environment changes from treeless alpine tundra of rocks, ice, and tiny wildflowers to treeless desert complete with prickly pear cacti. In recognition of this great geographic diversity, along with a similar diversity in scenery, wildlife, and cultural history, the United States Congress set aside the Hells Canyon National Recreation Area in 1975, a 652,500-acre preserve that Idaho shares with the neighboring state of Oregon.

Hundreds of miles of trails are in the recreation area, nearly all of which provide the visitor with eye-popping scenery. In the craggy heights of the Seven Devils Mountains, the trails visit snow-streaked cliffs of dark basalt towering above cirque lakes of stunning beauty. In addition to the nearby mountain scenery, these high trails frequently allow hikers to look down to the bottom of the canyon and, with binoculars, spot other hikers walking on paths that provide a radically different experience. Snow almost never falls down there, and July wildflowers, which bloom so profusely in the mountains, are replaced by grasses that are dried brown by the desert sun as soon as early May.

Hikers looking up from those river-level trails are awed by equally impressive scenery and neck-craning vistas. The view extends up a seemingly endless series of basalt cliffs and grassy terraces where elk and bighorn sheep often roam. Those hikers would be well advised to spend some time looking down as well, to avoid an unexpected encounter with a rattlesnake, an abundant resident in this area. Other hazards lurking near your boots include poison ivy, especially near watercourses, and ticks, which are at their bloodsucking worst in the spring.

Finding water is another problem in the lower canyon, because the river is not always accessible from the trail and, by late in the season, only major tributary creeks are still flowing. Carry at least 2 quarts of water and refill them at every opportunity. The final, and perhaps the most oppressive, problem faced by canyon hikers is the heat. While midsummer temperatures top out in the comfortable 70s in the mountains, highs are typically more than 100°F near the Snake River—and there is almost no shade. Spring and fall provide the most comfortable travel in the canyon. On the other hand, late June–early August is the best time to hike the trails in the Seven Devils Mountains. Thus, this remarkably diverse region provides great hiking for most of the year.

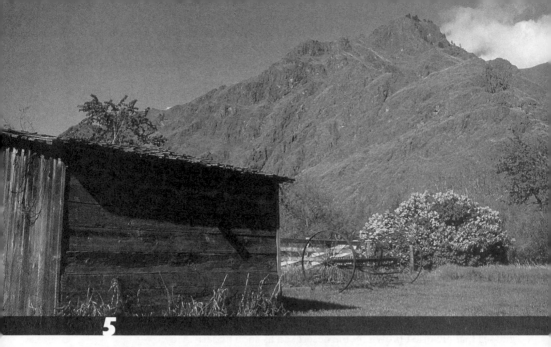

SNAKE RIVER TRAIL

RATINGS: Scenery 10   Solitude 6   Difficulty 6
MILES: 54
ELEVATION GAIN: 5,300'
DAYS: 4–7
MAP(S): USFS *Hells Canyon National Recreation Area and Wilderness*
USUALLY OPEN: Year-round (except during winter storms)
BEST: Mid-April–mid-May, October
PERMITS: None
RULES: All fires within 0.25 mile of the Snake River must be in a fire pan, and ashes must be packed out.
CONTACT: Hells Canyon National Recreation Area, Riggins Office, 208-628-3916

SPECIAL ATTRACTIONS ·

Jaw-dropping canyon scenery; whitewater rafters to watch; historic sites; wildlife

CHALLENGES ·

Rattlesnakes; ticks; extreme summer heat; poison ivy

Above: At Kirkwood Ranch

HOW TO GET THERE ·····························

From Grangeville, drive 18 miles south on US 95 to the bottom of the Salmon River Canyon, where you turn right (northwest) at a junction, following signs to Hammer Creek Recreation Area. (Coming from the south, this turnoff is about 28 miles north of Riggins.) After 0.9 mile, turn left, cross a bridge, and immediately turn left again onto Deer Creek Road. This road starts out paved, and then it turns to gravel and climbs 10.9 miles to the Hells Canyon National Recreation Area boundary at Pittsburg Saddle. The narrow road then goes steeply downhill for 6 miles to a major junction. Turn left, following signs to Upper Landing, and drive 1.3 miles on a single-lane paved road to the signed trailhead parking lot.

INTRODUCTION ·····························

No matter how much you've heard about it before you go, nothing can really prepare you for the awesome depth and breathtaking scenery of Hells Canyon. From river level, the view extends up a mind-boggling 8,000 feet to the craggy heights of Idaho's Seven Devils Mountains. Across the river, the Summit Ridge is not as high, but it's still more than a vertical mile up from the Snake River to Hat Point, the highest point on the Oregon side.

Spectacular views are only one of the area's attractions, though those alone would be more than enough reason to visit. If your schedule precludes taking a vacation during the summer months, Hells Canyon is an excellent alternative, because when most trails in Idaho are buried under several feet of snow, the low-elevation path along the Snake River provides excellent early- or late-season hiking. Spring is probably the best time to visit, because that is when the canyon is green and the wildlife is most abundant.

Wildlife isn't the only reason that spring is the best time for a visit. From mid-April to mid-May temperatures in Hells Canyon are relatively cool, the canyon is green, the flowers are blooming, and the seasonal tributary creeks provide reliable sources of water. Spring hikers, however, must also contend with a greater number of rattlesnakes and ticks, so watch your step and check yourself from time to time to remove any bloodsucking hangers-on.

Spring and fall are the best times to visit, mostly because, from late May to about mid-September, temperatures in Hells Canyon are so high that the Devil himself would feel at home. In addition, because the only trees at the bottom of the canyon are thorny hackberries and a few isolated ponderosa pines, shade is minimal. The best plan is to get an early start and do most of your hiking in the morning, when the trail is shaded by the canyon walls.

The fragile Snake River corridor sees a fair amount of use, especially by boaters. To minimize the impact, the U.S. Forest Service stresses the need for all visitors to practice Leave No Trace techniques. Jet boaters and rafters are required to pack out all human waste from the river corridor. Though this is unrealistic for backpackers, it is important that you properly bury your deposits as far away from the river as possible, and otherwise minimize your impact on the land.

DESCRIPTION ·····························

From the large trailhead parking lot, walk the remaining 0.3 mile of road to the picnic area at Upper Landing, where the official footpath begins.

Any thoughts you may have had about a gentle riverside hike are soon dashed as the trail almost immediately begins a series of short, rugged ups and downs. This roller coaster pattern, which will continue for most of the hike, is necessary because the trail must negotiate countless little rock outcrops. Sometimes the trail is simply blasted into the rock, but it usually is forced to go over or around these obstacles. The terrain becomes gentle and the trail relatively flat only on occasional riverside benches and at the outwash areas near the mouths of tributary creeks.

Your efforts are rewarded by the superb scenery, which features a continuous series of amazing views of the raging river, the ruggedly contorted canyon walls, and even occasional glimpses of the high Summit Ridge in Oregon. Closer at hand are the rocks, nearly all of which are covered with strange patterns of colorful lichens. Even the canyon's sounds are impressive, such as when the honking calls of a pair of Canada geese or the loud rattle of a belted kingfisher reverberates off the canyon walls and creates an echoing stereo effect. Unfortunately, the less pleasant roar of jet boats does the same thing, but these interruptions are fairly brief. After 1 mile, you pass a possible campsite about 200 yards before you hop over Corral Creek.

WARNING: Watch where you step and especially where you sit down to rest here, because rattlesnakes, black widow spiders, poison ivy, and prickly pear cacti are all common.

Shortly after the creek, the trail goes up a side gulch, and then out to a cliff-top overlook about 250 feet above the water, where you'll get your last good look back at the Pittsburg Landing area.

HELLISHLY WILD

From late winter through mid spring, animals seem to be everywhere in Hells Canyon, and they come in a wide variety of forms. The river teems with fish, including sturgeon, rainbow trout, catfish, bass, salmon, and steelhead. Canada geese and merganser ducks float on the water, and you will likely see elk, mountain goats, and bighorn sheep grazing on ledges that overlook the canyon. More secretive creatures include western fence lizards, which scurry away from you in rocky areas, furtive cottontail rabbits that seem to be afraid of anything that moves, and elusive mountain lions, which prowl throughout the canyon and keep the deer, elk, and bighorn sheep constantly on guard. You need to be alert as well, because at least once during your trip you can expect to be startled by the heart-stopping sound of a rattlesnake, warning you to keep your distance.

Chukars, members of the partridge family, are not nearly as dangerous but are equally nerve-racking. They have a habit of remaining out of sight until the last possible second, and then frightening unprepared hikers with a sudden squawk and furious flapping. Other common birds in the canyon include swooping white-throated swifts, perky canyon wrens, majestic golden eagles, and showy black-billed magpies.

The trail generally stays well above the river for the next few miles, crossing steep slopes and descending to river level only once, at about the 3.5-mile point. During the canyon's beautiful, but all-too-brief green season, these bunchgrass-covered slopes are tinged with green and sprinkled with colorful wildflowers. Look for the blues of *Brodiaea* and larkspur, the yellows of balsamroot and *Lomatium,* the cream color of death camas, the white of prairie star, and the pink of phlox, among many others. Unfortunately, the only water along the way comes where you cross the meager flow of Kirby Creek.

At about the 6-mile point, you descend six short, fairly steep switchbacks to Kirkwood Bar, a large, grassy, river-level flat. On the north end of Kirkwood Bar are several developed campsites complete with picnic tables, fire pits, and flush toilets. There is no potable water, however, so you will have to treat or filter the water from Kirkwood Creek, a boisterous little stream that crosses the flat through an oasis of dense riparian vegetation dominated by black hawthorns, red birches, chokecherries, and syringas.

Kirkwood Bar also holds the historic Kirkwood Ranch, which the U.S. Forest Service now runs as a museum. Even if you aren't camping here, try to schedule a minimum of half an hour to tour the ranch, look at old photos, read the interpretive signs, and examine the many outbuildings and scattered farm equipment. The friendly U.S. Forest Service volunteers, who are stationed here year-round, can answer any of your questions. Hidden just a short walk up the jeep track along Kirkwood Creek are several more historic sites, including a prehistoric Indian pit house and the old Carter homestead. Kirkwood Ranch is the usual turnaround point for this trail's relatively few day hikers, so from here on, the already uncrowded trail gets even more lonesome.

For the next mile past Kirkwood Bar, you make several small ups and downs to a bend in the river that opens up views of Oregon's Summit Ridge, which remains blanketed with snow into late May. The next major highlight is Suicide Point, a high overlook that you reach after a short, stiff ascent. The view from Suicide Point is dramatic, including not only the river and the canyon walls, but also the distant ramparts of Summit Ridge and a spur of Idaho's lofty Seven Devils Mountains. Suicide Point supposedly got its name from a Romeo and Juliet legend about a pair of young lovers who were members of two feuding tribes, the Nez Perce and the Shoshone. Lamenting their forbidden love, the couple leaped to their deaths from this point above the river.

From Suicide Point, you work your way down to Big Bar, a large, sloping, grassy bench that the trail crosses. On the Oregon side, you can see the fences, barns, and ranch house of Temperance Creek Ranch, an isolated but friendly place that is now leased to a hunting and fishing outfitter.

TIP: The grassy areas south of Temperance Creek Ranch are a particularly good place to see elk in the morning and evening.

At the south end of Big Bar, you make a brief climb, and then go into the twisting canyon of Myers Creek, where you can rest beside the splashing stream and refill your water bottles. The trail then crosses a small grassy area above Little Bar, which is visible below the trail and has some very good campsites, though the only nearby water is from the river (a questionable source, due to farm runoff in southern Idaho). Just past Little Bar, you come to the gully that holds the usually dry Caribou Creek, where you will see a small stone cabin about 75 yards above where you cross the gully.

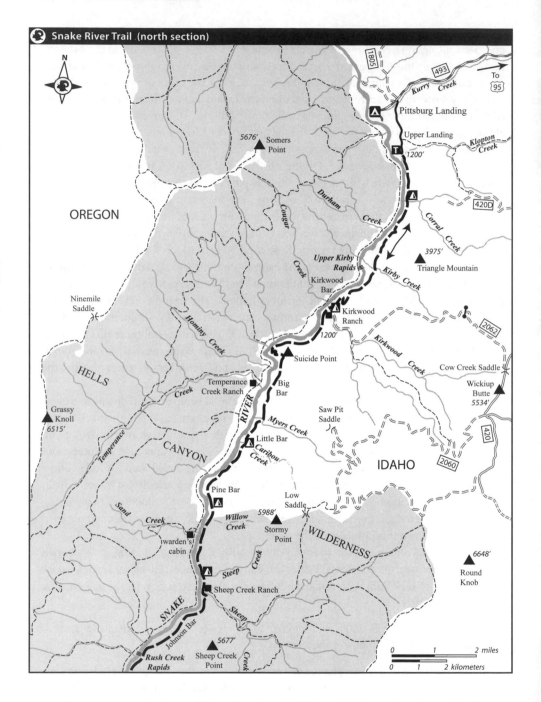

Snake River Trail (north section)

OREGON

5676' Somers Point

Durham Creek

Cougar Creek

1805

493

To 95

Kurry Creek

Pittsburg Landing

Upper Landing

T 1200'

Klopton Creek

420D

Corral Creek

3975' Triangle Mountain

Kirby Creek

Upper Kirby Rapids

Kirkwood Bar

Kirkwood Ranch

1200'

Kirkwood Creek

2062

Suicide Point

Cow Creek Saddle

Wickiup Butte 5534'

Ninemile Saddle

Hominy Creek

HELLS

Temperance Creek

Grassy Knoll 6515'

Temperance

CANYON

RIVER

Temperance Creek Ranch

Big Bar

Myers Creek

Little Bar

Caribou Creek

Saw Pit Saddle

IDAHO

420

2060

Pine Bar

Sand Creek

warden's cabin

Willow Creek

5988' Stormy Point

Low Saddle

WILDERNESS

6648' Round Knob

Steep Creek

Sheep Creek Ranch

SNAKE

Johnson Bar

Sheep Creek

Rush Creek Rapids

5677' Sheep Creek Point

0   1   2 miles

0   1   2 kilometers

The trail descends from Caribou Creek, travels close to the river for a little less than 1 mile, and then climbs to another grassy, tablelike bench where the river makes a sweeping turn to the south. After crossing this bench, you drop a bit and come to Pine Bar, where a patch of ponderosa pines provides a welcome area of shade. Below the trail here is a good

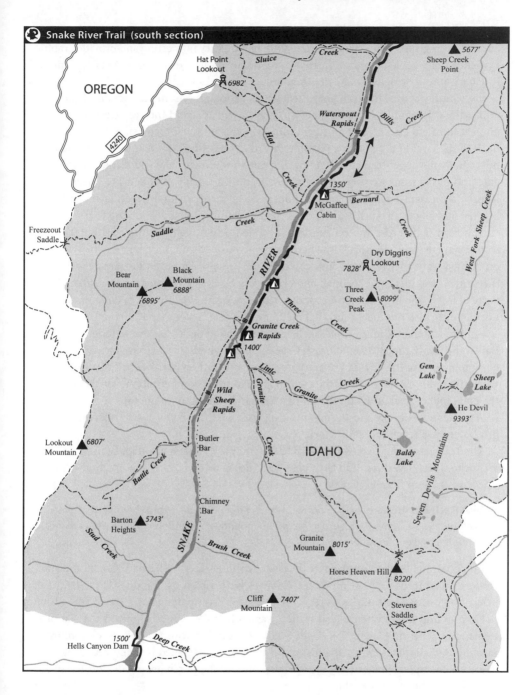

Snake River Trail (south section)

OREGON

Hat Point Lookout △ 6982'

Sluice

Creek

Sheep Creek Point ▲ 5677'

Waterspout Rapids

Bills Creek

4240

Hat Creek

1350'

McGaffee Cabin

Bernard Creek

Freezeout Saddle

Saddle Creek

Dry Diggins Lookout △ 7828'

West Fork Sheep Creek

Bear Mountain ▲ 6895'

Black Mountain ▲ 6888'

RIVER

Three Creek

Three Creek Peak ▲ 8099'

Granite Creek Rapids 1400'

Gem Lake

Sheep Lake

Little Granite

Granite Creek

He Devil ▲ 9393'

Wild Sheep Rapids

Lookout Mountain ▲ 6807'

Butler Bar

IDAHO

Baldy Lake

Seven Devils Mountains

Battle Creek

Chimney Bar

Barton Heights ▲ 5743'

Stud Creek

SNAKE

Brush Creek

Granite Mountain ▲ 8015'

Horse Heaven Hill ▲ 8220'

Cliff Mountain ▲ 7407'

Stevens Saddle

1500' Hells Canyon Dam

Deep Creek

campsite, while above the trail is a steep, exposed area of alum beds that are distinguished by colorful yellow and orange soils.

The trail then climbs over a rock outcrop, where there are fine views up and down the river, and then drops to tiny Willow Creek, which usually has water, at least in the spring.

History buffs might want to spend a little time exploring the rocks in this area for some ancient petroglyphs. They can be hard to find, but are very interesting and provide graphic evidence that people have lived in Hells Canyon for thousands of years. As always, never touch or otherwise deface this important archaeological site.

Continuing south, the trail goes through a particularly dramatic section of the canyon, where the trail makes a series of ups and downs to avoid the very steep walls. You go past the Sand Creek game warden cabin, which is on the Oregon side, and then drop back to the river and come to a possible campsite on a small, sandy beach near the tiny, but usually flowing, Steep Creek. A few more ups and downs take you through a wooden gate and past an incongruous mailbox (serviced by a weekly mail boat) to Sheep Creek Ranch, a pleasant oasis that features poplar trees, a surprisingly green lawn, and lilac bushes that bloom in April and May. Just past the ranch house is a junction.

You turn right, cross Sheep Creek on a wooden bridge, and then travel about 0.4 mile to the start of long Johnson Bar, where the canyon opens up. Large, grassy benches are on both sides of the river here, and you can look downstream into the narrow section of the canyon you just came through and crane your neck to gaze upward more than 5,700 vertical feet to the high, sometimes snowy ridgeline around Hat Point in Oregon. A sharp eye can even pick out the 90-foot-tall metal fire lookout tower atop Hat Point.

A little less than 2 miles of nearly level hiking take you across the waterless Johnson Bar to the roaring maelstrom of Rush Creek Rapids, where it's fun to watch rafters struggling to negotiate this Class IV whitewater. The canyon then narrows and turns south, to where intervening ridges block the view of Hat Point. As compensation, you can now see the even higher peak in Idaho that has Dry Diggins Lookout on the top.

Another mile of easy, mostly level walking leads to the remains of a collapsed stone hut just before you reach tiny Bills Creek.

The trail gets more rugged now as it takes you past Waterspout Rapids, makes a long ascent to a high overlook, and then goes back down to river level at a junction with the very faint trail up Bernard Creek.

WARNING: Beware of poison ivy, which seems to be everywhere in this area. Fortunately, the sumac, which also grows abundantly here and throughout the canyon, is not the poisonous variety.

You go straight, take a bridge over the clear, rushing waters of Bernard Creek, and soon come to the nicely restored McGaffee Cabin, where a sign on the door says WELCOME STRANGERS—COME ON IN. It's worthwhile to accept this invitation and spend some time poking around the old homestead, which was built in 1905 and is now on the National Register of Historic Places. The inside walls are papered with fascinating old *Saturday Evening Post* clippings, while the history of the cabin is detailed in interpretive signs. If you want to enjoy a longer visit, the upstairs loft and the porch are good spots to lay out your sleeping bag for the night.

WARNING: South of Bernard Creek the Snake River Trail gets less use than it does to the north, so it is even more overgrown with grasses and poison ivy, which is hard to avoid in places. If you are particularly allergic, you might want to stop at Bernard Creek.

To continue on to Granite Creek, follow the trail up the little slope just south of McGaffee Cabin and gradually gain about 200 feet before dropping back to the river. You pass the prominent Saddle Creek, coming in on the Oregon side, and then enter another narrow section of the canyon. Sheer cliffs on the Oregon side force the trail in that state to make a difficult detour some 1,500 feet above river level, but your trail makes it through this section very easily with almost none of the usual ups and downs. About 3 miles from Bernard Creek, you go right (downhill) at a potentially confusing fork (the left fork just dead-ends) and come to a grassy flat with possible campsites. The trail loops to the right around a boggy area here, and then climbs briefly to Three Creek, which is a good source of water if you camp at the flat.

You splash across Three Creek, and then go up and down past Granite Creek Rapids and through a 0.5-mile section that stays very close to the river's waters. Near the south end of this section the trail crosses an overhanging rock face, where it must have taken lots of dynamite to blast the trail into the rock. Immediately after this rock face, the path crosses a small, flat area with possible camps just before you reach the swift-flowing Granite Creek. The Snake River Trail goes a short distance up Granite Creek through an area of unusually lush riparian vegetation and comes to a meadow and a junction.

If you are interested in the canyon's history, bear left at this junction and hike a little less than 1 mile up the Little Granite Trail to an old homestead, whose history is detailed in the interpretive material at McGaffee Cabin.

WARNING: Though the homestead is worth exploring, the trail to it is overgrown with poison ivy and has an unusually high concentration of rattlesnakes.

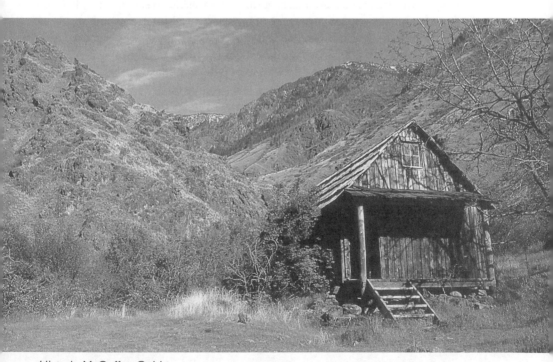

Historic McGaffee Cabin

If you are looking for a place to spend the night, turn right at the junction, cross Granite Creek on a sturdy bridge, and almost immediately come to a grassy flat with nice campsites.

Granite Creek is the recommended turnaround point for this trip. Some hikers continue another 2 miles to Butler Bar, but at that point the maintained trail ends. An old trail keeps going another 4 miles to Brush Creek, but the U.S. Forest Service cautiously describes this unmaintained section as "not really a trail anymore," partly because of periodic flooding by water releases from Hells Canyon Dam. So, unless you have arranged for some kind of boat transportation, it's time to turn around and hike back the way you came.

POSSIBLE ITINERARY

	CAMP	MILES	ELEVATION GAIN
Day 1	Little Bar	11.5	1,400'
Day 2	Bernard Creek	10.0	800'
Day 3	Bernard Creek	11.0	1,100'
	(day hike to Granite Creek)		
Day 4	Little Bar	10.0	700'
Day 5	Out	11.5	1,300'

BEST SHORTER ALTERNATIVE ·

Every step of this trail is outstanding, so it would be a shame to shorten it. Still, if you *must* do so, consider making arrangements in advance for a jet boat coming up from Lewiston to pick you up at Pittsburg Landing and drop you off somewhere around Johnson Bar. From there, simply make a one-way hike back downstream to your car. Alternatively, backpack past Kirkwood Ranch to a base camp at Little Bar, make a day hike to Johnson Bar or, if you have the energy, McGaffee Cabin, and then return the way you came. One reliable company that provides jet boat service is Beamers Hells Canyon Tours, 800-522-6966. The only reasonable day hike sampler of the canyon is to Kirkwood Bar and Museum—worthwhile, but you'll feel cheated if you don't have the time to see more.

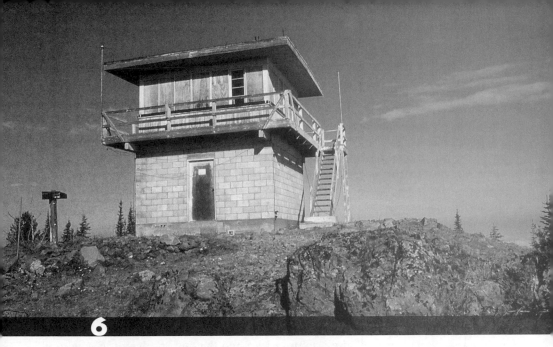

6

SEVEN DEVILS LOOP

RATINGS: Scenery 8   Solitude 6   Difficulty 5
MILES: 33 (43)
ELEVATION GAIN: 5,850' (8,500')
DAYS: 2–4 (3–6)
MAP(S): USFS *Hells Canyon National Recreation Area and Wilderness*
USUALLY OPEN: Late June–October
BEST: Late June–early August
PERMITS: None
RULES: Maximum group size of 8 people and 16 stock animals
CONTACT: Hells Canyon National Recreation Area, Riggins Office,
208-628-3916

SPECIAL ATTRACTIONS ·

Good mountain scenery; great views from Dry Diggins Lookout

CHALLENGES ·

Rough access road; numerous fire-scarred areas

Above: Dry Diggins Lookout

HOW TO GET THERE ·

From New Meadows, drive 34 miles north on US 95 to a junction exactly 0.3 mile south of the Hells Canyon National Recreation area office in Riggins. Turn left (west) on a gravel road, following signs to Seven Devils Campground, and go 1.8 miles to an unsigned fork. Turn left and begin climbing on Forest Service Road 517, a good gravel road that is suitable for passenger cars, but which is also narrow, steep, and bumpy, so trailers and recreational vehicles are not recommended. After 9.8 miles, go right (uphill) at a fork, where the route abruptly deteriorates to a slow, rocky dirt road. Exactly 4.8 miles later is another unsigned fork, where you veer right (uphill) and drive a final 0.5 mile to a junction at Windy Saddle. Turn left and go 100 feet to the well-signed trailhead parking lot on the right.

INTRODUCTION ·

The alpine meadows, green forests, and towering crags of the Seven Devils Mountains provide a welcome high-elevation contrast to the stark, bunchgrass-covered slopes of Hells Canyon. Unlike that sunbaked landscape, these high peaks provide all the usual mountain pleasures, including flower-covered meadows and trout-filled cirque lakes, plus the more unusual benefit of awe-inspiring views into the canyon's depths. A good trail goes all the way around the Seven Devils Mountains, but because the main loop bypasses almost all of the high lakes and many of the best viewpoints, you'll want to schedule extra time for plenty of side trips.

These mountains lie west of the great Idaho Batholith, so the geology of the Seven Devils is different from other mountains in central Idaho. Instead of the usual granite, these mountains are composed of dark-colored basalt, which has been uplifted and spectacularly eroded by water and glaciers into a wildly contorted assortment of cliffs, crags, and cirque basins.

DESCRIPTION ·

Most people hike this loop counterclockwise, but I prefer a clockwise tour as this saves the best scenery for last. So, go east across the dirt road directly opposite the trailhead parking lot and start hiking on Boise Trail #101, which makes a downhill traverse

ALL IN A NAME

The intriguing name Seven Devils comes from an American Indian legend about a lost Indian brave. While traversing this craggy terrain, the brave is said to have encountered a devil, from which he fled in fear only to come across a series of six more devils before finally making his way to safety. In honor of this legend, the highest peaks in this range carry sinister-sounding names such as He Devil, She Devil, Devils Tooth, Devils Thumb, Tower of Babel, The Ogre, and The Goblin. Fortunately, the landscape is much more appealing than those ominous names would suggest.

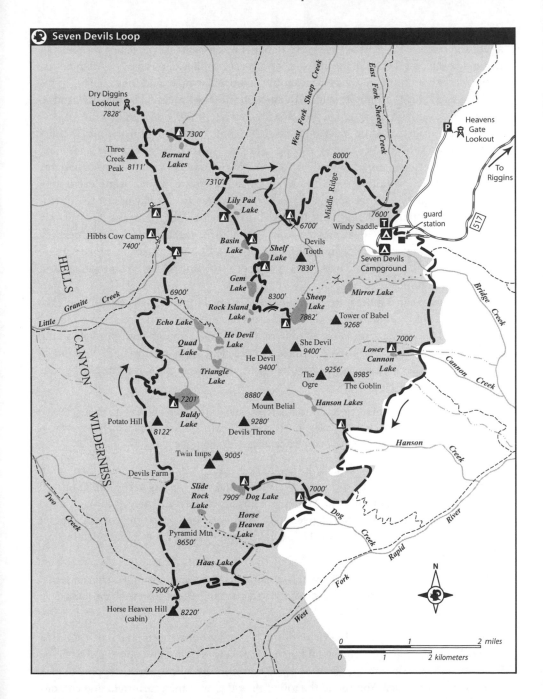

Seven Devils Loop

Dry Diggins Lookout 7828'
7300'
Three Creek Peak 8111'
Bernard Lakes
7310'
West Fork Sheep Creek
East Fork Sheep Creek
8000'
Middle Ridge
Heavens Gate Lookout
To Riggins
517
Lily Pad Lake
6700'
7600'
Windy Saddle
guard station
Hibbs Cow Camp 7400'
Basin Lake
Shelf Lake
Devils Tooth 7830'
Seven Devils Campground
HELLS
Granite Creek
6900'
Gem Lake
8300'
Sheep Lake 7882'
Mirror Lake
Bridge Creek
Little
Rock Island Lake
Tower of Babel 9268'
CANYON
Echo Lake
He Devil Lake
She Devil 9400'
Lower Cannon Lake
7000'
Cannon Creek
Quad Lake
He Devil 9400'
The Ogre 9256'
The Goblin 8985'
Triangle Lake
8880' Mount Belial
Hanson Lakes
WILDERNESS
7201'
Baldy Lake
Hanson
Potato Hill 8122'
Devils Throne 9280'
Hanson Creek
Twin Imps 9005'
Devils Farm
Slide Rock Lake
7909' Dog Lake
7000'
Two Creek
Horse Heaven Lake
Pyramid Mtn 8650'
Dog Creek
Rapid River
Haas Lake
7900'
West Fork
N
Horse Heaven Hill (cabin) 8220'

0   1   2 miles
0   1   2 kilometers

across a grassy slope. In July, this dry slope is brightened by colorful wildflowers like buckwheat, yarrow, aster, and paintbrush, while 4-foot-tall coneflower and groundsel are found in the wetter areas. In addition to the flowers, these meadows provide excellent views east to the endless, rolling mountains of central Idaho and southwest to the dark crags of the Seven Devils Mountains.

You descend two quick switchbacks to the bottom of the meadows, and then go through a gate and pass a U.S. Forest Service guard station. Look for small signs stating simply TRAIL that guide you past the buildings and over the dirt access roads of this facility. After the station, you descend through open forests mostly of lodgepole pines and subalpine firs to the wilderness boundary at another gate and a junction with the little-used Silvers Trail. You go straight, pass through the gate, and walk downhill for about 200 yards beside a tiny creek.

The trail finally levels off, curves to the right (south), and then for the next 2 miles maintains a nearly level course by zigging into side canyons with trickling creeks and zagging out to ridgelines with good views. Most of the way is through forests and large burn areas, where wildflowers such as birchleaf spirea, fireweed, and pearly everlasting have taken advantage of the sunlight to put on an impressive display of color. This display should continue for many years, because the regrowing lodgepole pines are still only a few feet tall. The burn areas provide good habitat for several species of woodpeckers, which pound away at the decaying snags, looking for grubs and insects. For hikers, these open areas provide nice views of the Tower of Babel, a distinctive high point with a dark, squared-off summit.

A little more than 3 miles from the trailhead is a signed junction with the Cannon Lake Trail. This 0.75-mile side trail makes a moderately steep climb up a fire-scarred hillside to the small Lower Cannon Lake, a lovely mountain gem rimmed with pink-blooming spirea. The lake has several good campsites and excellent views of Tower of Babel and its surrounding crags. Mountain goats are often seen on these crags, their white bodies contrasting nicely with the dark rock.

> **WARNING:** The Hells Canyon National Recreation Area map shows lots of ups and downs along the next several miles of the Boise Trail. The actual alignment is really very gentle. Do not rely on this map to calculate elevation gains and losses.

Go straight at the Cannon Lake junction, hop over Cannon Creek, and then climb a bit to a ridgeline and a junction with the Wurl Trail, which forks to the left. Your trail goes slightly right and for the next 2 miles remains nearly level as it travels through more burn areas and scattered patches of green trees. At the end of this section, you pass a good campsite on the right, just 75 yards before you step across the meager, but reliable, flow of Hanson Creek.

> **TIP:** Off-trail enthusiasts can scramble about 1 mile up this creek to the high cirque basin that holds the two Hanson Lakes, which are set impressively beneath the heights of The Ogre and Mount Belial.

After Hanson Creek, you climb a bit through another burn area on the north side of a spur ridge. In mid-August you should plan on making slow progress during this climb, because huckleberries are abundant here and you won't be able to resist stopping to pick and eat the juicy treats. You round the top of the ridge, and then turn right and contour for 0.5 mile to a junction with the Dog Ridge Trail. Go straight and continue on the level to yet another burn area and a crossing of the small Dog Creek. Just after the crossing, in a tiny patch of unburned spruce and fir trees west of the trail, is a good campsite. A superb side trip follows a steep, unmaintained boot path up Dog Creek to the beautiful Dog Lake, which has a couple of decent campsites and excellent views of the cliffs below Twin Imps.

WARNING: Dog Creek is the last reliable water source on the main trail for more than 9 miles, so stock up here and carry at least 2 quarts.

The Boise Trail continues south from Dog Creek, climbs to the top of another spur ridge, and then does some lazy ups and downs through yet another large burn area. Though rather stark and completely shadeless, these fire-ravaged areas have an eerie sort of beauty. This is especially true in July and early August, when the black and silver snags are mixed with vivid displays of fireweed and pearly everlasting. After leaving this burn area, the trail traverses a south-facing hillside with good views of the craggy Monument Peak and Black Imp in the southern Seven Devils, and then comes to Horse Heaven Creek, which is usually dry. An unsigned track heads uphill beside this creek toward Horse Heaven and Slide Rock Lakes in the remote talus-rimmed basin to the west.

Immediately after Horse Heaven Creek, the trail passes just above a shallow pond, which typically dries up by midsummer, and then comes to the base of a jumbled rockslide. Here you turn southeast, make an uphill traverse to the top of yet another spur ridge, and then turn sharply west and climb across the south side of the ridge through flower-spangled meadows with excellent views. The traverse ends with four switchbacks that go up a large talus slope to a four-way junction in a high saddle at the southern end of your loop.

Views from this saddle are restricted by trees, so take the time for a side trip to the old lookout site at Horse Heaven Hill. To reach it, go left (south) and climb four switchbacks in about 0.5 mile to a quaint log cabin at the top of Horse Heaven Hill. If you like great views, then this spot will be heaven for more than just horses. To the north are the contorted peaks of the Seven Devils Mountains, dominated by the distinctive pinnacle of He Devil, while to the south are Carbonate Hill and tall Monument Peak. The most impressive view, however, is to the west of the distant Wallowa Mountains in Oregon and down into the gaping chasm of Hells Canyon, which drops fully 6,700 feet from the top of Horse Heaven Hill to the Snake River. Bring your lunch and schedule extra time to do plenty of gawking.

To continue the loop trip, return to the junction in the saddle north of Horse Heaven Hill and go north, following signs to Hibbs Cow Camp. The well-graded trail begins with a gradual climb across steeply sloping meadows filled with brushy Douglas's knotweed and the silvery snags of a very old burn. You top out on a side ridge with fine views down the canyon of Devils Farm Creek, and then descend four switchbacks on a very rocky and exposed hillside. At the bottom of these switchbacks, you contour across a burned-over hillside, and then go through Devils Farm, a rocky and waterless little basin below the towering ramparts of a ridge south of Twin Imps. The trail then makes a gradual, 250-foot climb that turns out to be nothing but a waste of energy, because you immediately lose all of that elevation (and more) on a long downhill traverse of a partially burned-over slope on the west side of Potato Hill.

At the bottom of the traverse, the trail goes around a wide ridge and comes to a fork. The trail to the right goes uphill to the large Baldy Lake. This side trip is well worth doing, because the lake has a choice of excellent campsites and features superb views across the water to the dark mass of Devils Throne. The main trail veers left at the Baldy Lake junction and winds down through an old burn area that is now filled with regrowing pines.

At the bottom of this descent, use stepping-stones to cross two branches of Middle Fork Little Granite Creek, and then make two switchbacks and a lengthy traverse up a sun-exposed hillside, where you are treated to outstanding views west to Oregon's Black and Bear Mountains and down to the Snake River at Granite Creek. You then go up and down around a ridge and across a wooded basin to a small culvert over a seasonal creek. A few hundred yards past this creek is a junction with the dead-end trail to Echo and He Devil Lakes, yet another good side trip.

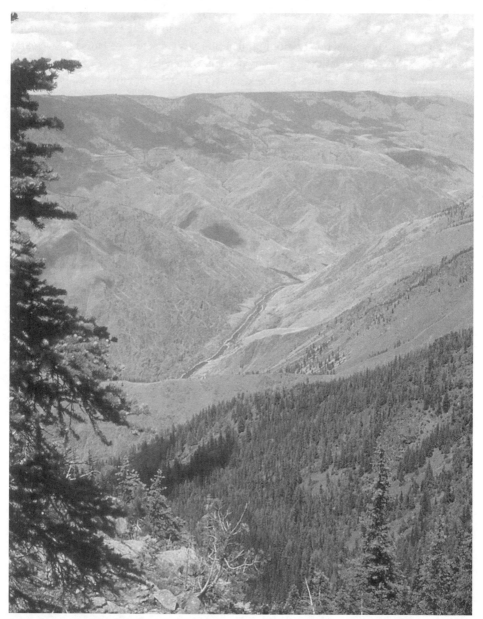

Hells Canyon from Dry Diggins Lookout

The main trail goes straight and climbs steadily for about 1 mile through a pleasant mix of forests and view-packed meadows to a very good campsite just after you step over the trickling headwaters of Little Granite Creek. A short uphill then takes you to a junction. About 100 yards west of this junction is Hibbs Cow Camp, where you will find a good (but equestrian-oriented) campsite, a trickling creek, and the chimney of a burned-down old cabin. A signed trail descends from this camp to the Snake River at Granite Creek.

You go straight at the junction and walk 0.5 mile up an increasingly dusty and horse-pounded trail to another junction in a sparsely vegetated hilltop meadow. The fastest way to complete the loop is to go right, but if you do that, you'll miss Dry Diggins Lookout, which has perhaps the best views in the state of Idaho. So bear left and walk slightly downhill for about 0.2 mile to an unsigned fork with a horse trail that goes left to an outfitter camp. You go straight and gradually gain elevation through forests and lovely meadows filled with the colorful blossoms of lousewort, yarrow, valerian, lupine, Jacob's ladder, and larkspur to a rocky viewpoint near the top of the 8,099-foot Three Creek Peak. There are superb views here, especially back to the peaks of the Seven Devils Mountains.

But the best views are yet to come, so follow the trail as it steeply descends from Three Creek Peak in three switchbacks to a junction just below a grassy saddle. Drop your pack here, grab your lunch and a camera, and take the trail to the left. In 0.5 mile this wildly scenic path winds up to the lookout building atop Dry Diggins. Though it has not been used for decades, this sturdy building is still in remarkably good condition and provides a nice platform for taking in the scenery.

And what scenery! Any credible list of America's greatest viewpoints *must* include Dry Diggins. The expected view southeast to the craggy summits of the Seven Devils Mountains is outstanding, as is the distant vista southwest to Oregon's snowy Wallowa Mountains. But the real breathtaking highlight is the look seemingly straight down over 6,500 feet to the raging whitewater of the Snake River at the bottom of Hells Canyon. It's one of those scenes that words, and even photographs, cannot adequately convey. You have to see it for yourself. Sharing the view with you may be a small band of surprisingly tame mountain goats, which wander around on the crags near the lookout.

After spending as much time at Dry Diggins as your schedule will allow, return to the junction 0.5 mile from the lookout and take the trail that goes downhill to the east. This path descends several rocky switchbacks, initially in meadows and then through forests, to Bernard Lakes. The first of this group of three lakes is only a pond, but it is immediately followed by a much larger body of water. Both of these lily pad–filled lakes have good views of Dry Diggins to the west and the craggy Three Creek Peak to the southwest.

TIP: The best camps are above the north shore of the third, least scenic lake, which is a short distance downhill from the second lake.

After the third Bernard Lake, the circuitous trail winds down through more forests and past a small, marshy pond to a usually dry gully at the head of Bernard Creek. From there, you walk through lush meadows and ascend nine moderately steep switchbacks to a prominent four-way junction in a large burn area.

A little-used trail goes left (north) along Dry Diggins Ridge, while the heavily used trail that bears slightly left (east) is your return route to Windy Saddle. First, however, take the time for a terrific side trip past a string of scenic, fish-filled mountain pools to the spectacular Sheep Lake. To do so, turn right on a dusty trail and walk about 0.4 mile to a trail fork, where you bear left and go past the aptly named Lily Pad Lake to a small, very green meadow with a good campsite near its north end. The trail then goes southeast, heading directly toward the ominous mass of He Devil, the highest point in the Seven Devils, and several lesser peaks that flank it on either side. Together they form an impressive skyline.

You soon pass just below Basin Lake, which has good campsites and a nice setting, and then cross the lake's trickling outlet creek and almost immediately turn left at an unsigned fork (the right branch just dead-ends at Basin Lake). You climb two switchbacks and ascend a bit more on a rocky tread to a ridge a little above the lovely Shelf Lake. This lake is a step up in both elevation and scenery from Basin Lake. A side trail drops left to some good campsites near the southwest shore of Shelf Lake.

More twists and turns in the trail take you up to an unsigned junction immediately before you cross a small creek. The trail to the right goes steeply uphill for about 250 yards to the deep and well-named Gem Lake, which features outstanding views of He Devil to the southeast and an unnamed craggy ridge to the west.

But don't stop here, because the array of increasingly impressive lakes is not yet over. The main trail goes left at the unsigned junction, crosses the small creek, and climbs the rocky hillside east of Gem Lake to Rock Island Lake, which is tiny but gorgeous. From there, you make a few more long switchbacks up to a wide saddle, where you can look southeast over the basin of Sheep Lake to the hulk of She Devil and east to the more dainty Tower of Babel. The trail then switchbacks down to some excellent, but rather popular, camps on Sheep Lake's southwest shore.

TIP: The best and most photogenic views of Sheep Lake are from its north end, which you can reach on a rough angler's path.

After this lengthy and rewarding side trip, return to the four-way junction north of Lily Pad Lake and turn right (east). The trail descends six irregularly spaced but well-graded switchbacks to the bottom of a large talus slope, and then goes up and down across a heavily forested basin. An abundance of huckleberries provides tasty treats if you are visiting in August or early September.

You splash across the bubbling creek that drains from Shelf Lake, and then take a log over West Fork Sheep Creek to a very good campsite just below a lovely cascading waterfall. In the next couple of miles the trail gains some 1,300 feet, beginning with four short switchbacks and then a long traverse across a talus slope.

TIP: As you climb, be sure to look behind you for great views of the sharp pinnacle of Devils Tooth.

The next 10 uphill switchbacks have long northward legs and short southward legs, so by the time you finally reach the top of the ridge you are at least 1 mile north of the falls on West Fork Sheep Creek. After completing this gently graded but tiring ascent, the trail rounds the north side of the wide Middle Ridge just above some impressive cliffs, from the top of which are fine views east to Heavens Gate Lookout and north down the rugged canyon of Sheep Creek.

You now make two gentle, downhill switchbacks and a long, curving traverse that take you to a junction near the base of a large rock formation. You go straight, and then climb five rounded switchbacks to Windy Saddle and your car.

VARIATIONS •

For the adventure of a lifetime (though with complicated transportation logistics), do the northern part of the loop, and then take the trail down Little Granite Creek from Hibbs Cow Camp to Snake River. From there, either walk down the Snake River Trail to Pittsburg Landing (see Trip 5), or arrange for a raft to pick you up and float the river to Pittsburg Landing or Lewiston.

POSSIBLE ITINERARY

	CAMP	MILES	ELEVATION GAIN
Day 1	Dog Creek	6.5	250'
	Side trip to Lower Cannon Lake	1.5	350'
Day 2	Baldy Lake	8.0	1,500'
	Side trip to Dog Lake	3.0	900'
	Side trip to Horse Heaven Hill	1.0	400'
Day 3	Sheep Lake	8.5	2,000'
	Side trip to Dry Diggins Lookout	4.5	1,000'
Day 4	Out	10.0	2,100'

BEST SHORTER ALTERNATIVE •

The northern part of this range is the most spectacular. For a shorter version of this trip, consider hiking directly from Windy Saddle to Dry Diggins Lookout, which is truly not to be missed. With an extra day, make the side trip to Sheep Lake. If you are experienced with cross-country travel, it is possible to loop back from Sheep Lake by hiking to the north end of this lake, and then angling uphill to the east-northeast to a rocky pass before dropping steeply to the beautiful Mirror Lake, which is situated right beneath the crags of Tower of Babel. From there a sketchy boot path drops down to the maintained trail south of the Seven Devils Guard Station and then back to your starting point.

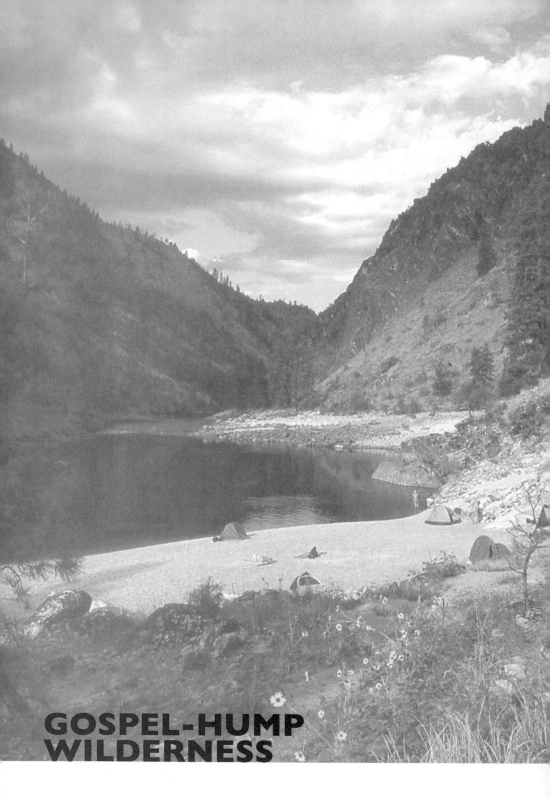

GOSPEL-HUMP
WILDERNESS

Rafters along Salmon River

Covering some 206,000 acres of rugged topography, Gospel-Hump Wilderness protects a remarkably diverse territory along the lower Salmon River in west-central Idaho. The scenic terrain here ranges from the contorted, low-elevation landscape of the Salmon River Breaks in the south to the rolling, high-elevation mountains, meadows, and plateaus in the north. As you would expect, the changes in altitude and terrain create a wide range of climates and vegetation types. The wilderness includes everything from steep, sunbaked hillsides covered with bunchgrass and scattered ponderosa pines to flower-covered mountain meadows surrounded by dense forests of lodgepole pines and subalpine firs.

What you will not encounter anywhere in this wilderness is crowds. As one of the least visited parts of the state, Gospel-Hump Wilderness remains an excellent option for those looking to "get away from it all." Believe me, when you are in Gospel-Hump Wilderness, "it all" is *really* a long way away. Only in October, when hunters arrive hoping to bag a trophy deer or elk, do very many people visit the backcountry. Of course, spring and summer hikers can also appreciate the wildlife, and they can expect to see more than just deer and elk. Bighorn sheep, for example, are common amid the rugged Salmon River Breaks, and you stand a good chance of seeing moose or mountain goats in the high country.

With all these crowd-pleasing attributes, you may be wondering why there aren't any crowds. The answer lies in access problems. The wilderness is a long way from the nearest population center, requiring several hours of driving from either Boise or Spokane to Grangeville, the small farming and lumber town nearest to the wilderness. And the drive isn't over there, because it's at least another hour and a half from Grangeville to the nearest wilderness trailhead.

Once you get out of the car, you soon discover another price hikers must pay to enjoy the solitude of Gospel-Hump Wilderness. Many of the trails here are rarely, if ever, maintained. Every trail shown on the map exists, at least in a theoretical sense, but it takes experience, and a bit of luck, to navigate the lesser-used routes.

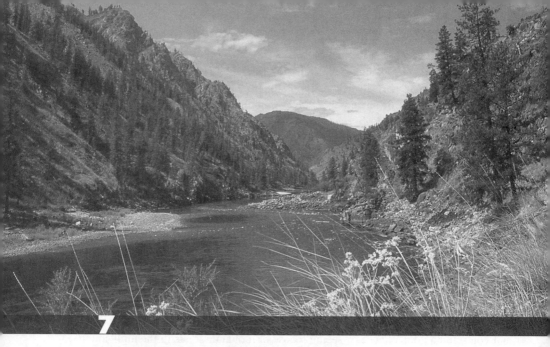

GOSPEL-HUMP LOOP

RATINGS: Scenery 7   Solitude 8   Difficulty 10
MILES: 68 (70)
ELEVATION GAIN: 12,150' (13,600')
DAYS: 5–8 (5–8)
MAP(S): USFS *Gospel-Hump Wilderness*
USUALLY OPEN: July–October
BEST: Early to mid-July, if you can stand the sometimes intense heat in the
   Salmon River Canyon; otherwise September
PERMITS: None
RULES: Maximum group size of 20 people and 20 stock animals
CONTACT: Red River Ranger District, 208-842-2245 and Salmon River Ranger
   District, 208-839-2211

SPECIAL ATTRACTIONS •

Solitude; great views of the Salmon River Canyon; whitewater rafters to watch

CHALLENGES •

Rattlesnakes and poison ivy in the Salmon River Canyon; some brushy and poorly
maintained trails

Above: Salmon River near Crooked Creek

HOW TO GET THERE •

From US 95 in Grangeville, turn east onto ID 13 and drive 1 mile through town to a junction directly across from the Nez Perce National Forest headquarters. Turn right (south), following signs for Snow Haven Ski Area, and drive 0.8 mile on this paved road to a junction, where you go straight. Just 1.5 miles later, veer right at another junction and stay on the road as it goes past the ski area and enters national forest land, where it becomes Forest Service Road 221. At 24.2 miles from the Grangeville turnoff is a four-way junction, signed as Four Corners. Turn left, staying on the paved FS 221, and drive 6.8 miles to a junction, where you turn left again, following signs to Gospel-Hump Wilderness and Sawyer Lookout.

You are now on FS 444, which is steep, but otherwise is a good gravel road with a relatively smooth surface. This road is also wildly scenic, with outstanding views that make it one of the most spectacular drives in Idaho. After 6 miles the surface gets rougher, but it remains a reasonably good gravel and dirt road that passenger cars can easily travel. Several signed trailheads are along the road. The one you want is 11.8 miles from FS 221, directly opposite the single log building of the Moores Guard Station.

INTRODUCTION •

Diversity is the defining characteristic of Gospel-Hump Wilderness, with its amazing variety of landforms, vegetation, and wildlife. This ruggedly difficult loop samples all of the wilderness's diverse scenery, including view-packed subalpine ridges, high mountain lakes, and the great depths of the Salmon River Canyon. The flora along the route is equally diverse, with everything from subalpine forests and wildflower meadows at higher elevations to parched grasses and scattered ponderosa pines in the near desert, at the bottom of the Salmon River Canyon. Wildlife is common in all of these environments, including black bears, elk, moose, and bighorn sheep. Except for boaters on the Salmon River, however, your chances of seeing very many people on this hike are slim.

The hike is unabashedly difficult, with many steep ups and downs over extremely rugged terrain. Take this hike only if you are in top physical condition, and even then you will need to take it slow.

DESCRIPTION •

The trail begins as a narrow jeep track that gradually descends through lovely bear grass meadows in a high-elevation forest of subalpine firs. You soon cross a small burn area and come to the end of the road, where you bear right on a foot trail and drop to a crossing of a trickling tributary of Anchor Creek. From here, you contour through pleasant forests to a junction at the east end of Anchor Meadows, a beautiful group of small, subalpine meadows that are covered with wildflowers in July. You bear right, hop over the main stem of the small Anchor Creek, and then go up a moderately steep incline for about 1 mile to a grassy saddle on the east shoulder of Sheep Mountain. The trail then descends to another small meadow before climbing rather steeply to the top of a ridge that extends south from the 7,917-foot-tall Plummer Point.

About 2 miles south of Plummer Point, the rolling trail takes you across burned-over slopes on the east and south sides of the rounded Marble Butte, a little above small Porcupine Meadow, where you actually stand a better chance of seeing deer or elk than porcupines. The

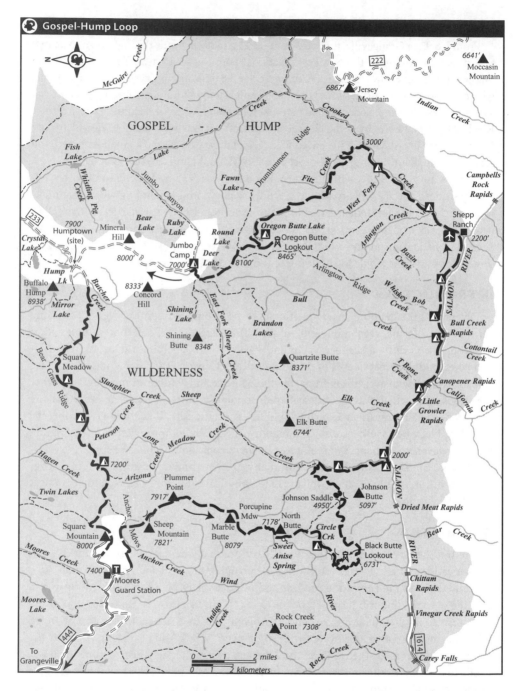

Gospel-Hump Loop

trail then descends 700 feet through a lovely forest untouched by the fire to the small but reliable Sweet Anise Spring, which has good water but no campsite.

After the spring, you make a steady downhill through lodgepole pine forests to a junction with the Johnson Butte Trail. By taking this steep route you can shorten the loop distance by about 5 miles, but you'd also miss some terrific canyon scenery and the view from Black Butte. So I recommend that you turn right, go fairly steeply downhill for 0.5 mile; then travel up and down through an area of large erratic boulders to a very good campsite about 200 yards beyond the crossing of the tiny Circle Creek. More steep little ups and downs then take you to a second creek crossing, where a much smaller campsite has room for only a single tent.

The trail makes a short but very steep climb away from Circle Creek to a viewless saddle on the east side of Black Butte, followed by an uphill traverse of the densely forested north side of the peak. At the end of this traverse is a junction with the short and not-to-be-missed spur trail to the top of Black Butte. This side trail makes 10 short switchbacks to the brushy summit, which is graced with a sturdy-looking, but unstaffed, wooden fire lookout building that sits atop a solid stone base. The view from this lofty grandstand is stupendous, especially south to the gaping Salmon River Canyon, which drops 4,700 feet down to the raging river. You can also look northeast over the forested mountains, ridges, and canyons of the Gospel-Hump Wilderness, and north to the Gospel Peaks and Square Mountain, near where you started this hike.

Back on the main trail, the elevation rapidly falls and the temperature quickly rises as you switchback steeply down the relatively dry and sunny southwest side of Black Butte. The vegetation changes to suit the new environment, with lots of brushy ceanothus bushes beneath open stands of fire-scarred ponderosa pines. A little more than 1 mile down from the Black Butte Lookout Trail is a junction with a trail that heads west (right) to the Wind River Bridge and the Lower Salmon River Road. You veer left and make a long, view-packed, up-and-down traverse of the steep slopes of the Salmon River Canyon. Views down into the canyon and up to several granite rock outcrops above the trail are almost constant and always outstanding. The rugged, 3-mile traverse ends at Johnson Saddle with a reunion with the Johnson Butte Trail.

WARNING: Rattlesnakes are abundant in the Salmon River Canyon. Though they are not aggressive, they will defend themselves if they feel threatened or if you inadvertently get too close. Few hikers make it through the upcoming section without seeing at least one or two of these chunky, venomous reptiles.

Brace your knees now, because it's all downhill from Johnson Saddle as the trail makes several, often steep switchbacks and long traverses that take you down 2,500 feet in 3 miles to an unsigned fork just above rushing Sheep Creek. Your trail veers right (downhill), switchbacks a few more times, and then turns downstream and follows a brushy and somewhat overgrown course beside the large Sheep Creek. You soon pass a good campsite with a rock-lined fireplace, after which the steep-sided canyon gets increasingly scenic with impressive walls and an interesting forest of ponderosa pines and Douglas-firs. The poorly maintained trail through this area stays on the west bank of the stream, alternating between traveling beside the water, where you have to fight through areas of thick brush, and traversing drier hillsides above the creek, where the going is much easier. In a few places the trail has been blasted into steep rock faces several dozen feet above the water. About 2.5 miles down this trail is a large wooden bridge over Sheep Creek, just before the creek's confluence with the Salmon River. Some very good, boater-oriented campsites are on either side of the bridge.

The trail turns left (east) and goes up the Salmon River's scenic canyon, generally staying on open, rocky slopes with scattered ponderosa pines, bunchgrass, and late-summer-blooming sunflowers. The wetter, north-facing slopes on the opposite side of the river have more trees, but they also show evidence of large fires with many burned-over areas.

WARNING: Poison ivy is very common along this section of the trail, so despite the often hot temperatures, shorts are a poor clothing choice.

However, it won't be easy for you to concentrate on avoiding ground-level menaces like poison ivy and rattlesnakes, because your attention will naturally be drawn to the scenery. Of particular interest are the river's numerous sandy beaches, which are covered with water early in the season, but make great lunch spots or campsites in late summer. At other points, the trail climbs to rocky overlooks about 100 feet above the river, where the views up and down the river corridor are outstanding.

About 1.5 miles from Sheep Creek you make an easy ford of Elk Creek, and then walk past Little Growler Rapids to a good campsite at the small T-Bone Creek. The rapids come fast and furious above this point, and you walk past four major rapids in the next 3 miles. It is fun to spend some time in this section watching whitewater rafters struggle through these rapids, especially when so many of them get wet or overturned in the process.

WARNING: The canyon's wild character is often disturbed by noisy jet boats. Fortunately, these boats go by quickly and the canyon soon resumes its quiet appeal.

The next major landmark is Bull Creek, a tributary that flows out of an impressive side canyon. Several good campsites are located near the log crossing of this creek, the best ones being on the west side. The river has fewer rapids above Bull Creek, as the greenish water flows through gentle riffles and quiet eddies for the next 4 miles. Two good campsites are along the way, the first just before the crossing of the often-dry Whiskey Bob Creek, and the second, 1 mile later, near Basin Creek, which is also dry. This very scenic section ends where the trail enters the mouth of the large canyon of Crooked Creek.

The trail goes a few hundred yards up Crooked Creek Canyon to the south end of a small landing strip, where the route turns right and crosses a segmented bridge to the privately owned Shepp Ranch, a comfortable-looking guest facility. *Note:* The area around this ranch, and for about 1 mile up Crooked Creek, is private property. Hikers are allowed to walk through but not camp.

After crossing the bridge, you turn left, walk past the ranch's horse pens, and then take a jeep road that parallels Crooked Creek. When the road ends, you make a knee-deep ford of the creek, and then pick up the foot trail heading up the canyon.

TIP: To avoid this ford, instead of crossing the bridge at Shepp Ranch, simply walk to the north end of the landing strip, and then wander through open forests to the trail.

Shortly after the ford is a junction with the trail up Arlington Ridge, where you go straight and soon pass a sign identifying the end of private land. Less than 0.5 mile later, you splash across Arlington Creek near a fair campsite on a small flat beside Crooked Creek.

You climb briefly to a junction with Trail #202, where you go straight, and then walk slowly uphill on the open, ponderosa pine–studded hillside a little above Crooked Creek. After about 2 miles, the trail descends from the hillside and follows the stream to a log crossing of West Fork Crooked Creek. A good campsite is on the north side of this crossing.

Not quite 1.5 miles from West Fork Crooked Creek, the trail enters an area devastated by fire, and then comes to a junction just 50 yards after crossing the small Fitz Creek. You turn left and head up the canyon of this tributary stream on a miserably brushy trail that crosses the creek five times in the next mile.

TIP: Be sure to fill your water bottles at the last crossing, because it's 4 tough miles, and almost 3,000 feet up, to your next water source.

After the last crossing, the trail leaves the dense shrubbery near Fitz Creek, goes up two switchbacks on a fire-scarred hillside, and then makes a steep uphill traverse on the northeast side of a forested ridge. The traverse ends at a ridgetop saddle, where you can rest and enjoy the view. You'll need that rest because the ascent is far from over, as the trail now winds steeply up burned-over and sunbaked slopes on the southwest side of the ridge. The climb is long and very tiring, but rewards you with a fine view south to the Salmon River Canyon and to the forested hills of the distant Frank Church–River of No Return Wilderness.

The seemingly endless climb goes through more charred areas of blackened snags and lots of deadfall as the ridgeline completes a long curve to the north. This curve causes the trail to lose its view of the Salmon River Canyon, but it offers new vistas to the northwest of Oregon Butte with its distinctive, white lookout building on top. The poorly maintained trail leaves the ridgecrest near a charred trail sign and makes a tough, up-and-down traverse on the west side of the ridge.

WARNING: Careful navigation is important here, because it is very easy to lose the route amid all the tough-limbed brush and deadfall.

After a little more than 0.5 mile of this difficult traverse, you hop over a tributary of West Fork Crooked Creek (your first water since Fitz Creek), and then switchback steeply over a small, rocky ridge. The trail reenters unburned forest here and follows the main stem of West Fork Crooked Creek up a woodsy canyon. Though the trail is still maddeningly brushy in places, at least it's mostly in the shade and reasonably easy to follow.

You soon make a rock-hop crossing of the creek, and then go steeply uphill for another mile. Exactly 160 yards after you cross the second of two tiny, trickling creeks, look for an

WORLD-CLASS VIEWS

From the meadows and fire-scarred forests atop this high ridge you'll be treated to fabulous views of a vast, wild landscape that only a state like Idaho can still offer. To the east are Oregon Butte, the distinctive Buffalo Hump, and several other destinations that are yet to come on this hike. To the northwest are the jagged Gospel Peaks, while in the distance to the southwest are the even more rugged Seven Devils Mountains. Dropping off to the south are the deep canyons of the Salmon River and its tributaries. And through all of this incredible scenery, there isn't a single sign of human beings!

orange survey tape tied to a small tree on your left that marks the start of a terrific side trip to Oregon Butte Lake. Though not an officially maintained trail, this faint angler's path is marked with orange survey tapes, so it's reasonably easy to follow. The 500-yard trail travels around a meadow and through dense woods to a great campsite beside the small lake, where you can enjoy both good trout fishing and a great view of Oregon Butte.

Back on the main trail, another 0.5 mile of moderately steep uphill through increasingly open forests takes you to the junction with the trail to Oregon Butte Lookout and a highly recommended side trip. This side trail goes left and ascends a rocky ridge for a little more than 0.5 mile to the staffed lookout building. The views from this facility are outstanding; you can see most of this hike's route as well as seemingly endless peaks and ridges in all directions.

The main loop trail goes right and wanders gradually uphill through lovely forests and meadows in a subalpine environment. Several side trails meet your route in this area and many are worth exploring. The first side trail goes to the right and follows Drumlummen Ridge to the remote Fawn Lake, which is a favorite hangout for moose. The main trail makes a short, steep climb away from this junction to a meadow-studded ridgeline, and then goes about 100 yards down from the top of this ridge to a junction with the Arlington Ridge Trail. A side trip along this trail will take you in a little more than 1 mile to some fine viewpoints along the mostly open west slopes of Oregon Butte.

The main trail goes straight at the Arlington Ridge junction and wanders generally downhill on this beautiful, view-packed ridge to a sign pointing to Deer Lake, which you can reach by following a hard-to-find angler's trail. The next junction is with the Brandon Lakes Trail, an obscure path that goes about 3 miles to these tiny and rarely visited lakes. You bear slightly right (downhill) and, a few hundred yards later, reach the junction with the Sheep Creek Trail. About 0.5 mile down this trail is the junction with a scenic side trail to the lovely Shining Lake, which has lots of big fish, though they are hard to catch.

Your route goes straight at the Sheep Creek junction, and then winds steeply down several short switchbacks to a log over the clear and slow-moving Jumbo Creek. Immediately past this log the trail ends at Jumbo Camp, a remote campground at the end of a primitive, four-wheel drive road. Here you will come across an outhouse as well as several nice (but often buggy) campsites, which you only rarely have to share with car campers.

To continue past Jumbo Camp, go north on the narrow and very rocky jeep road that goes up and down past lovely meadows and several isolated miners' cabins. (*Note:* These cabins are private property. Stay on the public roadway and do not trespass near the buildings.) The road climbs above the end of a large meadow, and then makes a high traverse across the west side of Mineral Hill, where you'll have outstanding views northwest to Buffalo Hump and west to the distant Square Mountain and the Gospel Peaks. Even though this is technically a road walk, something I try to avoid, the road is so primitive and the views are so exceptional that you will not find the walk at all tedious. About 4.5 miles from Jumbo Camp is the former site of Humptown, in a wide, meadowy saddle with great views of the massive Buffalo Hump. A signed jeep road goes left (downhill) here on its way to Hump Trail #313 and the continuation of your loop.

Before going that way, however, take some time for a scenic side trip to the nearby Hump Lake and, if possible, continue on to the larger Crystal Lake and the small but gorgeous Mirror Lake. To get to these places, stay on the main road for 50 yards, and then turn left on a jeep road. About 200 yards down this road is a very nice log cabin, from which you can saunter a short distance north to the shore of the long, meadow-rimmed Hump Lake. There are some exceptionally photogenic views across this lake of the imposing Buffalo Hump.

TIP: Look for moose browsing near the shore of this lake.

To make the 1.5-mile hike to Crystal Lake, follow the unsigned trail that goes around the east shore of Hump Lake, walk past a mine, and then go steeply down a ridge to the east end of Crystal Lake.

To find Mirror Lake, which may be the most scenic pool in the entire Gospel-Hump Wilderness, go almost due west from the south end of Hump Lake on a narrow old jeep track. After crossing the south shoulder of Buffalo Hump, look for a sketchy route going to the right (mostly downhill). This leads about 0.5 mile to Mirror Lake, which is tucked in a very scenic little cirque on the west side of the towering Buffalo Hump.

To complete the loop, return to the site of Humptown and hike 0.5 mile along the previously mentioned side road to the wilderness boundary and the start of Hump Trail #313. You will follow this scenic route for the remainder of your hike, generally staying on a high ridgeline that goes constantly up and down through lovely subalpine meadows and forests. Though there is plenty of elevation gain and loss, the grade is rarely steep, in part because much of the way follows segments of a long-abandoned jeep road.

The first mile gradually descends to a tributary of Butcher Creek, and then you climb around the edge of some rocky bluffs, which offers great views of Concord Hill and both Shining and Quartzite Buttes to the south. Immediately after this uphill, you leave the rocky old road and angle downhill to the left on an obvious foot trail. This trail takes you to a step-over crossing of the headwaters of Slaughter Creek and down to a reunion with the old road. You follow this road as it contours briefly, and then climbs to an unsigned fork near the scattered openings of Squaw Meadow. You veer left, staying on the more obvious route, and, less than 0.5 mile later, come to the unsigned junction with Boundary Creek Trail.

You go straight and gradually curve to the southwest along the gentle, open slopes of the appropriately named Bear Grass Ridge. After 1.5 miles, you pass a good campsite beside a tiny, shallow pond, and then do more ups and downs and follow the trickling headwaters of Peterson Creek. You hop over the creek shortly before a decent campsite, and then gradually pull away from the water to the signed junction with faint Trail #315 to Johns Creek. Go straight, make a moderately steep ascent to a high point on the ridge, and then go down to a small meadow with a very tiny trickle of water and a nice campsite. Another moderate uphill (this trail never stays level for long) takes you to a cairn marking a junction that is not shown on the wilderness map. You go straight (uphill) and do still more ups and downs for about 1 mile to a signed junction.

The main trail goes left and returns to the trailhead via Anchor Meadows. For a different route that provides better views with almost no added mileage, go straight, descend to a little meadow, and then climb fairly steeply up the east side of Square Mountain to a junction with Square Mountain Trail #383. You bear left and finish the hike with a scenic traverse across the view-packed slopes on the south side of Square Mountain. The trail ends at a gravel road, where you turn left and walk downhill to the Moores Guard Station.

CENTRAL IDAHO SHUTTLE SERVICES

The mountains and canyons of central Idaho form a vast wilderness complex that covers an area larger than the state of New Jersey. Lovers of true wilderness delight in the fact that no paved roads cross this area and trailhead access is often limited to long drives on rugged dirt roads. From US 12 in the north to ID 21 and ID 75 in the south, a distance of 150 miles, only one rutted, dirt road crosses central Idaho. For wildlife, this allows for unrestricted travel without the disturbance of highways. For people, however, this situation has a downside, because circling around from a trailhead on one side of the wilderness to a different trailhead on the other side entails a tedious and time-consuming drive of as many as 300 miles. This means that on point-to-point backpacking trips, your hiking time will be shortened by two full days because you have to shuttle cars back and forth at each end of your trip.

One way to avoid a long car shuttle is to take a loop hike, and several are recommended on the following pages. Because this is not always feasible, you might want to look into other alternatives. Commercial car-shuttle services cannot make enough money if they cater only to hikers, but whitewater rafters floating down Idaho's famous rivers need transportation as well, and these people are numerous enough to keep shuttle companies in business. Hikers can also use these services, and many companies will gladly take you not only to and from river put-in and takeout sites but also to most area trailheads, whether or not the stop is on their regular itinerary. It isn't cheap, but many hikers think that it is well worth it.

POSSIBLE ITINERARY

	CAMP	MILES	ELEVATION GAIN
Day 1	Circle Creek	12.0	1,500'
Day 2	Salmon River at Sheep Creek	10.0	500'
	Side trip to Black Butte Lookout	1.0	700'
Day 3	Arlington Creek	11.0	1,800'
Day 4	Oregon Butte Lake	10.0	4,900'
Day 5	Hump Lake	10.0	1,250'
	Side trip to Oregon Butte Lookout	1.0	750'
Day 6	Out	15.0	2,200'

One reliable company is River Shuttles, located in Salmon, 208-756-4188. It will happily transport you to any reasonably accessible trailhead in the Sawtooth National Recreation Area, the Salmon River country, or along the Selway River. Another advantage is that it keeps your car at its facility, which is more secure than a trailhead, and it only takes the car to your planned exit point on the day you are scheduled to return. You must have reservations for this service, and it is fairly expensive, but splitting the fee with a group makes it reasonable.

Another option for getting into or out of the backcountry is by bush plane. Dozens of remote airstrips are scattered around the wilderness where you can be dropped off and left to hike out to your car. Alternatively, you can hike in and be picked up on a prearranged date, or pay for two plane rides and hike from one airstrip to another. Two good companies that operate throughout the state but specialize in central Idaho's wilderness areas are McCall Air Taxi, 800-992-6559, and Arnold Aviation, 208-382-4844. The price of a trip depends on the size of the plane required to transport your group, how much gear you have, and the distance of the flight(s). A typical trip that transports two people and their backpacks to one of the remote airstrips along the Middle Fork Salmon River costs almost $500, as of 2015. That is expensive, but you have to weigh the cost against the time saved, the unique views you'll enjoy from the air, and the hair-raising fun and excitement of landing or taking off in a small plane from one of these tiny dirt airstrips.

VARIATIONS

You can also access this hike from the Wind River trailhead off the Lower Salmon River Road out of Riggins. From there, it's a long, tough, often hot climb to the junction below Black Butte Lookout.

BEST SHORTER ALTERNATIVE

The only realistic shorter option involves putting yourself and your car through the torture of driving the mining track (Road 233) to Humptown (see map). From there you could make excellent day hikes to Crystal Lake and Oregon Butte.

From the much-easier-on-your-car Moores Guard Station trailhead, you might consider a quick overnighter to Black Butte Lookout, which is worthwhile, though this still misses too much to be considered a satisfying alternative to the full loop.

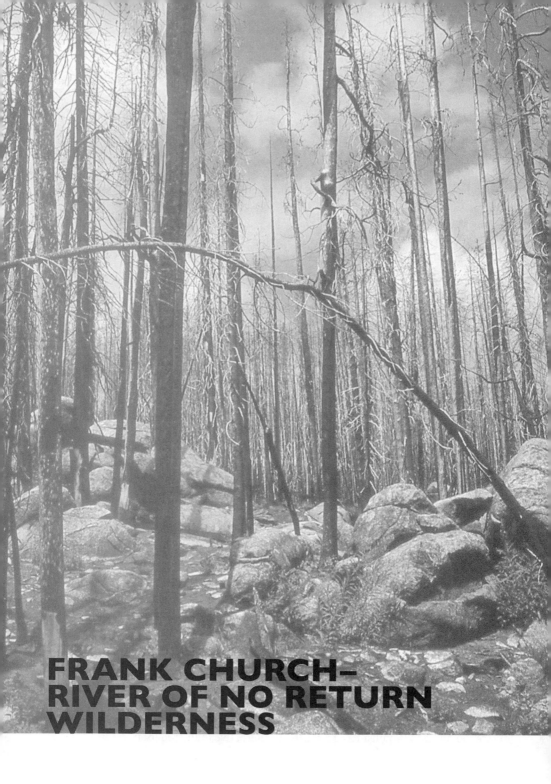

FRANK CHURCH–RIVER OF NO RETURN WILDERNESS

Burn area near Flossie Lake (Trip 8)

The Frank Church–River of No Return Wilderness isn't just big—it's positively enormous. At more than 2.3 million acres, this is the second-largest designated wilderness area in the contiguous United States. Amazingly, this seemingly endless expanse of rugged canyons, rolling mountains, and high plateaus feels even larger than it is, because the protected land is flanked by hundreds of thousands of acres of wild country that is not officially designated as wilderness (but should be). In addition, this wilderness is separated from the almost equally large Selway-Bitterroot Wilderness only by a primitive dirt road.

The average backpacker cannot reach the vast interior of this wilderness by ordinary means. It takes several days to hike into the center of this preserve from one of the outer trailheads. Access is made easier by methods that are very unusual in a designated wilderness. Much as in the wilds of Alaska, small bush planes provide regular service to several dirt airstrips scattered around the wilderness. These planes bring mail and supplies to remote wilderness ranches and guard stations, and provide convenient, if rather expensive, access for hunters, anglers, hikers, and other outdoor lovers.

Another common way of accessing the interior of this wilderness is to float its streams. Rafters joyfully descend some of North America's most exciting whitewater on the Middle Fork and the main stem of the Salmon River. A great way to see this wilderness is to pay a river operator to take you down the river, and then offload and enjoy a long hike back to your car. Thus, if you can afford the price of a plane ride or a raft trip, almost every part of the wilderness is accessible, even for the average backpacker.

Regardless of how you choose to make your way into this wilderness, your efforts will be richly rewarded. Though the scenery is generally more subdued than in the higher mountains to the south and east, the area's lakes, forested plateaus, and ridges are still very attractive, and the river canyons are both deep and spectacular.

Perhaps more impressive than the scenery is the abundance of wildlife. Big-game animals like deer, elk, black bears, and bighorn sheep seem to be everywhere. The wilderness is especially appealing to species like the mountain lion, gray wolf, and wolverine, which require large territories without the intrusion of human beings.

Probably the greatest attribute of Frank Church–River of No Return Wilderness is the simple thrill of knowing that you are hiking through the wildest land remaining in the Lower 48 states. To the true wilderness lover, just knowing that the nearest road is more than 30 miles away adds an indefinable sense of adventure and satisfaction to your trip.

The U.S. Forest Service sells two four-color contour maps that separately cover the north and south halves of the wilderness. Hikers, however, should not rely on these maps. To display all of this enormous wilderness requires that the maps be huge, two-sided, foldout sheets, which are ungainly and awkward to use in the field. In addition, because the area is so big, even after breaking down the wilderness into these four large sections, the maps are still at a scale of 1:100,000, which is too small to be useful for hikers. So carry the U.S. Forest Service map for updated information about roads and trails, but bring U.S. Geological Survey (USGS) maps for greater detail.

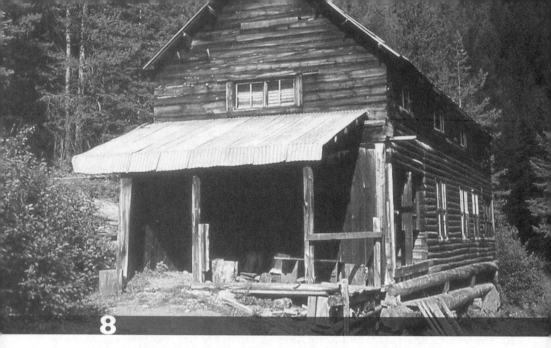

8

CHAMBERLAIN BASIN LOOP

RATINGS: Scenery 5   Solitude 7   Difficulty 7
MILES: 50 (51)
ELEVATION GAIN: 10,300' (10,600')
DAYS: 4–7 (4–7)
MAP(S): USGS *Big Creek,* USGS *Chicken Peak,* USGS *Lodgepole Creek,*
   USGS *Meadow of Doubt,* USGS *Mosquito Peak,* USGS *Sheepeater Mountain,*
   USGS *Wolf Fang Peak*
USUALLY OPEN: Mid-June–October
BEST: Mid-July–September
PERMITS: None
RULES: Maximum group size of 20 people and 20 stock animals; fires must be
   in approved fire rings near Chamberlain Airfield.
CONTACT: Krassel Ranger District, 208-634-0600

SPECIAL ATTRACTIONS •

Wildlife; solitude

CHALLENGES •

Long, rough road access; extensive burn areas

Above: Old Golden Hand Mine

HOW TO GET THERE •

There are several possible approaches to this trailhead, all of which require long drives on bumpy gravel roads. The most direct access starts from a junction on ID 55, 27 miles south of McCall or 0.8 mile north of Cascade. Turn east onto Warm Lake Road, which becomes Forest Service Road 22, and drive 34.8 miles on this winding, paved road past Warm Lake (where the road becomes FS 579) and over Warm Lake Summit to the junction with Johnson Creek Road just before the pavement ends. Turn left (north) onto FS 413 and go 25.4 miles on this sometimes bumpy gravel road to a junction at the isolated mining settlement of Yellow Pine. Turn right (east) onto FS 412, following signs to Big Creek Station, and, after 4.9 miles, turn left (north) onto FS 340, following signs to Big Creek. Drive 18.4 miles on this narrow gravel road over Profile Gap and down to a junction with FS 371, where you turn right. Follow this moderately rough road for 2.7 miles to the signed Big Creek trailhead, which is a possible alternate starting point if your car does not have good ground clearance.

To reach the recommended starting point, drive through the Big Creek trailhead parking area, cross a bridge, and then follow rough and bumpy Smith Creek Road. This primitive road is badly rutted and has some big rocks, but it remains passable for most cars if you go slowly. After 3.7 miles look for a tiny brown sign on a tree on your left stating SMITH CREEK CUTOFF TRAIL. Park here.

INTRODUCTION •

Close your eyes and try to picture what the American mountain west looked like 200 years ago. You know what I mean: one of those scenes sometimes pictured in Western movies showing vast forests, an endless series of lonesome ridges and peaks, pristine lakes, and lots of wildlife. Now open your eyes and head for the Frank Church–River of No Return Wilderness to see how well you did. There is no better place in America to run this experiment because this is the second-largest wilderness area in the contiguous 48 states, and it is perhaps the last place where you can still hike for days, weeks, or even months, and never even come close to a road.

The hike into Chamberlain Basin, actually a high, forested plateau, is one of the more enticing trips in this wilderness because it has a particular abundance of wildlife, several lakes, excellent views, and reasonable trail access. Of course, *reasonable* is not the same as *easy*—it's still a long walk—but at least you don't have to start your trip under a back-bending load of two or three weeks' worth of supplies, which is necessary for most other trips in this huge wilderness.

Though reasonably good, the scenery on this hike does not compare to the grandeur of most of the other trips in this book. Instead, this trip's appeal lies in the feeling of being in a true wilderness, a feeling that does not show up in pretty pictures.

WARNING: Much of this hike goes through fire-scarred areas with little or no shade. It can be very uncomfortable during hot weather.

DESCRIPTION •

The Smith Creek Cutoff Trail heads north (uphill) from the small parking area, passes two broken-down log cabins, and then makes 11 short, steep switchbacks up a wooded slope. At the top of these switchbacks, you enter an area with an unusual abundance of bear grass, which in some years puts on an impressive show of tall, white blossoms in early to mid-July. Later in the year you may catch sight of a black bear digging up the roots of this grasslike lily, which was named after the hungry bruins.

After a short traverse, you come to a jeep road and the still occasionally occupied buildings of the Werdenhoff Mine. (*Note:* If you have a rugged, high-clearance, four-wheel drive vehicle, it is possible to drive to this point, but for most people it's better to be on foot.) You bear right (uphill) on the rough jeep road, cross a small creek, and, immediately thereafter, reach a fork. Veer right and steadily climb the jeep road for a little more than 1 mile to a hunter's camp and the start of the poorly signed Mosquito Ridge Trail, which angles off to the left. This is the beginning of your loop.

In order to avoid a long, tough uphill at the end of your trip, and to save the better scenery for the end, I recommend doing the circuit counterclockwise. So go straight, staying on the jeep road as it crosses the trickling North Fork Smith Creek and gradually climbs for another mile to the wilderness boundary at Pueblo Summit, where the road ends at a gate.

The view from Pueblo Summit is inspiring. As far as the eye can see to the north and east are rolling, forested mountains and canyons with no roads or any other signs of human beings. This is the perfect place to test how well you did on that visualization experiment I suggested earlier.

Stepping out now into true wilderness, you go around the gate and follow an abandoned jeep track that has now deteriorated into a wide, rubbly trail. For the next 2 miles this old track slowly descends through forests of subalpine firs and lodgepole and limber pines to the interesting old buildings and remains of the Golden Hand Mine, which are worth investing some time to explore.

The old jeep road goes right (downhill) at an unsigned junction beside the mine's largest building, crosses the small Coin Creek, and then traverses a hillside for several hundred yards to an unsigned junction. You leave the old jeep road here and take an obvious foot trail that switchbacks downhill to the right and steeply descends for about 1 mile along Coin Creek. At the bottom of the downhill you cross Beaver Creek on a log just downstream from a horse ford, and then walk 150 yards up the opposite bank to a junction with the well-used Chamberlain Trail. Bear left and, a few yards later, come to the spacious Hand Creek Camp, which has room for at least a dozen tents if you have a large party.

From Hand Creek Camp, you go 80 yards northeast on the Chamberlain Trail to a small sign identifying the Ramey Ridge Trail, which, according to the wilderness map, heads off to the right, though there is no evidence of this unmaintained route on the ground. The Chamberlain Trail goes straight and, for a little more than 1 mile, wanders uphill through viewless but pleasant forests to a crossing of Hand Creek. In early summer this ford is chilly and calf-deep, but by mid-August the water will barely get above the tops of your boots. The trail steadily ascends from the ford and follows a pleasant course under the shady canopy of Douglas-firs and Engelmann spruces. The trail never takes you far from Hand Creek, so you can count on the soothing sound of "river music" as a constant companion.

Eventually, the pace of your climb quickens and the forest cover thins as lodgepole pines come to dominate at higher elevations. These more open forests have less shade, but reward you with frequent views of the forests and rock outcrops on the ridge west of Hand Creek. Not quite 2 miles from the ford, the trail takes a little wooden bridge over a tributary stream. This is a lovely spot to rest or eat lunch, which gives you the time to appreciate the groundsel, grass of Parnassus, Queen Anne's lace, wild carrot, and other colorful wildflowers that grow on the banks of the little creek.

The trail follows the tributary creek briefly, and then makes one switchback and returns to its course beside the larger Hand Creek. The climbing abates 0.5 mile later, after which you lazily wander through open pine forests above a grassy area bordering Hand Creek to a signed junction with the Crane Meadows Trail. Bear right and, about 250 yards later, pass a very good, but easily overlooked, campsite below you on the left, just above a small meadow on Hand Creek.

Now the trail, which has been significantly rerouted from what is shown on the wilderness map, makes a long and very unsatisfying climb through viewless forests on the hillside to the northeast. This realignment was done so the trail would bypass the lovely but fragile Hand Meadows, which was once a scenic highlight of this trip and a good place to see wildlife. The new trail stays in less attractive forests and burn areas and misses the meadows altogether.

After topping a woodsy ridge, the trail skirts the edge of an old burn area, and then curves to the right and makes a downhill traverse to a four-way junction. You go slightly left, staying on the Chamberlain Trail, and for the next 2.5 miles make a rather monotonous and shadeless passage through a large burn area. Deadfall is a constant problem here and in most of the other burn areas along this trail. Not quite 2 miles into this burn area is a fair campsite beside a trickle of water at the head of Lodgepole Creek.

TIP: Refill your water bottles here, because this is the last water for the next 5.5 miles, and the majority of that distance has no shade.

For the next few miles the trail gradually descends along a wide, rolling ridge. The route includes a couple of lazy switchbacks, but for the most part it's a straightforward

BIOLOGY OF A BURN

The scenery for much of the area south of the Chamberlain Basin is a perfect classroom for studying the effects of natural fire on a wild forest. Though some areas were completely scorched from ground to treetop, most of the forest looks more like a patchwork quilt. Some trees, seemingly at random, were left unscathed, while their neighbors, just a few inches away, are now blackened snags. Many trees have singed trunks, but their crowns are still intact.

The different fire ages on display here allow you to observe the stages of how a forest recovers from a fire. Initially, only grasses poke up through the charred remains. After this, wildflowers like fireweed and bear grass take over, to be followed a few years later by young evergreens. The first trees to grow are usually lodgepole pines, because the cones of this evergreen require the heat of a fire to release their seeds, an evolutionary adaptation that gives the young pines an advantage in capturing the sunlight in a new fire scar. As for wildlife, elk are especially common in the most recent burn areas, feeding on the succulent young grasses that grow in disturbed areas.

downhill. Most of the distance goes through a fascinating mix of old fire scars, recent burn areas, and some pockets of trees that have, so far, been totally untouched by flames. In a wide saddle about 2 miles from Lodgepole Creek is a sign pointing to the very faint trail that goes to your right down Little Lodgepole Creek.

TIP: The wilderness map also shows a trail that goes left to Moose Jaw Meadow, but there is no sign of this trail on the ground.

You go straight on the main trail, descend two gentle switchbacks, and then go up and down along the top of the wide, fire-scarred ridge. About 1 mile from the Little Lodgepole turnoff, the rolling section of the ridge ends and the trail goes more consistently downhill. In this area you will probably begin to hear the occasional sound of small airplanes taking off and landing at the Chamberlain Airfield. This is an unusual sound for most designated wilderness areas, but it is fairly common in the large wilderness areas of Idaho, where several active landing strips provide access to these remote regions.

The ridge gradually peters out and drops off more steeply, but the trail compensates with a couple of well-graded switchbacks, so the downhill is never overly steep. Soon after the trail levels off, you come to a junction with the Cold Meadows Trail, which goes to the right. About 200 yards from this junction is a bridge over Chamberlain Creek—which is actually the size of a small river—where you can restock your water supply or spend a few hours trying to catch some of the creek's hungry trout.

TIP: The only approved campsites in this area are on the south side of the airfield, a few hundred yards north of the creek. Do not camp near the bridge.

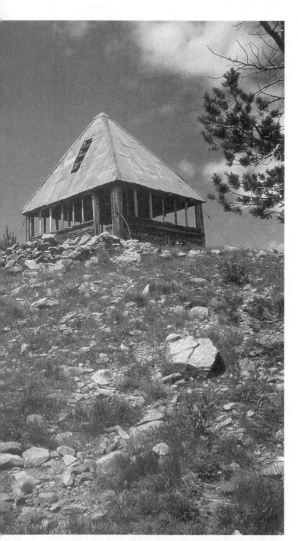

Remains of Chicken Peak Lookout

On the top of the low bank north of Chamberlain Creek is a poorly signed junction just before the long, east–west landing strip at Chamberlain Airfield. Go straight, cross the dirt landing strip, and walk a short distance through forests to an unsigned junction. Bear right, cross the clear waters of the small Ranch Creek, and soon come to the scattered buildings of the Chamberlain Guard Station. The two isolated U.S. Forest Service personnel who spend their summers here are happy to provide a greeting.

To continue the hike, go east across a north–south landing strip in Chamberlain Airfield and pick up the trail that goes north through the forest. At the end of the landing strip is a meadow where the trail splits. You veer left, following signs to Flossie Lake, and once again walk through partially burned forests. Much of the rest of the trip, in fact, is in burned areas, which is an interesting and unique ecosystem, though the scenery won't appeal to everyone.

For the next 1.5 miles the trail travels beside Ranch Creek, where lush, grassy meadows host a wide variety of wildflowers. The peak bloom is in July and early August, when the most common varieties are yarrow, aster, and cinquefoil. Later in the summer, goldenrod and gentians keep the color show going. Something else to look for in this area, and for some time to come, is signs of wolves. These large canines find good habitat in this area and you will probably see the scat and tracks of the small pack that calls this place home. If you are really lucky, you may even see the animals or hear them howling at night. One evening I lay in my sleeping bag for almost an hour listening to wolves howl—a classic wilderness experience that I will not soon forget.

You hop over Ranch Creek about 2.5 miles from the Chamberlain Guard Station; then the pace of your climb increases as eight switchbacks take you up a hillside that is badly charred by fire. After this, you wander up and down through a mix of green forests and burned woods, and then make a rather long and tiring climb around a series of rounded, rocky knolls, and drop about 100 feet to the shimmering Flossie Lake. This attractive lake sits in a small basin beneath a rocky butte, but the scene is less than perfect, because most of its shoreline is scarred by fire. Some of the trees on the south and west sides of the lake escaped the blaze, but in the designated camping area on the north side, which all visitors are required to use, there is nothing but blackened snags.

The trail continues slowly, climbing beyond Flossie Lake, first rounding the lake's basin, and then going up four switchbacks under the welcome shade of unburned spruce and pine trees. You pass a lovely little pond with a grassy shore and the appropriate name of Frog Pond, after which the rocky trail wanders up a half dozen switchbacks to a junction atop the viewless Highline Ridge.

You turn left (south) and follow the wide ridgeline for a little more than 1 mile to another junction on a severely fire-scarred hilltop with expansive views of Chamberlain Basin. The obscure and unsigned trail to the left heads down to Chamberlain Creek, but you turn right and walk slowly downhill through this bleak, charred landscape to a wide saddle. The trail then curves to the left (south) and makes an uneven descent to the south shore of the meadow-rimmed Fish Lake. Some excellent campsites are at this lake, though they tend to be plagued by mosquitoes.

TIP: The best campsites are under some large, unburned trees near an inlet creek on the southwest shore of the lake.

Not far above the southeast shore of Fish Lake is a junction, where you turn right and go steadily uphill for 1 mile to Sheepeater Lake. This beautiful lake sits in a cirque on the side of Sheepeater Mountain and is surrounded by lovely, unburned forests and scenic talus slopes. Sharp-eyed hikers will be able to spot the lookout building atop Sheepeater Mountain to the northwest. Excellent campsites are on the north shore of Sheepeater Lake, which allows you to savor a wonderful night at this mountain gem. The name *Sheepeater* is the Anglicized version of the name for a powerful tribe of local American Indians who called themselves meat eaters, and who preferred to hunt and eat bighorn sheep.

The trail now makes a moderately steep, 1-mile climb that winds up to a junction atop the ridge west of Sheepeater Lake. The short, not-to-be-missed trail to the right climbs 500 yards to the staffed lookout building atop Sheepeater Mountain. The friendly staffer, who told me that she has enjoyed this view for 17 summers, claims that her location is now the most isolated staffed fire lookout in the Lower 48 (as measured by its distance from the nearest road). In an average year she logs about 50 visitors, a number she thinks makes the place overly crowded.

To continue the hike, head south along the ridge trail, following signs to Chicken Peak, and walk mostly uphill for a few hundred yards to the signed junction with the little-used, 6.5-mile trail to Lemhi Point. This rather long side trip is worth the time, because from the heights of Lemhi Point you'll enjoy a great view almost straight down into the depths of the gaping Salmon River Canyon. The main trail goes straight at the junction and wanders up and down along the gently undulating ridge. It's an easy and very enjoyable walk with frequent views, lots of bear grass, and plenty of wildlife. Keep an eye out especially for nimble bighorn sheep near the rocky areas, and shy black bears, chubby spruce grouse, and swift mule deer in the forests. Not quite 1 mile from the Sheepeater Mountain turnoff is a small, marshy pond on your left, with permanent water and possible campsites.

About 3 miles south of Sheepeater Mountain the trail makes a steady descent to a woodsy saddle with the self-explanatory name of Fourway Junction. Go straight at the junction and climb eight short switchbacks; then begin a long, gradual ascent of the southern half of Sheepeater Ridge. Most of the way is in recent burn zones a short distance away from the rock outcrops and cliffs on the east side of the ridge.

TIP: Be sure to leave the trail from time to time to check out these rocky areas, both to enjoy the views and to look for bighorn sheep.

Not quite 1.5 miles from Fourway Junction, you lose about 100 feet of elevation and come to the welcome water of a tiny spring at the base of a small rockslide. You then go up five switchbacks and make a rugged, up-and-down traverse across the rocky east face of Sheepeater Ridge, passing four more tiny springs along the way. Eventually, you climb back up to the top of the ridge at a rocky, windswept saddle. If you look southwest from here, you should be able to spot the anomalous, bright orange roof of the old lookout building atop Chicken Peak.

The trail switches to the scenic west side of Sheepeater Ridge and climbs on a rocky tread to a high point on the eastern shoulder of Chicken Peak. It's easy and worthwhile to make the short side trip to the rapidly decaying lookout building on the summit of Chicken Peak. Though it is no longer staffed, this quaint building is worth a visit to examine the old-style architecture with its log cabin base and steeply sloping metal roof. If that doesn't interest you, then just sit back and admire the view, which includes more ridges, canyons, and mountains than I could possibly list here.

The trail makes a few lazy switchbacks down from the shoulder of Chicken Peak to a junction beside the reliable flow of Chicken Spring. Unfortunately, the lack of flat ground near this spring means that camping is not a realistic option. Go straight at the junction

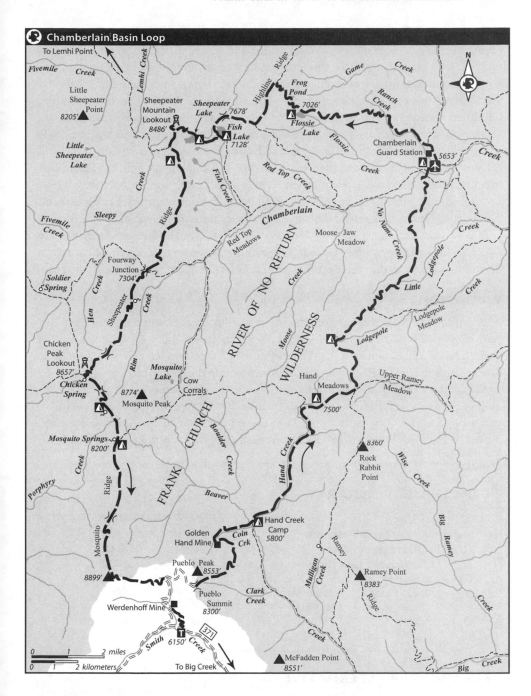

Chamberlain Basin Loop

and walk a short distance along the southwest side of the ridge; then switch to the northeast side at a little saddle. After this, you make a short, stiff climb above an intensely green meadow and pass a very pleasant campsite beside a couple of small springs.

TIP: If you plan to camp in this vicinity, do so at these springs rather than at the smelly outfitter camp near Mosquito Springs, which is larger and 0.5 mile ahead.

The now-gentle trail climbs a bit to an unsigned fork where a trail drops to the right to the outfitter camp at Mosquito Springs. You bear left and, just 50 yards later, come to a signed junction with a trail that goes left to a place with the uninviting name of Cow Corrals. You go straight, making your way south along the wide and very scenic Mosquito Ridge, and soon leave the last of the fire-damaged areas. The remainder of the hike goes through green, unburned meadows and forests that perfectly complement the excellent, distant views.

The scenic tour begins with a long, gradual ascent, mostly on the partly forested west side of the ridge, where gnarled whitebark pines add a nice touch to the scenery. You go around the west side of a high, rounded knoll, and then drop to a saddle and climb once again. This uphill starts with two switchbacks, and then makes a long, gentle ascent on the west side of the ridge nearly to the top of an 8,899-foot-high point. The trail then curves to the east and descends five moderately graded switchbacks to a nice ridgetop viewpoint, where you can look all the way north to Sheepeater Mountain. The final 1.5 miles takes you down 20 more switchbacks all the way to the Mosquito Ridge trailhead. Bear right and retrace your steps down the jeep road to the Werdenhoff Mine, the Smith Creek Cutoff Trail, and your car.

VARIATIONS

If you'd rather not drive the rough road to the Smith Creek Cutoff trailhead, then start your hike at the Big Creek trailhead instead. From there, walk about 3 miles down the Big Creek Trail to its junction with the Chamberlain Trail; then turn left and walk 7 miles up Beaver Creek to Hand Creek Camp and the junction with the described loop.

Yet another option is to turn this into a long, one-way adventure by continuing north on the Chamberlain Trail all the way to the Salmon River. From there, you can either have prearranged for a rafting party to pick you up and float you back to civilization, or be picked up by an airplane, perhaps from the remote Campbells Ferry Landing Field.

POSSIBLE ITINERARY

	CAMP	MILES	ELEVATION GAIN
Day 1	Lower Hand Meadows	10.0	3,900'
Day 2	Chamberlain Basin	10.0	400'
Day 3	Sheepeater Lake	11.0	2,700'
Day 4	Mosquito Springs	11.0	2,600'
	Side trip to Sheepeater Mountain	0.5	200'
	Side trip to Chicken Peak	0.5	100'
Day 5	Out	8.0	800'

BEST SHORTER ALTERNATIVE

The only realistic way to shorten this hike is expensive but fun. Begin by hiring a small plane to take you into Chamberlain Airfield. From there, make a loop that goes past Flossie and Fish Lakes to Sheepeater Mountain, hike south along Sheepeater Ridge to Fourway Junction, and then turn east on the trail along Chamberlain Creek to a scheduled pickup at the airfield by another small plane.

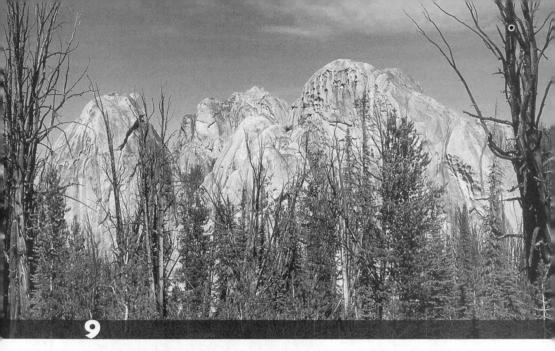

9

BIGHORN CRAGS

RATINGS: Scenery 9   Solitude 4   Difficulty 6
MILES: 46
ELEVATION GAIN: 9,000'
DAYS: 3–6
MAP(S): USGS *Hoodoo Meadows*, USGS *Mount McGuire*
USUALLY OPEN: July–mid-October
BEST: Mid-July–mid-August
PERMITS: None (just register at the trailhead)
RULES: Maximum group size of 20 people and 20 stock animals
CONTACT: Salmon/Cobalt Ranger District, 208-756-5200

SPECIAL ATTRACTIONS •

Spectacular granite domes and peaks; stunning alpine lakes; wildlife

CHALLENGES •

High altitudes with no chance to acclimate; poor access road

HOW TO GET THERE •

From Challis, drive 8 miles north on US 93, and turn left onto Morgan Creek Road, following signs to Cobalt. Stay on this good gravel road, which becomes Forest Service Road 55, for 33.2 miles as it climbs over Morgan Creek Summit and descends into the valley of

Above: Along the eastern part of the Crags Trail

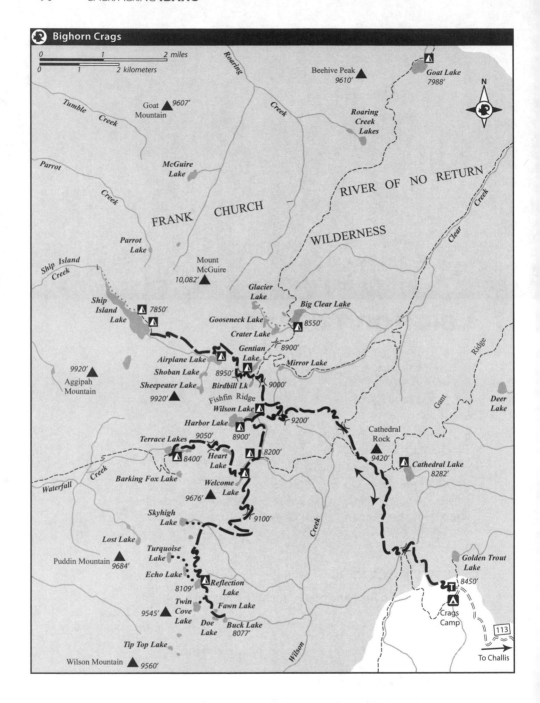

Bighorn Crags

Panther Creek to a junction. Turn left onto FS 112, following signs to Bighorn Crags and Yellowjacket, and climb 7.1 miles on this bumpy gravel road to a saddle and a four-way junction. Turn right onto FS 113, and drive carefully for 8.6 miles on this rough dirt-and-gravel route to another junction. Turn right onto FS 114 and drive 2.2 difficult but passable miles to Crags Campground and the signed parking lot for the hiker's trailhead.

INTRODUCTION •

The Bighorn Crags feature the most spectacular peaks and lakes in Frank Church–River of No Return Wilderness. And *spectacular* is definitely the right word. The scenery is absolutely delightful, with craggy granite spires, high peaks, and dozens of gorgeous alpine lakes tucked into glacial cirques. In addition to scenery, lucky hikers sometimes see elk, mountain goats, and bighorn sheep. The Crags, in fact, were named for a small band of nimble-footed sheep that live amid the spires.

Though uncrowded by comparison to similarly scenic backcountry in other parts of the American West, by Idaho standards the Bighorn Crags get a lot of visitors. The U.S. Forest Service, therefore, asks hikers to tread lightly and follow all Leave No Trace principles.

WARNING: At 8,456 feet, the Crags trailhead is one of the highest in the state. Those not accustomed to the altitude will have no warm-up period in which to get acclimated.

Also, there is no water along the first 7 miles of this ridgeline trail, so you should start with at least 2 quarts.

DESCRIPTION •

The trail begins with a series of short uphill switchbacks, followed by a long traverse across a mostly open slope with views down to Golden Trout Lake. The high-elevation forests here, and for nearly all of this hike, consist primarily of whitebark pines and sub-alpine firs with a few lodgepole pines. Many of the trees are dead, creating a forest of scenic, silvery snags. After about 1 mile those dead trees help to frame a wonderful view where the trail rounds a high ridge and you get your first sweeping vistas of the many impressive granite domes, cliffs, and spires of the Bighorn Crags.

A little less than 2 miles from the trailhead is a four-way junction in a little saddle. Two trails come in from the left here—the wide stock trail from Crags Campground, and a narrower trail that leads to Yellowjacket Lake. You go straight, climb a bit, and follow a scenic ridge with lots of polished granite towers and outcrops that rise from the ridgetop. Though the trail has many ups and downs, it is gently graded, and cool breezes often waft over the ridge, so the hiking is enjoyable.

About 2.5 miles from the Yellowjacket Lake turnoff is a junction near the base of Cathedral Rock, a prominent granite monolith. The Gant Mountain Trail goes to the right. This path drops fairly steeply for a little less than 0.5 mile to Cathedral Lake and a nearby marshy meadow with a very photogenic view of Cathedral Rock. This side trip provides you with the first chance for water and possible campsites.

The main Crags Trail bears left at the junction at the base of Cathedral Rock, descends about 150 feet, and then traverses around the south side of the rock. The open forests here provide good habitat for Clark's nutcrackers, a striking gray, black, and white relative of the crow, and the most common bird at these altitudes. The species was named after its discoverer, Captain William Clark, of the Lewis and Clark expedition.

Not quite 0.5 mile from the Gant Mountain Trail turnoff is a junction with the Water-fall Trail, which heads left on its way to Welcome Lake and the southern Bighorn Crags. You turn right (uphill) on the shorter and more popular trail to the Crags, which quickly ascends to a saddle on a windy ridge, where you can look northeast down the forested valley of Clear Creek.

At the northwest end of the saddle is a junction with the Clear Creek Trail, where you go straight and make a fairly steep climb up the shoulder of a rounded ridge. After savoring the fine views from atop this ridge, you descend a bit, and then traverse a hillside above a tiny, shimmering pond in a basin on your left. The trail makes two switchbacks up to a high, often windy pass where you get your first up-close look at the rugged Bighorn Crags. The high, jagged, and very narrow ridgeline directly to the west is Fishfin Ridge, while in a shallow, but very scenic basin to the southwest you can see Wilson and Harbor Lakes. These enticing lakes are surrounded by a series of high peaks and polished granite domes.

The trail descends from the pass in one moderately long switchback to a junction just a few feet above a rocky gap in Fishfin Ridge. The Crags Trail to Ship Island Lake goes to the right, but for the nearest water and camps go straight on the Harbor Lakes Trail. This path descends one switchback, and then contours to the shores of the beautiful Wilson Lake. Unless you made the side trip to Cathedral Lake, this is the first reliable water since the trailhead, almost 7 miles back. Several good campsites are near the outlet, and an excellent campsite is hidden in the trees beside the inlet on the southwest shore.

To visit the equally beautiful Harbor Lake, stay on the trail as it goes around the south shore of Wilson Lake to a switchback; then leave the official trail and go straight on an obvious footpath. This path climbs briefly through a low, grassy swale to Harbor Lake, a deep mountain gem with scenic peninsulas and shores that are rimmed with heather, grasses, and boulders.

TIP: Three or four very good campsites are amid the subalpine firs near the lake's outlet.

Either Harbor or Wilson Lake makes an excellent central location for a base camp from which to explore the rest of the Bighorn Crags. There are enough worthwhile destinations to keep you busy for a wonderful week of exploring. The three most rewarding day hikes are described below.

To visit Ship Island Lake, the largest and best known lake in the Crags, return to the junction on Fishfin Ridge and turn north on the Crags Trail. This well-built path descends three very gradual switchbacks on a steep talus slope to the base of the cliffs on the north side of Fishfin Ridge. From here, you traverse gradually uphill on open, rocky slopes to the top of a narrow ridge, and then descend three gentle switchbacks to a junction near unseen Birdbill Lake.

The trail to the right goes past a pond below Gentian Lake, and then switchbacks steeply over a pass and drops to the appropriately named Big Clear Lake, a worthy destination in itself. For Ship Island Lake, however, you turn left and drop to the popular camps around Birdbill and Gentian Lakes. The trail goes west, between the two lakes, and then climbs seven switchbacks to a pass, where you can look northwest to Airplane and Ship Island Lakes, and north to Mount McGuire, the highest peak in the Crags at 10,082 feet. The very gently graded route now goes down three short switchbacks, and then turns right and descends 15 irregularly spaced switchbacks to a signed junction above unseen Airplane Lake. A short side trail goes left to some good campsites on the northeast shore of this lovely lake.

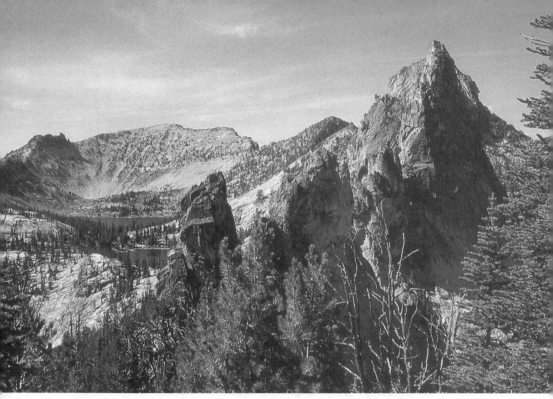

View west from Fishfin Pass to basin of Wilson and Harbor Lakes

TIP: If you are feeling adventurous, you can scramble southwest from Airplane Lake to Shoban and Sheepeater Lakes, which don't have trails but do have secluded camps and good fishing.

To continue to Ship Island Lake, hike west for 1.5 miles down a woodsy valley with lots of bear grass to some excellent campsites at the southeast end of this long and very scenic lake. The lake is surrounded by high peaks, the most dramatic being a group of tall, jagged, granite spires above the northwest shore. The lake has a small island, but it takes a lot of imagination to envision this low, forested bit of land as a "ship."

TIP: In mid- to late September the huckleberry bushes near this lake's shoreline turn bright red, adding a touch of color to the scenery.

A maintained trail continues about 0.5 mile along the lake's northeast shore past some scenic peninsulas and superb campsites. Beyond this point, adventurous hikers can follow a rough game trail all the way to the lake's outlet, and then carefully scramble down steep granite slabs to an impressive waterfall on Ship Island Creek.

WARNING: The granite rock face beside this fall provides good footing when it is dry, but it can be dangerously slippery when wet.

From the top of this waterfall are excellent views to the bottom of the Middle Fork Salmon River Canyon, almost 5,000 feet below.

Another excellent day hike from your base camp at Wilson or Harbor Lake goes south to Reflection Lake and a string of smaller lakes in the southern Bighorn Crags. To visit this area, start from the switchback on the south shore of Wilson Lake and go south on the official trail. This path contours briefly, and then descends a steep hillside of granite slabs, where the trail is marked by small cairns and your knees take a pounding on the unyielding rock. At the base of this section is a small campsite with unreliable water. You then go fairly steeply downhill, beside a tiny creek in a slot canyon on your left, to a junction with the Waterfall Trail and a nice, woodsy campsite beside Wilson Creek.

You turn right, hop over the creek, and then gradually ascend a few lazy switchbacks to a junction with the trail to the Terrace Lakes (see the recommended day hike on the next page). For Reflection Lake, you go straight and, 100 yards later, pass a short, unmarked spur trail to the right. This path leads to some nice campsites beside the shallow Welcome Lake, which is surrounded by large meadows and has a good view of a high, unnamed mountain to the west.

WARNING: In July, this lake hosts the worst concentration of mosquitoes in the Bighorn Crags.

To continue to Reflection Lake, bear left at the junction with the Welcome Lake spur trail and climb a series of nine, long, well-graded switchbacks to the top of a ridge. Views from this ridge extend all the way east to the mountains of Montana. As you gradually round this ridge to the right (southwest) you also gain fine perspectives of Reflection Lake and its surrounding lake-dotted basin to the southwest.

To reach this basin, you go down two very long switchbacks to a pretty meadow, and then wind downhill in the trees to a small creek. You hop over the creek and then, for the next few miles, wander up and down through this forested basin on a very gradual and

Airplane Lake

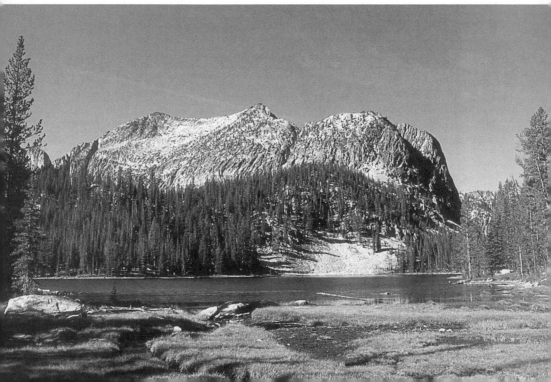

extremely circuitous trail. You eventually pass a small, marshy pond filled with lily pads, and then climb a bit more and finally reach the deep Reflection Lake, which offers a couple of good campsites.

Beyond Reflection Lake the trail goes over a minor ridge and dead-ends at the marvelously named family grouping of Fawn, Doe, and Buck Lakes. For even more scenery, leave the trail and explore the scenic basin surrounding Reflection Lake. Of the many off-trail lakes in this vicinity, the prettiest are Twin Cove, Turquoise, and Skyhigh, all of which can be reached via reasonable scrambles by those skilled with map and compass.

Yet another outstanding day hike from your base camp at Harbor or Wilson Lake goes to the Terrace Lakes, a string of four, jewellike bodies of water on the west side of the Bighorn Crags divide. To reach them, take the route described above to the junction near Welcome Lake and turn right (west). This trail climbs in long switchbacks to Heart Lake, a curved pool in a scenic basin, and then ascends two more long switchbacks to a narrow, rocky divide where you can see the Terrace Lakes strung out in the basin to the west.

The recently rerouted trail makes one switchback, then a sloping traverse to another switchback, and reaches the first lake in this chain. All four of these deep lakes have fish and adequate campsites, but the final Terrace Lake is the largest and arguably the most scenic.

TIP: The campsites at these lakes provide more solitude than most others in the Bighorn Crags, because they are somewhat off the main trails.

If you still have some energy and are looking for a secluded spot, try Barking Fox Lake. To reach it, hike south on the Waterfall Trail, which goes gradually downhill from the last Terrace Lake on its way to the Middle Fork Salmon River. After about 0.5 mile, you round the end of a ridge and come to the first switchback and a junction. Turn left here on an obvious but unsigned boot path and follow it for about 0.1 mile to the tiny, meadow rimmed Barking Fox Lake. Once you've had your fill, return to your car the way you came.

VARIATIONS ·

You can make a semiloop out of this trip by returning from the southern Bighorn Crags on the Waterfall Trail, between the junction beside Wilson Creek, northeast of Welcome Lake, and the junction near Cathedral Rock.

If you want to extend this hike into an area with more solitude, then leave the main Bighorn Crags at the junction near Birdbill Lake and hike 7 miles northeast, past Big Clear Lake, to remote Goat Lake, in a scenic basin beneath Beehive Mountain.

POSSIBLE ITINERARY

	CAMP	MILES	ELEVATION GAIN
Day 1	Harbor Lake	7.0	1,200'
Day 2	Harbor Lake		
	(day hike to Ship Island Lake)	11.0	2,300'
Day 3	Harbor Lake		
	(day hike to Buck and Reflection Lakes)	13.5	2,700'
Day 4	Harbor Lake (day hike to Terrace Lakes)	7.5	2,200'
Day 5	Out	7.0	600'

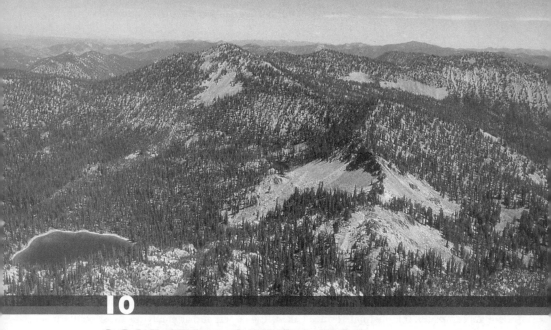

SOLDIER LAKES LOOP

RATINGS: Scenery 7   Solitude 6   Difficulty 7
MILES: 40 (42)
SHUTTLE MILEAGE: 4
ELEVATION GAIN: 7,500' (8,300')
DAYS: 3–5 (3–5)
MAP(S): USGS *Big Soldier Mountain,* USGS *Cape Horn Lakes,*
   USGS *Soldier Creek*
USUALLY OPEN: July–October
BEST: July–September
PERMITS: None
RULES: Maximum group size of 20 people and 20 stock animals
CONTACT: Yankee Fork Ranger District, 208-879-4100; Middle Fork Ranger
   District, 208-879-4101

SPECIAL ATTRACTIONS ·

Easy road access; lots of small but pretty lakes; fine views from lookouts

CHALLENGES ·

A few rattlesnakes in the Middle Fork Salmon River Canyon

Above: View north from Ruffneck Peak Lookout

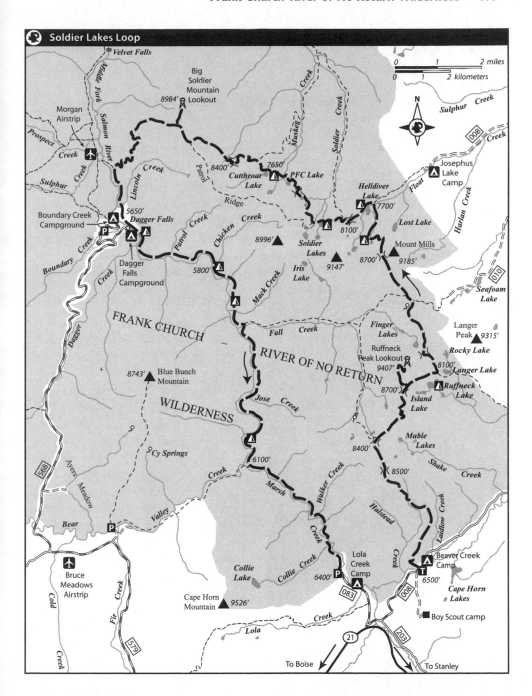

Soldier Lakes Loop

Velvet Falls

Big Soldier Mountain Lookout 8984'

Morgan Airstrip

Prospect Creek

Sulphur

Boundary Creek Campground

5650' Dagger Falls

Dagger Falls Campground

Boundary Creek

FRANK CHURCH

Patrol Ridge

8400'

Cutthroat Lake

7650' PFC Lake

Helldiver Lake 7700'

Lost Lake

8100'

Mount Mills 8700' 9185'

Soldier Lakes

8996' 9147'

Iris Lake

5800'

Mack Creek

Chicken Creek

Fall Creek

Finger Lakes

Ruffneck Peak Lookout 9407'

8700'

RIVER OF NO RETURN

Blue Bunch Mountain 8743'

WILDERNESS

Jose Creek

Cy Springs

6100'

Marsh

Creek

Valley

Bear

Bruce Meadows Airstrip

Cold Creek

Fir Creek

579

Collie Lake

Cape Horn Mountain 9526'

Lola

Collie Creek

6400'

083

Lola Creek Camp

Walker Creek

8400'

8500'

Island Lake

Mable Lakes

Shake Creek

Halstead

Creek

Laidlow Creek

Beaver Creek Camp

6500'

Cape Horn Lakes

Boy Scout camp

Langer Peak 9315'

Rocky Lake

8100' Langer Lake

Ruffneck Lake

Seafoam Lake

Josephus Lake Camp

Sulphur Creek

008 Creek

Float

Harlan Creek

010

To Boise 21

To Stanley

203

0 1 2 miles
0 1 2 kilometers

N

HOW TO GET THERE

From Stanley, drive 18.4 miles northwest on ID 21 to a junction just after the highway makes a sweeping turn southwest. Turn right (north), following signs to the Seafoam Area and Lola Campground, and go just 30 yards to a junction. If you have two cars, take one of them 1.6 miles down the road to the left to the large trailhead parking lot for the Middle Fork Trail.

To reach the recommended starting point, turn right at the junction and drive 0.4 mile to a fork. Bear left, following signs to Seafoam, and proceed 1.7 miles on this smooth, oiled-gravel road to the trailhead parking lot immediately after a bridge over Beaver Creek. The trail starts next to the creek, just past a large livestock tie-off area.

INTRODUCTION ·

This is a nice sampler of the huge Frank Church–River of No Return Wilderness that avoids the long, bumpy drive on dirt and gravel roads required to reach most other trailheads in this wilderness. In addition to good road access, this loop gives you a taste of all the varied environments here, including forested ridges, high mountain lakes, tall viewpoint peaks, and a deep river canyon. Though the loop does not take you to the *best* the wilderness has to offer of any of these features, it's a good choice if you want to get a bit of everything in one compact package.

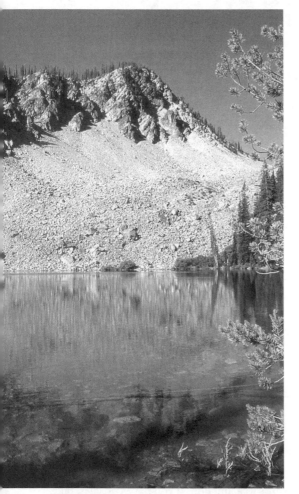

Cutthroat Lake

DESCRIPTION · · · · · · · ·

The trail follows Beaver Creek downstream for about 100 yards, and then curves to the right through a grassy meadow rimmed with lodgepole pines. The first 1.5 miles are nearly level and provide a nice warm-up that gets you into the swing of backpacking. You will need that warm-up, because the trail then makes a long climb that, despite being moderately graded, is quite tiring. The route takes you up a partly forested hillside, where the trees are almost all lodgepole pines, with just a few Douglas-firs sprinkled in for variety. Where the trees break at forest openings, the vegetation is dominated by grasses, sagebrush, and the blossoms of yarrow and lupine. Though the climb provides little in the way of views, you probably will see plenty of wildlife.

About 2.5 miles from the trailhead, you step over a small creek, and then make a long climb up a steep hillside. Fortunately, the ascent includes a half dozen switchbacks, so the grade remains reasonable. Not quite 5 miles from the trailhead, you top out at a pass on a small ridge, from which you get your first view north to the rocky hump of Ruffneck Peak, which is 9,407 feet high, and several nearby mountains. The trail then makes a curving descent to a small meadow, losing about 150 feet, followed by an uneven climb to a junction at a pass on top of a second ridge.

Your trail angles to the right and makes a view-packed, slightly uphill traverse across the rocky southeast side of an unnamed knoll. The views here encompass some of Idaho's best-known and most spectacular areas, including much of the Sawtooth Range, the White Cloud and Boulder Mountains, and the broad Sawtooth Valley. The views get even better when the traverse ends and two switchbacks take you up to a high ridgeline, where you can look down on several small, greenish lakes in the forested basins on either side. You can also admire new vistas of the many rugged ridges and peaks in this corner of the wilderness, all of which are composed of whitish or light-tan rocks.

The trail follows the undulating ridgeline north on a course that heads directly for Ruffneck Peak. This distinctive summit is easy to recognize, because it has a gently sloping, forested west side and a much steeper, rocky east face. At a junction in a saddle just south of the peak, it's time to drop your pack and make an excellent side trip. So grab your camera and bear left on a trail that goes up three long switchbacks in a moderately steep, 0.5-mile climb to the summit of Ruffneck Peak. At the top is a green-roofed fire lookout, which despite being a bit run-down is still staffed and has extensive views. In addition to the previously described views south toward the Sawtooth Valley, you can enjoy sweeping vistas north and west into the vast heart of Frank Church–River of No Return Wilderness and look east to the rugged peaks of the Yankee Fork country.

From the junction in the saddle south of Ruffneck Peak, the main trail goes right, descends two switchbacks, and then makes a long downhill traverse across the rocky east face of the peak. Near the bottom of the traverse, you pass a tiny pond with a good view back up to Ruffneck Peak, and then come to a junction not far above the shore of Langer Lake.

> **TIP:** It's worth your time to visit Langer Lake and to go south on obvious boot paths to the nearby Ruffneck and Island Lakes, which are both backed by impressive rocky buttes and have good campsites.

You turn left at the junction and soon regain much of your previously lost elevation. The trail goes uphill at a moderately steep grade through partial forest to a pass on the

BIG SOLDIER MOUNTAIN SIDE TRIP

To visit Big Soldier Mountain, go straight at the junction on Patrol Ridge and walk 0.5 mile up the view-packed ridgeline to the mountain's abandoned lookout building. The historic old wooden building is interesting to look at, but the walkway around it is so deteriorated it's probably not safe to walk on. The view, however, remains unimpaired and is glorious. The enormity of Frank Church–River of No Return Wilderness spreads out to the north, west, and east, while to the southeast you can look over much of the rugged terrain that you have already traversed on this loop. To the southwest you can look 3,400 feet down to the bottom of the Middle Fork Salmon River Canyon, your next destination.

northeast side of Ruffneck Peak, from which you can see the lookout on the top of the peak and a deep, blue lake in the basin to the west.

The trail, which has been significantly rerouted from the one shown on the U.S. Geological Survey (USGS) and U.S. Forest Service wilderness maps, descends a bouldery slope on the northwest side of the pass to a murky, tea-colored pond. From there, you lose about 200 feet on a steep, rocky tread, and then go up and down across the west flank of an unnamed peak. Eventually, you pass just above a spring and, 100 yards later, reach a junction with the trail to Seafoam Creek. You go straight and descend to a second junction, where you once again go straight and tackle the next climb, a 700-foot, 1.5-mile ascent to a high pass on the west shoulder of Mount Mills. Most of this climb is evenly graded, but the final 150 feet are quite steep.

You make two moderately steep switchbacks down from the pass, and then wind down to a scenic little lake near the base of a rockslide. A little above the lake's northeast shore is an excellent campsite.

TIP: Though this lake is too shallow for fish, the campsite here is much more private than those at the popular Helldiver Lake, ahead.

You hop over the lake's trickling outlet creek, and then turn downstream and follow the intermittent flow through an open forest. After crossing the creek a second time, you descend to a log crossing of Float Creek and almost immediately reach a junction. Turn left and soon come to the lovely Helldiver Lake, which has several good campsites and nice views of Mount Mills.

WARNING: This lake is accessible by a short, 2-mile walk from a trailhead at Josephus Lake, so it is fairly crowded, especially on weekends.

From Helldiver Lake, the trail climbs 400 feet to a heavily forested divide, and then goes down seven short switchbacks to a junction beside a marshy pond. You turn left and traverse a slope with an almost even mix of subalpine fir woods and talus fields to an excellent, but rather crowded, campsite beside the first of the Soldier Lakes. For more privacy, take an unsigned angler's path to an isolated campsite on the lake's southwest shore.

This lovely subalpine pool will naturally generate an appetite to see more lakes, and fortunately, there are plenty nearby to satisfy that hunger. The most attractive destinations are the two largest and most scenic Soldier Lakes. Though these lakes are off-trail, they can be reached by rugged angler's paths that head south and southwest from the first Soldier Lake. In addition to better scenery and good fishing, these lakes provide more privacy than the first lake.

The main trail goes about 0.4 mile from the first lake to a junction shortly after you cross the cascading outlet of Colonel Lake, a narrow gem with nice campsites. Here you have a choice. If you're looking for views, turn left and take the high route along Patrol Ridge, where you'll enjoy magnificent panoramas down into the Middle Fork Salmon River Canyon and over the rugged peaks and ridges of the southern part of Frank Church–River of No Return Wilderness. Because that trail passes no water or campsites, however, most people will prefer to follow the right fork. This rocky, up-and-down route soon goes past a pair of scenic, unnamed lakes, both of which sit below impressive rock outcrops, and then climbs three switchbacks to a low divide. From here, you descend past a pond at the base of a talus slope, and then continue downhill to an obvious side trail that leads to P.F.C. Lake. This deep lake sits beneath the crags of Patrol Ridge and, despite having a lower rank than the other Soldier Lakes, is arguably the most spectacular member of the troop.

After P.F.C. Lake, the trail switchbacks down to a log over Muskeg Creek, and then goes up and down for not quite 0.5 mile to Cutthroat Lake. True to its name, this lake has cutthroat trout, as well as good campsites and excellent views of the jagged Patrol Ridge. After crossing the outlet creek of Cutthroat Lake, the trail curves to the right and climbs fairly steeply to a junction. You turn left and go gradually uphill past a shallow pond, and then switchback twice and go up a hillside with a mix of flower-filled meadows and open, high-elevation forests. The climb ends with five steep switchbacks that take you up to a saddle at the top of a spur ridge. The grade eases here as the trail goes up and down through a lovely alpine meadow below the main line of Patrol Ridge.

TIP: Fill your water bottles at one of the two small creeks in this meadow, because this is your last water source until Lincoln Creek, at the bottom of the Middle Fork Salmon River Canyon about 6 miles ahead.

Once the trail leaves the meadow, it climbs across the top of a huge talus field and steeply ascends to a ridgetop junction amid a field of August-blooming lupines. This is where you reunite with the trail along Patrol Ridge.

You turn right, contour around the southwest side of a rounded knoll, and come to a rather faint junction. The loop continues downhill to the left. The rewarding side trip to Big Soldier Mountain begins here.

To tackle the long descent to the bottom of the Middle Fork Salmon River Canyon, make a rather gentle downhill on a spur ridge, where whitebark pines thrive and alpine wildflowers such as pink heather brighten the slopes. The trail then gets very steep as it goes down through a shadeless burn area, quickly leaving the high-elevation environment in favor of mid-elevation grassy slopes and forests of Douglas-firs and lodgepole pines.

WARNING: The trail here has lots of dangerously loose rocks and pebbles that require careful footing.

The steepness of the descent lessens briefly, and then resumes on a relentless down-hill that requires plenty of rest stops for sore knees and jammed toes. The difficulty is increased because the trail receives only sporadic maintenance, so there are usually sig-nificant amounts of deadfall along the way. Also, relatively few switchbacks relieve the steep grade, and most of those are concentrated near the bottom.

TIP: Going up this steep, waterless slope is extremely arduous, which is why I recommend a counterclockwise loop.

The trail abruptly levels off on the flats near the Middle Fork Salmon River and comes to a junction. You turn left, following signs to Dagger Falls, and soon climb away from the crystal-clear river, making a rough traverse of a talus-and-scree slope well above the water. A little more than 1 mile from the junction, you cross the small but very welcome Lincoln Creek, where you can finally refill your water bottles and soak your tired feet in cool water.

The trail now makes a series of short but very steep ups and downs for 0.5 mile to a junc-tion beside a large bridge over the Middle Fork Salmon River just above rampaging Dagger Falls. You go straight, staying on the east side of the river, and soon pass a riverside campsite.

The now-gentle trail spends most of the next few miles either crossing nearly level riv-erside benches peppered with lodgepole pines and quaking aspens, or contouring across dry slopes with lots of sagebrush and wildflowers. The two most showy flowers here are balsamroot, which blooms yellow in June and early July, and rabbitbrush, which also blooms yellow, but not until mid-August and September. Just 2 miles above Dagger Falls the trail crosses Patrol Creek on a wooden bridge, and then does more gentle ups and downs as it follows the curves of the meandering river. About 2 miles past Patrol Creek is a bridge over Chicken Creek and a very good, large camp just past the bridge.

For the next few miles the trail crosses several small side creeks on bridges, climbs over rock outcrops with canyon views, and goes across forested flats about 50 to 100 feet above the river. The hiking isn't spectacularly scenic, but it's easy and attractive, especially in the cool of the morning.

WARNING: On hot afternoons you will often be bothered by large horseflies, which follow you for miles and are almost impossible to swat.

A little less than 1 mile from Chicken Creek is a good riverside campsite just below a well-preserved log cabin. As in so many similar old cabins, the doorway into this one is only about 4 feet high, which leaves you to wonder about the stature of all those early pioneers and miners.

You go a short distance into the major side canyon of Fall Creek and soon reach a junction with the Fall Creek Trail. Go straight, cross the creek on a large bridge, and then return to your course above the river. The trail soon goes through a recent burn area, and then makes a long climb through forests and up a talus slope to an overlook about 400 feet above the river. From this high point, you gradually descend back to river level and go through a particularly dramatic section where the trail has been blasted into the rock just a few feet above the water.

TIP: Excellent fly-fishing opportunities abound in this area.

As the trail climbs away from the river, it passes two fine campsites, and then climbs over a rocky overlook and comes to a fork.

The trail to the right goes up Bear Valley Creek, but your trail goes left and follows Marsh Creek. It is the merging of these two large creeks that forms the Middle Fork Salmon River. Above this point the canyon is wider and the slopes are less steep than they were farther downstream, which allows Marsh Creek to meander lazily over gravel bars and through small meadows. The trail is also gentle, spending most of its time climbing gradually through forests and crossing small tributaries. About 3 miles from the Bear Valley Creek turnoff is a large bridge over Marsh Creek, after which you take a bridge over Collie Creek, and then make a gentle, 1-mile walk to the Middle Fork trailhead. If you were not able to leave a car here, then you will either have to hitchhike or make the easy, 3.7-mile road walk back to your car.

POSSIBLE ITINERARY

	CAMP	MILES	ELEVATION GAIN
Day 1	Ruffneck Lake	8.0	3,000'
	Side trip to Ruffneck Peak Lookout	1.0	500'
Day 2	Cutthroat Lake	10.5	1,800'
Day 3	Chicken Creek	11.0	1,800'
	Side trip to Big Soldier Mountain Lookout	1.0	300'
Day 4	Out	10.5*	900'*

* This excludes the 3.7-mile road walk to close the loop.

BEST SHORTER ALTERNATIVE ·

If your vehicle can manage the rough drive to Josephus Lake Camp (see map), then start at the trailhead here and hike past Helldiver Lake and the Soldier Lakes to Big Soldier Mountain Lookout. From there loop back along the top of Patrol Ridge to your starting point. Be sure to ask about road conditions before considering this alternative.

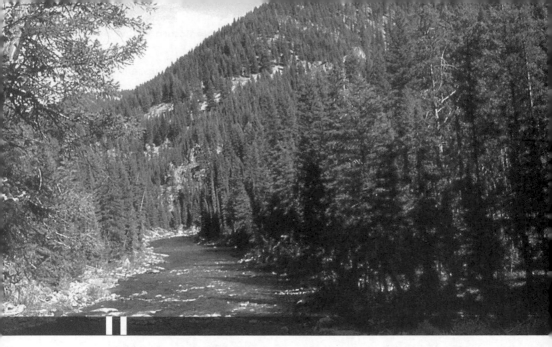

MIDDLE FORK SALMON RIVER

RATINGS: Scenery 7   Solitude 6   Difficulty 6
MILES: 67
SHUTTLE MILEAGE: 89
ELEVATION GAIN: 4,200'
DAYS: 6–8
MAP(S): USFS *Frank Church–River of No Return Wilderness: South Half*
USUALLY OPEN: May–November
BEST: September and October
PERMITS: None
RULES: Maximum group size of 20 people and 20 stock animals; all fires within 0.25 mile of the Middle Fork Salmon River must be in fire pans; you are required to pack out all human waste from a corridor 0.25 mile on either side of the Middle Fork Salmon River (easy enough for boaters, but not realistic for backpackers).
CONTACT: Middle Fork Ranger District, 208-879-4101

SPECIAL ATTRACTIONS ·

Whitewater rafters to watch; terrific canyon scenery; numerous excellent hot springs

CHALLENGES ·

Long car shuttle; rattlesnakes; hot summer temperatures; rough road access to the eastern trailhead

Above: Middle Fork Salmon River near Rams Horn Creek

HOW TO GET THERE •

To reach the recommended exit point, drive 13.2 miles northeast of Stanley on ID 75 to a junction just before a bridge over Yankee Fork Salmon River. Turn left (north) onto Yankee Fork Road and drive 8.7 miles on this paved (then good gravel) road past an interesting assortment of mining equipment and exhibits to a fork just after the bridge over Jordan Creek. Turn left onto Forest Service Road 172 and drive 4.4 miles to an unsigned fork. Go straight (uphill) and proceed 16 miles over scenic Loon Creek Summit and down to the Loon Creek Guard Station. Continue 0.7 mile past the guard station to a fork, where you bear right, now on Road 007, and drive the final 4.4 miles to the good-size parking lot for the Loon Creek trailhead at the end of the road.

WARNING: The road from the unsigned fork before Loon Creek Summit all the way to the trailhead is rocky and quite rough. Passenger cars can make it, but you must drive slowly and carefully.

To reach the starting point, return to Stanley and drive 21.8 miles northwest on ID 21 to a junction just before Banner Creek Campground. Turn right, following signs to Cascade and Bruce Meadows, and drive 9.6 miles on the gravel FS 198 to a prominent junction. Turn right on Road 568, following signs to Dagger Falls and Boundary Creek Campground, and proceed 9.8 miles to a fork, where you bear left and go 0.6 mile to the large trailhead parking area.

INTRODUCTION •

Over countless millions of years the Middle Fork Salmon River has been busy carving a spectacular, deep canyon into the granite rock of central Idaho. From the top of the canyon looking down, this massive gash in the Earth is impressive, but it pales in comparison to the awe-inspiring views enjoyed by visitors at the bottom of the canyon who look up at towering walls that rise thousands of feet above the remarkably clear river. One hundred years ago, most of the people who saw these views were trappers and prospectors who established remote homesteads in the canyon. In recent years, the vast majority of visitors have been rafters and kayakers, who are drawn not only to the scenery but also to the challenge of one of America's most legendary whitewater rivers.

Hikers are only beginning to discover the wonders of this canyon, but their numbers are sure to increase as word gets out about the excellent scenery and the canyon's other great attribute, its hot springs. The trail passes numerous excellent hot springs, ranging from tiny seeps to huge springs where large volumes of hot water come bubbling out of the ground. Almost all of the springs provide excellent bathing opportunities, which makes the Middle Fork Salmon River Trail perhaps the best extended backpacking trip for hot-springs lovers in the American West.

TIP: The Middle Fork Salmon River is managed as a catch-and-release fishery; single barbless hooks are required and no live bait is allowed.

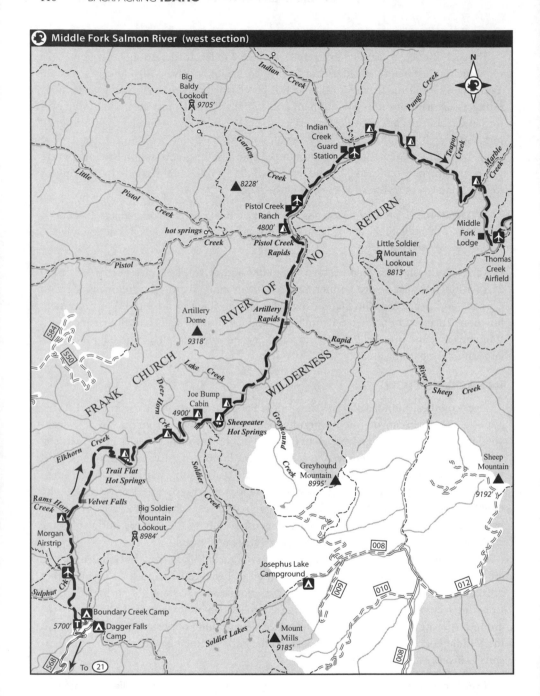

Middle Fork Salmon River (west section)

DESCRIPTION

You set off on a wide and dusty trail in an old burn area that is now covered with a regrowing forest of lodgepole pines, a few quaking aspens, and some Douglas-firs. The trail goes up and over a minor ridge, and then drops to a junction with a trail to the Boundary Creek boat launch. Just 100 yards later, you meet the lightly used Trail #215,

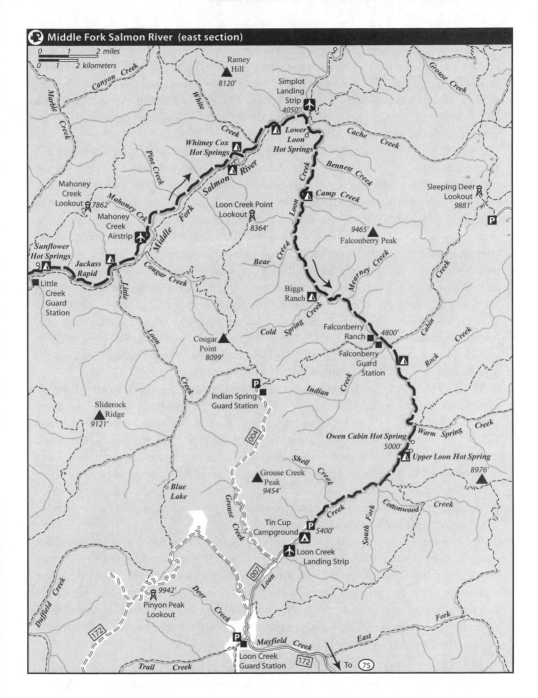

Middle Fork Salmon River (east section)

which angles left. The main trail goes straight at both junctions and wanders up and down through forest well away from the Middle Fork Salmon River for the next 1.5 miles. As the trail slowly gets closer to the river, it skirts the privately owned Morgan Landing Strip, which is prominently labeled with several NO TRESPASSING signs.

At the end of the private property, the trail crosses the fairly large Sulphur Creek on a sturdy, metal bridge, and then comes to an easy rock-hop crossing of Prospector Creek and a junction with the trail of the same name. You bear right and walk a short distance to a second junction, this time with a lower spur of the Prospector Creek Trail. You go straight, cross a forested shelf about 30 feet above the river, and then hop over a tiny creek a little before the wooden bridge over Rams Horn Creek. A good (but very small) campsite is about 50 yards past this bridge.

Downstream from Rams Horn Creek the trail closely follows the lovely, green-tinted river as it cascades merrily along past rock outcrops, steep hillsides, and talus slopes. One particularly rugged stretch of whitewater on the river here goes by the name Velvet Falls, though it is really more of a rapid. The trail goes around these obstacles with numerous ups and downs on the forested hillside above the river. Individually, these sections aren't particularly difficult, but together they add up to a fair amount of elevation gain and loss. A prominent rocky ridge soon forces the river to make a wide turn to the southeast. The trail follows suit, though in a more rugged fashion than the river, as you are forced to climb over a high rock outcrop, and then switchback down a rough talus slope back to river level. Just before the river turns north is an excellent, large camp area above Trail Flat Hot Springs, an inviting group of pools at the edge of a rocky gravel bar by the river. Like all of the hot springs in this canyon, this is a great place to spend some time soaking sore muscles and enjoying the scenery. Bring a swimsuit if you're concerned about modesty.

The trail climbs gradually away from the hot springs, and then makes three downhill switchbacks to a bridge over the rushing Elkhorn Creek. After this, it's more up and down near the river as the canyon becomes increasingly narrow with steeper walls and lots of rough talus slopes. In addition to getting steeper, the terrain also gets drier, so the forests are less dense and consist almost entirely of Douglas-firs and ponderosa pines. You pass a nice campsite where the winding river makes a sharp bend to the right, and, shortly thereafter, rock-hop over Deer Horn Creek. More curves in the river then lead you through a particularly steep-walled part of the canyon to several good campsites on a lightly forested flat near the small Joe Bump Cabin.

Just 100 yards beyond Joe Bump Cabin is a tiny wooden sign pointing to the Soldier Creek Trail on the other side of the river (no bridge). This is soon followed by the grave site of Elmer "Set-Trigger" Purcell, whose headstone informs you that he was a prospector and trapper who died in 1936. About 1 mile later is the excellent camp area beside the wonderfully warm waters of the large Sheepeater Hot Springs. The rotten egg smell from sulfur in the water makes camping here a bit aromatic, but the opportunity to luxuriate in such warm water more than makes up for the unpleasant odor.

TIP: Because Sheepeater Hot Springs is often crowded, especially during the boating season, you might prefer to set up your tent at a good boater's camp about 0.5 mile past the hot springs.

For the next several miles the trail crosses increasingly barren and brushy slopes that are exposed to the sun and can be very hot in midsummer. Fortunately, though you rarely have easy access to the river, there are several small side creeks along the way, so finding water is never a problem. The next significant landmark is the narrow canyon of Rapid

Though it isn't a desert, the Middle Fork Salmon River Canyon is noticeably hotter and drier than the surrounding mountains. As a result, the area's spring wildflowers soon wilt under the relentless sun, and trees are scarce in the lower reaches of the canyon. During July and August it can be oppressively hot in the canyon, so this trip is best done in the "shoulder" seasons of spring and fall. Spring is beautiful, but in May and June the river is often crowded with boaters. On the other hand, September is idyllic, because most of the boaters have gone home for the season and you will generally have the canyon and its hot springs all to yourself.

River, which joins the Middle Fork just below Artillery Rapids. A trail comes down that canyon, but instead of crossing the Middle Fork here, that trail follows the river downstream, paralleling your route for the next several miles. The trail on your side of the river spends most of those miles traveling through a partial burn area, where many of the trees are either dead or fire-scarred, so shade is at a premium.

About 3 miles past Rapid River you take a large bridge over Pistol Creek to a junction near several good campsites on the creek's north bank.

TIP: For a nice side trip, turn left and hike 3 miles up the Pistol Creek Trail to a secluded hot spring.

The main trail goes right and soon takes you past the log buildings and private landing strip at Pistol Creek Ranch. Several confusing jeep roads cross the trail near the ranch. To find the correct route, walk straight through the ranch property to the northeast end of the landing strip, where a sign saying INDIAN CREEK WAY marks the resumption of the trail.

The gentle trail now takes you to a rock-hop crossing of small Garden Creek and, immediately thereafter, a junction with the trail to Big Baldy Lookout. You bear slightly right (staying level) and closely follow the river for 1 mile to a fork just before the Indian Creek Landing Strip. The main trail goes right, but if you want to visit the Indian Creek Guard Station, bear left and soon reach the isolated station, with its quaint log buildings, friendly personnel, and piped water.

The trail goes through the guard station property and continues to the end of the landing strip, where you reunite with the trail that bypassed the station. Another 0.5 mile of gentle walking takes you to a good campsite just before the bridge over the large Indian Creek. Immediately after this bridge you turn right at an unsigned junction and walk 1 mile to Pungo Creek, which has several good campsites on either side of the hop-over crossing.

The Middle Fork Salmon River Trail now wanders merrily along at a gentle grade, slowly going down into an ever-drier and increasingly barren landscape. The only trees here are a few ponderosa pines, while twisted big sagebrush grows near the water, and the higher canyon slopes are covered with nothing but bunchgrass and rocks. In early

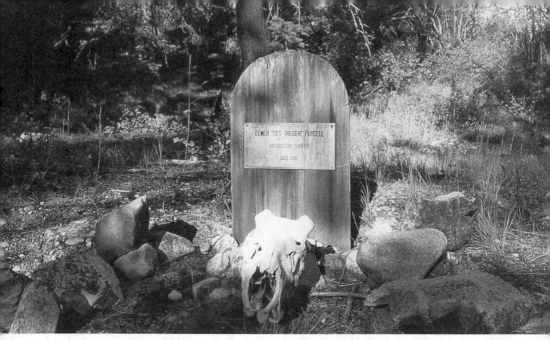

Grave of Elmer Purcell in the Middle Fork Salmon River Canyon

summer these slopes support wildflowers such as balsamroot and skyrocket gilia, but by later in the season they dry out and take on a golden-brown appearance.

About 1.5 miles from Pungo Creek you hop over the splashing Teapot Creek, and then go around a sharp bend in the river to a large and excellent campsite on a ponderosa pine–dotted flat just above the river. Shortly after this campsite is a junction, where you turn right and immediately cross a bridge over Marble Creek. The trail then heads south, following another of the river's many twists and turns, to a junction with a faint trail that goes uphill and left on its way to Mahoney Creek Lookout, which is now abandoned. Immediately after this junction is a large bridge across the Middle Fork Salmon River that provides access to Middle Fork Lodge. This modern guest lodge comes complete with several cozy bungalows, a manicured lawn, and views from the porch that will take your breath away.

The bridge is open only to lodge guests, so others must stay on the east side of the river and follow a narrow road around a bend in the river to the Thomas Creek Airfield. The trail goes around the right side of the landing strip and soon comes to a split. To the right is Trail #001.1, which crosses the Middle Fork on a bridge, passes Little Creek Guard Station, and then follows the south bank of the river for 10 miles before rejoining the main trail at White Creek Bridge. You go left on Trail #001, staying on the north side of the river, pass the end of the landing strip, and soon come to a good campsite beside a picturesque log cabin. Just 150 yards beyond this cabin is Sunflower Hot Springs, which bubbles out of the ground and invites an extended stay.

The canyon is largely devoid of trees below this point, so summer temperatures can be oppressive on these sun-exposed slopes. A more comfortable season is late August and September, when temperatures start to fall and the blossoms of sunflowers and rabbit-brush add spots of yellow to the increasingly desertlike environment.

WARNING: Rattlesnakes are very common in this dry environment, so watch your step.

About 2.5 miles from Sunflower Hot Springs is a good campsite directly opposite where Little Loon Creek joins the Middle Fork. After this, you make a moderate, 300-foot ascent to the Mahoney Creek Landing Strip, which rarely receives many airborne visitors. About halfway down the airstrip the Middle Fork Salmon River Trail angles left at an unsigned but obvious foot trail.

The canyon scenery remains impressive as the trail goes over barren slopes, crosses a few trickling side creeks, and passes high overlooks with outstanding views of the river and canyon. Almost 5 miles from the Mahoney Creek Landing Strip is Whitey Cox Hot Springs. Good campsites are about 300 yards beyond the small spring. Though there is a meager flow on the north side of the river, the main spring is on the south side of the stream, which also has several good campsites. Unfortunately, it is only feasible for hikers to cross the river in very late summer or fall of dry years.

TIP: Another option for visiting these springs is to continue hiking another 1.3 miles to the White Creek Bridge; then backtrack on the trail that follows the south side of the river to the camping area and rock-lined springs.

Not far from Whitey Cox Hot Springs you hop over White Creek and immediately bear right at an unsigned junction. The trail then goes over White Creek Bridge—a large, metal span across the Middle Fork Salmon River—and reunites with Trail #001.1. You turn left at this junction and walk downstream across a north-facing slope that supports many more trees than the drier environment on the other side of the canyon. You soon pass a good campsite and continue another mile to the mouth of Loon Creek Canyon.

The trail goes several hundred yards up Loon Creek Canyon to a junction, where the Middle Fork Salmon River Trail turns left and immediately crosses a bridge over the bois-terous Loon Creek. Your route goes straight at this junction, leaving the Middle Fork and heading up Loon Creek's narrow, partly forested canyon for 0.5 mile to Lower Loon Hot Springs. These springs are the perfect temperature for hours of soaking, but you'll have to pull yourself out of the water well before sunset because there is no flat ground nearby for camping. A little more than 1 mile upstream from Lower Loon Hot Springs, the trail takes a bridge over Loon Creek and begins an uneven, 2-mile ascent to a nice campsite on a small flat near the hop-over crossing of Camp Creek.

Above Camp Creek, the trail goes through a dramatic gorge, where the cascading Loon Creek has carved a deep chasm with towering rock pinnacles and impressively tall cliffs. After the canyon widens, you make an easy, 1-mile walk, and then pass a grassy flat on the opposite side of the creek that was once the site of Biggs Ranch. The only thing left of this old homestead is the dilapidated remains of a log cabin, but the grassy flat still has plenty of good places to camp, if you don't mind making the cold, calf-deep ford of Loon Creek to get there.

About 1 mile above Biggs Ranch the trail goes through another dramatic, cliff-walled chasm; then the canyon widens once again, and you walk across a hillside overlooking a mile-long grassy flat that is on the southwest side of Loon Creek. At the southeast end of this flat you pass an old landing strip and recently abandoned Falconberry Ranch. Soon you come to a junction with a trail that takes a bridge over the creek to Falconberry Guard Station.

You go straight, staying on the northeast side of Loon Creek, and go a short way up the brushy canyon of Cabin Creek to an unsigned and easy-to-miss junction. The main trail seems to go straight along the north bank of Cabin Creek, but you turn right and make a rock-hop crossing of the creek. The trail then crosses a grassy flat, passes above an excellent campsite (complete with a seemingly out-of-place picnic table), and climbs steadily to a bridge over Rock Creek. It's another 2 miles from here to a junction just before the bridge over the large Warm Springs Creek. You bear right, cross the bridge, and, 300 yards later, reach Owen Cabin Hot Springs, which is followed less than 0.5 mile later by Upper Loon Hot Springs, the last of the hot springs you pass on this trip. The best campsites and bathing pools are near an old log cabin at Upper Loon Hot Springs.

About 1.5 miles beyond Upper Loon Hot Springs is a junction with the Cottonwood Trail, where you go straight and soon cross a bridge over Loon Creek. The trail's final 3 miles take you gently to an easy hop over Shell Creek, followed by a passage through an impressive, steep-walled gorge to the Loon Creek trailhead.

VARIATIONS

This trip lends itself nicely to several imaginative variations. If you have only one car, consider turning this into a huge, 120-mile loop by hiking back from the Loon Creek trailhead via Loon Creek Guard Station, Trail-Beaver Divide, Beaver Creek, and Marsh Creek. This loop involves some road walking and adds three full days of hiking to an already long trip, but the scenery is good throughout.

Another option is to skip the Loon Creek Trail and keep hiking downstream on the Middle Fork Salmon River Trail to the Big Creek Pack Bridge. From there, you can either hike out via the 26-mile trail up Big Creek (see Trip 32) or climb the Waterfall Trail and exit via the Bighorn Crags (see Trip 9).

POSSIBLE ITINERARY

	CAMP	MILES	ELEVATION GAIN
Day 1	Trail Flat Hot Springs	8.0	600'
Day 2	Pistol Creek	13.0	700'
Day 3	Sunflower Hot Springs	13.0	300'
Day 4	Whitey Cox Hot Springs	9.0	400'
Day 5	Camp Creek (after a long soak in Lower Loon Hot Springs)	7.0	600'
Day 6	Upper Loon Hot Springs	12.0	1,100'
Day 7	Out		

BEST SHORTER ALTERNATIVE

The only realistic alternatives are to either hire a small plane to take you into one of the airstrips along this route or join a float trip that drops you off partway along the trail. In either case you would then hike back upstream to your starting point. For a weekend backpacking trip, Trail Flat Hot Springs makes a good goal.

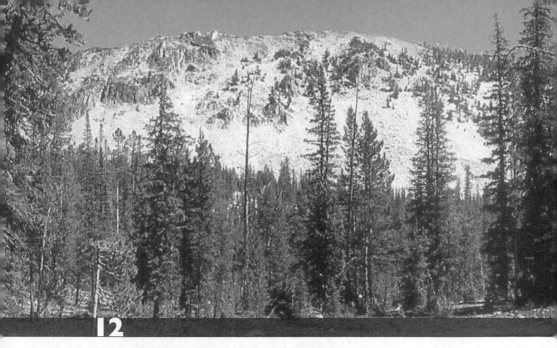

12

LOON CREEK LOOP

RATINGS: Scenery 8   Solitude 8   Difficulty 7
MILES: 27
ELEVATION GAIN: 6,100'
DAYS: 3–4
MAP(S): USGS *Casto,* USGS *Knapp Lakes,* USGS *Mount Jordan,*
   USGS *Pinyon Peak*
USUALLY OPEN: July–mid-October
BEST: Mid-July–September
PERMITS: None
RULES: Maximum group size of 20 people and 20 stock animals
CONTACT: Middle Fork Ranger District, 208-879-4101

SPECIAL ATTRACTIONS •

Solitude; colorful mountain scenery

CHALLENGES •

Fairly long and moderately difficult cross-county section; rough road access; rough trail through burn area

Above: Pond in the upper part of the Knapp Lakes Basin

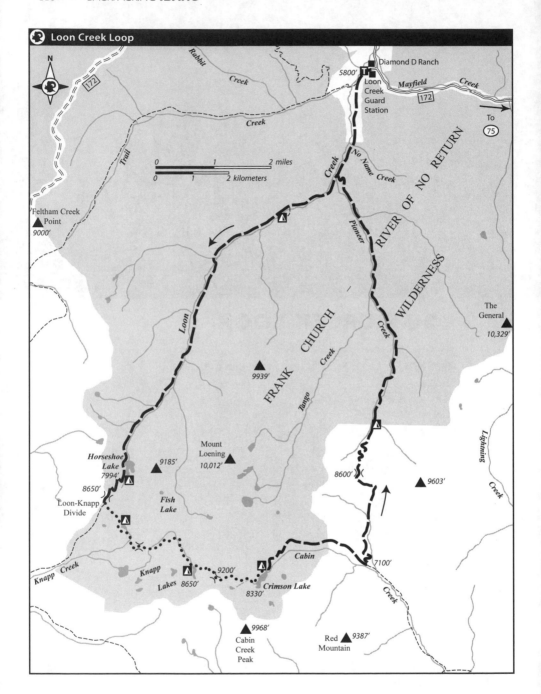

Loon Creek Loop

N
172

Rabbit
Creek

Diamond D Ranch
5800'
Loon
Creek
Guard
Station

Mayfield
Creek
172

To
75

Creek

No Name Creek

Creek

Pioneer

RIVER OF NO RETURN

Trail

Feltham Creek
Point
9000'

0   1   2 miles
0   1   2 kilometers

Creek

Loon

FRANK
CHURCH
WILDERNESS

Tango
Creek

9939'

The
General
10,329'

Lightning
Creek

Horseshoe
Lake
7994'
8650'

9185'

Mount
Loening
10,012'

8600'

9603'

Loon-Knapp
Divide

Fish
Lake

Knapp Creek

Knapp
Lakes
8650'

9200'

Cabin

Crimson Lake
8330'

7100'

Creek

9968'
Cabin
Creek
Peak

Red
Mountain
9387'

HOW TO GET THERE ●

From Stanley, drive 13.2 miles northeast on ID 75 to a junction just before a bridge over Yankee Fork Salmon River. Turn left (north) on Yankee Fork Road and drive 8.7 miles on this paved (then good gravel) road past an interesting assortment of mining equipment and exhibits to a junction just after the bridge over Jordan Creek. Turn left onto Forest Service Road 172 and drive 4.4 miles to an unsigned fork. Go straight (uphill) and proceed 16 miles on this narrow road as it climbs over the scenic Loon Creek Summit and down to the Loon Creek Guard Station. The road from the unsigned fork before Loon Creek Summit all the way to the guard station is rocky and quite rough. Passenger cars can make it, but you must drive slowly and carefully. Parking is not allowed inside the guard station property, so park near the fence outside.

INTRODUCTION

Though mining roads separate the protected headwaters of Loon Creek from the rest of Frank Church–River of No Return Wilderness, this small appendage contains some of the most scenic terrain in the entire wilderness. The jagged peaks here rise above 10,000 feet and are made up of a stunningly beautiful collage of gray, white, and reddish rocks. When you add this colorful geology to the area's cirque lakes, clear streams, and flower-covered meadows, you have a great place to go for a backpacking vacation.

DESCRIPTION

To locate the unsigned trailhead, walk past the guard station and go through a gate at the southwest corner of the property. You then walk diagonally 250 yards to the southwest corner of a livestock enclosure, which has another gate and a trail register box. The trail starts on the other side of the gate. The trail is in good shape and easy to follow, though it's a bit dusty due to horse use out of the adjacent Diamond D Ranch.

The trail goes about 500 yards across a nearly level plain, only populated by scattered sagebrush and a few Douglas-firs and lodgepole pines, to the signed junction with the Beaver–Trail Creek Trail. You go straight, briefly descend to the willow thickets beside Loon Creek, and then climb back up to the plain and pass through a mile-wide burn area. After this, the trail does some small ups and downs to a fork and the start of your loop.

The trip is easier to navigate if you go counterclockwise, so bear right at the fork and immediately drop to Pioneer Creek. The trail crosses the creek on a log, and then heads southwest up the scenic canyon of Loon Creek, following that stream for about 0.4 mile before coming to a knee-deep ford of the cold, clear water. You climb the opposite bank and walk through a partially burned area where deadfall is often a problem, but which affords your first good views of the steep and rugged walls on either side of the canyon.

WARNING: About 0.5 mile past the ford the trail appears to cross the creek, but this is actually just a side path that goes to a campsite on the other side of the creek.

Your trail remains on the northwest side of the stream and slowly climbs under the shade of a relatively dense Douglas-fir forest. The trees block any decent views, but the trail is never tedious and you stand a good chance of seeing elk. After 2 miles, you rock-hop an unnamed tributary creek, and then ford the main stem of Loon Creek, which is now somewhat smaller.

The canyon soon curves to the south and the forest cover changes to relatively small and widely spaced lodgepole pines, which allows you to catch tantalizing glimpses of the surrounding mountains. Those glimpses become unobstructed views about 1 mile later, when you cross an avalanche chute with lots of wildflowers and stunted quaking aspen trees. You reenter forest and come to another crossing of Loon Creek, this time on a convenient log. After this crossing, the trail climbs at a noticeably steeper grade for 1 mile to where a tall, pointed mountain splits the canyon in two.

TIP: The U.S. Forest Service wilderness map shows a primitive trail going up the left fork of the canyon to the tiny Fish Lake, but there is no sign of this trail on the ground.

You stick with the main branch of the cascading Loon Creek and climb fairly steeply for 2 miles until the grade levels off not far before Horseshoe Lake, which is large but shallow. This scenic pool has pleasing views of a rocky ridge to the east and some good campsites near its southwest shore.

From Horseshoe Lake, the trail winds steeply uphill for about 1 mile to the 8,650-foot Loon-Knapp Divide, where there are wonderful views northeast over the Horseshoe Lake Basin. On the other side of the divide you descend for 300 yards to a small, waterless gully, and then look for a sketchy path that angles uphill to the left. This is where you leave the trail and rely on your skills with map and compass. The open forests make the walking relatively easy, but trees block the views, so navigation can be difficult. Occasional game paths help keep you on course and you may even find a few cut logs indicating sections of a long-abandoned trail. Nonetheless, novice hikers should not attempt this section without experienced leadership. On the other hand, veteran route-finders will find it fairly easy and enjoyable. Of necessity, the description here is rather general, but those who are good at cross-country travel need only a general description.

The best route goes southeast, gradually losing elevation for about 0.5 mile to a lovely, meadow-rimmed lake with a good campsite on its northwest shore. You then follow this lake's seasonal outlet creek to the second of two shallow ponds, veer left, and climb over a tiny divide. From here, you angle downhill to a small creek; then turn upstream and follow this intermittent creek past a series of very scenic ponds and small lakes that are collectively called the Knapp Lakes. At the top of the drainage you come to the highest of the Knapp Lakes, a long, kidney-shaped pool that sits beneath a craggy ridge of light gray and tan rock. Plenty of flat ground around this lake means that you have a choice of very good campsites with almost guaranteed solitude. Unfortunately, there are no fish in any of these lakes.

The cross-country travel to this point has been relatively easy, but now you must make a short, very steep, and quite difficult climb. Your goal is a low point in the ridge due east of the lake at the top of a long, tannish-orange scree slope. The easiest way to reach the pass is to avoid the loose rock of the scree slope and head instead up a hillside just north of the pass, where the soil is stabilized by scattered whitebark pines. It's only a 600-foot climb, but plan on taking at least an hour to accomplish this steep ascent.

WARNING: Do not go over the inviting lower pass south of the lake. It leads to a small, unnamed lake that is worth visiting, but there is no reasonable access beyond that to Crimson Lake.

Things get a lot easier at the pass, as you descend a moderately steep slope of rocks and alpine wildflowers, where you soon catch sight of Crimson Lake in the basin to the east. The route down goes past a scenic tarn in an area of highly colorful rocks and follows this tarn's dry outlet creek all the way down to the large and irregularly shaped Crimson Lake.

The name of this lake obviously does not refer to the color of the water, but it does accurately describe the bright reddish-orange rocks and mountains that surround the lake. In addition to views of these colorful summits, the lake features fine reflections of the gray spires of Cabin Creek Peak to the south. An excellent campsite is on the west shore of

Crimson Lake, and another one is at the northeast end near the lake's outlet. The continuation of your loop leaves as a maintained foot trail from just above the outlet creek.

TIP: If you have the time, spend an extra day or two scrambling up to several scenic, trailless lakes in the colorful cirque basins south and north of Crimson Lake.

It's all downhill from Crimson Lake, both figuratively in terms of scenery, and, for a while at least, literally in elevation. The trail first goes over a rounded knoll and drops very steeply down a rocky hillside. At the bottom of the hill, you hop over a small side creek in a gully and then do a little steeper downhill until the trail's grade eases off. For the next 1.5 miles the trail goes through open forests, crosses avalanche chutes, and travels over rockslides in the canyon of Cabin Creek. Most of the way is downhill, but a few short, uphill pitches keep things interesting. About 2.5 miles from Crimson Lake is a junction with the Pioneer–Cabin Creek Trail.

You turn left, make two uphill switchbacks, and then begin a long, stair-step ascent where short, nearly level stretches are interspersed with moderate-to-steep uphills. This pattern continues all the way to a high pass, which has a good view to the south of the striking, red-topped pyramid of Red Mountain.

From this pass, the trail steeply descends six switchbacks, and then goes more moderately downhill through subalpine fir forests to a good campsite just before you hop over a clear tributary of Pioneer Creek. About 0.5 mile below this camp, you cross Pioneer Creek on a log, and then closely parallel the creek downstream for several hundred yards to a flood-damaged area where part of the creek flows directly down the bed of the trail. It's very easy to lose the route here, so you'll probably have to bushwhack. To relocate the trail, look on the opposite (east) bank about 200 yards downstream from the start of the flooded area.

The next mile is a relatively straightforward downhill walk through the forest above Pioneer Creek until the trail is obscured again, this time by both flood damage and a fire scar with large amounts of blowdown. You'll have to fight your way through this short section to where the trail becomes obvious again.

Below this point, the trail makes a rocky, sometimes steep descent through intermittent burn areas. The rugged and difficult trail is constantly in need of maintenance and should probably be rebuilt, but at least it's mostly downhill. Along the way, you pass the impressive side canyon of Tango Creek, coming in from the southwest, and then do another 2 miles of rough and, frankly, not-much-fun hiking to a rock-and-log crossing of a moderate-size side creek. You close the loop by contouring for about 0.5 mile, and then descending four switchbacks to the reunion with the Loon Creek Trail. To finish the trip, turn right and retrace the 2 miles back to the Loon Creek Guard Station.

POSSIBLE ITINERARY

	CAMP	MILES	ELEVATION GAIN
Day 1	Horseshoe Lake	8.0	2,300'
Day 2	Crimson Lake		
	(most of this distance is cross-country)	6.0	1,800'
Day 3	Out	13.0	2,000'

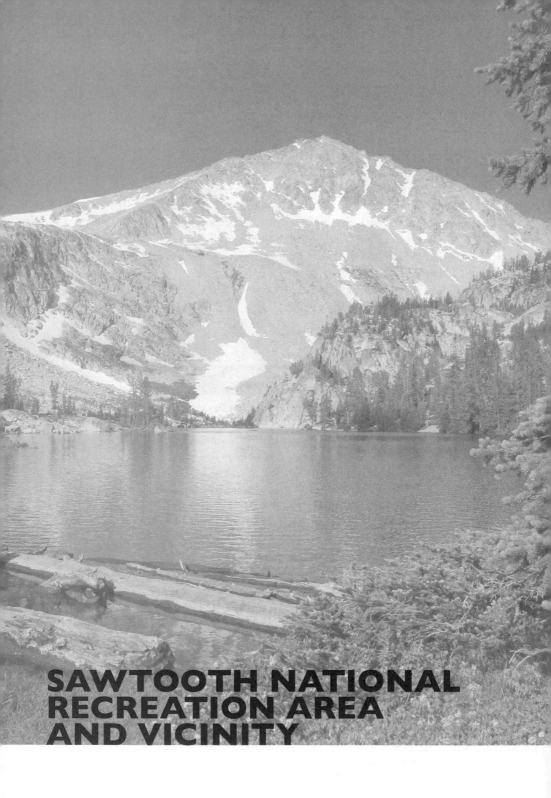

SAWTOOTH NATIONAL RECREATION AREA AND VICINITY

Peak 11,272 over Island Lake (Trip 17)

S mack in the middle of Idaho—if such an irregularly shaped state can be said to have a middle—sits the 754,000-acre Sawtooth National Recreation Area, justifiably the most popular outdoor playground in the state. Within the borders of this area are many of Idaho's most outstanding outdoor attractions. Here you will discover part or all of four major mountain ranges—the Boulder, Sawtooth, Smoky, and White Cloud Mountains. Another important range, the Pioneer Mountains, sits just outside the southeast side of the preserve. The recreation area also includes the headwaters of the world-famous Salmon River and the spectacular Sawtooth Valley, one of the most stunning mountain valleys in North America. Best of all, there are enough trails and hiking destinations to keep you happily exploring for decades.

In 1972 Congress set aside the Sawtooth Valley region as a national recreation area, with the stated purpose of assuring "the preservation and protection of the natural, scenic, historic, pastoral, and fish and wildlife values and provide for the enhancement of the recreation values." While this farsighted act did not provide the full protection of a national park, which many conservationists would have preferred, it did put a check on the impending development of subdivisions, indiscriminate logging, and rampant road building that would have destroyed the unique qualities of this area.

Only 217,000 acres of the national recreation area are protected as wilderness, and all of that is in the Sawtooth Mountains. Therefore, hikers traveling in other areas must be prepared to encounter jeep and mining roads, motorbikes on the trails, and mining activity. The mining is allowed because thousands of claims existed before the national recreation area was established, and these were grandfathered in by the enabling legislation.

The mountain scenery here ranks with the best in North America, in no small part because of the unique geology. The most noteworthy rock is the beautiful, pinkish granite of the Sawtooth Mountains. This unusual intrusion of granite formed during volcanic activity that took place only 50 million years ago and is distinct from the massive, 350-million-year-old Idaho Batholith, which underlies most of the mountains of central Idaho. In addition to being a different age and color, this rock fractures more easily, which made it especially susceptible to erosion by Ice Age glaciers. The ice left behind sharply serrated ridges and more than 400 stunningly beautiful cirque lakes, which are often the destinations of hikers today.

Though the Sawtooths draw the crowds, the lesser-known mountain ranges in the Sawtooth National Recreation Area also offer outstanding scenery. The White Cloud Peaks are particularly spectacular, with dozens of stunning lakes, lots of multicolored rock, countless high peaks, and some of the most scenic trails in Idaho. The adjacent Pioneer Mountains contain scenery that is quite similar to the Sawtooths, but without the crowds. To the south, the Smoky and Boulder Mountains are made up of porous rock, where water does not usually collect into lakes. Instead, you'll find view-packed ridges and plenty of wildflowers.

As is true in almost all the mountains of Idaho, the Sawtooths and their neighboring ranges have plenty of biting insects. Flies are an annoying problem, especially on sunny afternoons, but these pests can only survive below about 8,000 feet. Mosquitoes are abundant at all elevations, but these invertebrate vampires generally disappear by about mid-August. So, if you plan a trip to the high lakes late August–October, you should enjoy blissful, bug-free evenings.

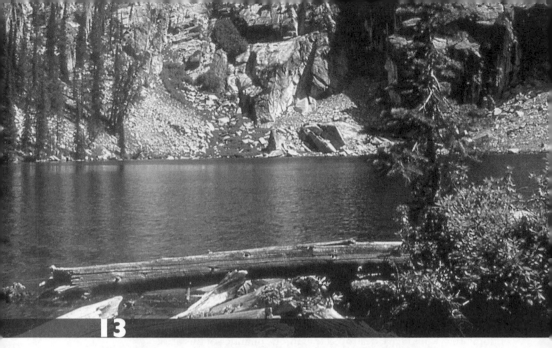

13

GRAND SAWTOOTHS LOOP

RATINGS: Scenery 9   Solitude 3   Difficulty 6

MILES: 65

ELEVATION GAIN: 12,700'

DAYS: 6–10

MAP(S): Earthwalk Press *Hiking Map & Guide: Sawtooth Wilderness, ID*

USUALLY OPEN: July–mid-October

BEST: Mid-July–mid-August

PERMITS: Yes (free at the trailhead)

RULES: Maximum group size of 12 people and 14 stock animals; all fires must be in fire pans or on fire blankets; no fires allowed within 200 yards of Sawtooth Lake or Alpine Lake; dogs must be on leash July 1–Labor Day.

CONTACT: Sawtooth National Recreation Area, 208-727-5000

SPECIAL ATTRACTIONS

Gorgeous ridgetop wildflower gardens; outstanding mountain scenery; good fishing

CHALLENGES

Relatively crowded in places

Above: Lower Trail Creek Lake

HOW TO GET THERE ●

From Boise, take exit 57 off I-84 and drive northeast on the Ponderosa Pine Scenic Highway (ID 21) to a junction near milepost 93 just before a large snow gate that is used to close the highway in winter. Turn right onto Forest Service Road 524, following signs to Sawtooth Lodge, and drive 8 miles on this good gravel road to the signed backpacker trailhead near Grandjean Campground. The trail starts next to a large signboard and permit station at the east end of the parking area.

INTRODUCTION ●

The Sawtooth Mountains contain some of Idaho's most beautiful scenery. Though the famous views from the road are superb, if you really want to appreciate all that this range has to offer, you have to leave your car and hit the trails. This long and magnificent loop visits many of the range's most outstanding locations and is the premier backpacking tour of the Sawtooth Mountains. It is possible to shorten this hike at several points, but every part of the trip is glorious, so it would be a shame to miss even 1 mile of this circuit.

DESCRIPTION ●

You start by walking 80 yards to an unsigned junction with a horse trail, which begins at a separate equestrian trailhead and loading ramp. You turn right, walk 120 yards to a bridge over Trail Creek, and then come to a junction and the start of your loop.

Hikers who want to shorten this trip should go straight on the South Fork Payette River Trail for 1.5 miles, turn left onto the Baron Creek Trail, and climb 2 miles to a junction with the North Baron Creek Trail. Unfortunately, this shortcut misses some of the finest scenery in the Sawtooth Mountains, so if you have the time, it's better to take the longer route up Trail Creek.

Note: In 2006, the large Trailhead Fire burned nearly all of the Trail Creek drainage and into the McGown Lakes area at the start of this trip. Expect lots of burned snags, deadfall, and almost no shade for the next several years as the land recovers.

The Trail Creek Trail goes left at the junction and switchbacks up a dry slope of grasses and low brush punctuated with a few scattered ponderosa pines, quaking aspens, and Douglas-firs. As the elevation increases the ponderosas are replaced by lodgepole pines, and these are later joined by Engelmann spruces and subalpine firs. About 1 mile from the South Payette junction, you cross Trail Creek on a narrow log and gradually ascend an open, south-facing slope, which supports a huge population of unusually large crickets. The steady uphill continues for the next few miles, but several dozen short switchbacks ensure that the grade is never overly steep. Along the way you make three easy crossings of Trail Creek, each time using rickety logs to keep your feet dry. About 4.3 miles, and 2,400 feet up, from the trailhead is a junction with a trail to the spectacular Trail Creek Lakes, a highly recommended side trip.

To visit these lakes, turn right at the junction, contour briefly, and hop across a small creek. From here, the rocky trail climbs steeply for a little less than 1 mile to the shore of Lower Trail Creek Lake, a picturesque mountain pool tucked in a steep-walled cirque at the base of a craggy granite peak. The lake is surrounded by scenic talus slopes and open subalpine fir forests, with several good-to-excellent campsites near the lake's outlet and more good camps along the north shore.

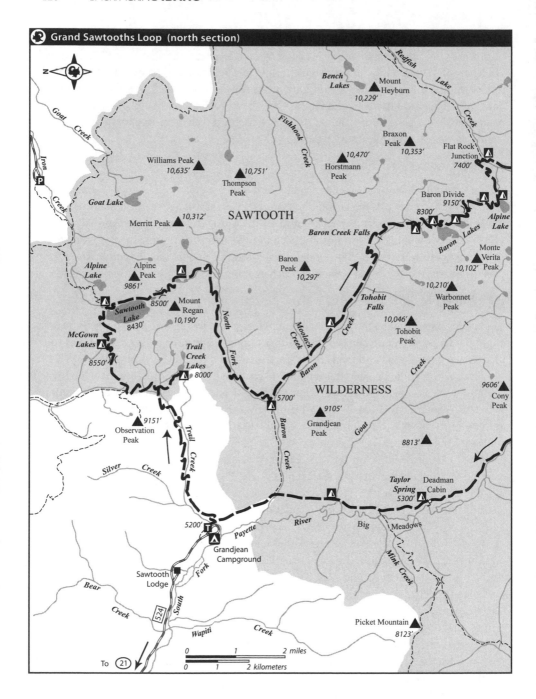

Grand Sawtooths Loop (north section)

Bench Lakes

Mount Heyburn
10,229'

Redfish Lake

Fishhook Creek

Braxon Peak
10,353'

Flat Rock Junction
7400'

Goat Creek

Iron Creek

Williams Peak
10,635'

10,751'
Thompson Peak

10,470'
Horstmann Peak

Baron Divide 9150'
8300'

Alpine Lake

SAWTOOTH

Baron Creek Falls

Monte Verita Peak
10,102'

Goat Lake

Merritt Peak
10,312'

Baron Peak
10,297'

10,210'
Warbonnet Peak

Alpine Lake

Alpine Peak
9861'

8500'

Mount Regan
10,190'

North Fork

Moolack Creek

Tohobit Falls

Baron Creek

10,046'
Tohobit Peak

Sawtooth Lake
8430'

McGown Lakes

8550'

Trail Creek Lakes
8000'

5700'

WILDERNESS

9105'
Grandjean Peak

9606'
Cony Peak

8813'

Observation Peak
9151'

Trail Creek

Baron Creek

Goat Creek

Silver Creek

Taylor Spring
5300'

Deadman Cabin

5200'

Payette

River

Big Meadows

Grandjean Campground

Mink Creek

Sawtooth Lodge

South Fork

Bear Creek

524

Wapiti Creek

Picket Mountain
8123'

To 21

0   1   2 miles

0   1   2 kilometers

Though the maintained trail ends at this lake, it's worth the effort to visit an equally scenic lake in the upper basin. To make this steep cross-country scramble, climb the slopes
east of the lower lake and follow the terrain as it naturally leads you to a trickling creek
and a small pond just below Upper Trail Creek Lake.

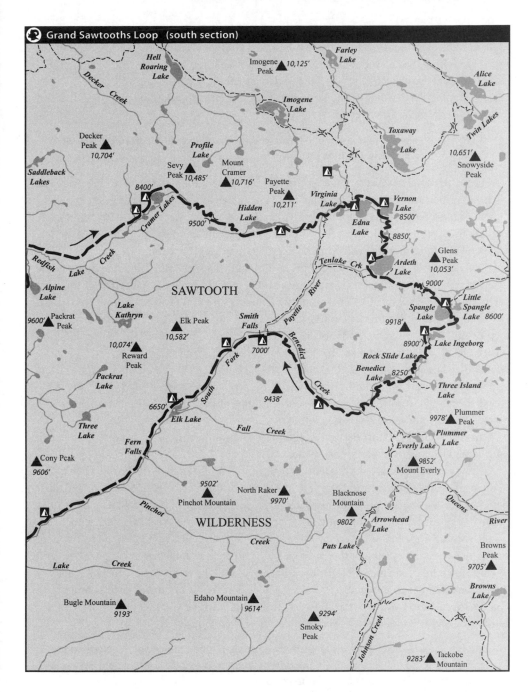

Grand Sawtooths Loop (south section)

To resume the loop, return to the Trail Creek Trail, turn right, and ascend a series of short, well-graded switchbacks to a four-way junction in a little notch.

TIP: For a fun side trip, turn sharply left and climb 1 mile to the top of the aptly named Observation Peak, where views extend over the entire northern Sawtooth Mountains.

You bear right at the four-way junction and climb several gentle switchbacks through open, high-elevation forests to the top of a small ridge. From there, you descend about 150 feet, climb over a second low ridge, and enter the lovely basin holding several bodies of water that are collectively called the McGown Lakes. After passing several ponds, you reach the last lake, which is the largest and most scenic, in addition to having the best campsites of the McGown chain.

TIP: The campsites here are much less crowded than those at the popular Sawtooth Lake, which is just over the next pass.

From the final McGown Lake, you make a relatively easy ascent to a high pass just below timberline, where you get your first view of Sawtooth Lake, the largest alpine lake in the range. No single superlative could do justice to this spectacular lake, but it's safe to say that it is one of the most beautiful and photogenic alpine lakes in North America. Several towering granite peaks rim the deep, azure waters, but Mount Regan, which rises directly above the lake's southwest shore, commands the spotlight. The route down to the lake starts with a gradual traverse across a view-packed, rocky slope north of the lake. The trail then descends two fairly long switchbacks and enters an open forest of twisted whitebark pines that frame countless great views. Finally, the path winds down to the lake's outlet, where some badly overused campsites should be avoided, and a junction with a trail that is heavily used by day hikers coming in from the east.

You go straight, hop across the lake's bubbling outlet creek, and climb to a rocky overlook. For the next mile, the trail goes up and down across an open talus slope above the east shore of Sawtooth Lake. At the southeast end of the lake you climb through a low, grassy saddle and pass a small lake below the steep slopes of Mount Regan. You then go over a rocky pass and descend a bouldery slope to a tiny basin holding two small, unnamed lakes with mediocre campsites.

Now you begin the long descent into the canyon of North Fork Baron Creek. The downhill starts by wandering through the forest beside the newborn stream, and then makes a dozen short, woodsy switchbacks to an easy crossing of the creek, which cascades down a steep slope on your right. After splashing across the creek, you descend a hot, south-facing slope that is covered with sagebrush and stunted trees kept small by frequent avalanches. At the bottom of this deep canyon, you enter a shadeless 1990s burn area and wind down to a crossing of North Fork Baron Creek. The trail crosses the creek on logs and rocks, and then descends several switchbacks through unburned forests and grasslands to a junction with the Baron Creek Trail. This is where you meet the shortcut route from the South Fork Payette River Trail mentioned previously.

TIP: If you are looking for a campsite, two excellent ones are about 70 yards to the right, where the trail fords North Fork Baron Creek, and a good one is about 50 yards to the left, in the shade of some large fir trees.

To continue the trip, turn left and hike up the canyon of Baron Creek on a gradual trail that travels through open forests and grassy meadows. Not quite 1.5 miles from the North Fork junction, you hop over the small Moolack Creek and walk another 0.6 mile to an excellent campsite beside Baron Creek. In early to mid-July the open, parklike meadows near this campsite support a wealth of wildflowers, especially spirea, which features aromatic clusters of tiny pink blossoms. Above this campsite you climb gently past Tohobit Falls, which cascade down the canyon wall on your right, and soon reach your first good view of veillike Baron Creek Falls dropping over a cliff in front of you.

Near the base of Baron Creek Falls, the trail curves left and begins a series of 22 tiring switchbacks. The first few switchbacks are under the shade of a pleasant forest, and the next several go up a brushy slope covered with ceanothus bushes. The remainder of the switchbacks ascend a sunbaked talus slope, where your frequent rest stops are rewarded with excellent views across the canyon to the jagged granite spires of Tohobit and Warbonnet Peaks.

TIP: Try to tackle this long climb in the cool shade of the morning.

A final set of four short switchbacks takes you around the base of a bulbous granite knob near the top of Baron Creek Falls. The trail then levels off and goes gently up the scenic upper valley of Baron Creek. It is interesting to observe how the granitic rocks in this upper valley display the smooth, polished surface typical of rocks shaped by the movement of glaciers. Apparently the ice did not reach the lower valley, because the rocks down there do not show this aspect.

You cross the creek where a bridge used to be, and then wind uphill for about 0.4 mile to a second crossing, possibly on narrow logs, if they still exist. Immediately on the other side of the creek is a superb campsite.

TIP: If you prefer solitude for the night, stay at this scenic campsite because it is less crowded than the camps at Baron Lake.

Above the campsite you climb several gentle switchbacks, and then cross the creek a final time on a bridge and come to the shores of the dramatic Baron Lake. Views are superb across this deep lake, especially of the towering Warbonnet and Monte Verita Peaks, with their numerous granite spires and cliffs. Several large but usually rather crowded camps are near the outlet of the lake.

The trail crosses a logjam at the outlet of Baron Lake, follows the east shore for a short distance, and then veers away from the lake and climbs past good viewpoints to Upper Baron Lake, which is smaller. Though very attractive, this pool will seem rather tame in comparison to the spectacular lower lake, and the single campsite here is less inviting than the ones at Baron Lake. After skirting the east shore of Upper Baron Lake, the trail climbs 30 short, moderately steep switchbacks to the top of the 9,150-foot Baron Divide, where a rest stop and lots of gawking are in order.

Views from this grandstand extend over much of the central and eastern Sawtooth Mountains. To the west and northwest are Monte Verita Peak, the Baron Lakes, and the valley you just ascended. To the east is the serrated eastern edge of the Sawtooths, an impressive display of craggy, pink granite. It looks very different from this angle than it does from the better-known Redfish Lake side, because the foreground here isn't flat with lakes, but instead is a sea of jagged peaks and valleys. Below you to the south is the basin holding the teardrop-shaped Alpine Lake, your next destination. Beyond that, to the southeast, is the upper canyon of Redfish Lake Creek.

After taking in all of these views, put your pack back on and descend a few moderate switchbacks to a small pond. Then the trail loops down to a larger, more attractive lake in a partly forested basin.

TIP: The campsites near this lake are usually less crowded than those at Alpine Lake.

You descend rather steeply along this lake's tiny outlet creek, cross it twice, and then climb briefly to the top of a side ridge. Four long switchbacks take you down to the shore of the popular Alpine Lake, with its overused campsites and decent views of Packrat Peak to the west.

Beyond Alpine Lake the heavily used trail traverses a hillside above the lake's outlet stream to a nice viewpoint of Redfish Lake Creek canyon. The trail then descends a series of irregularly spaced switchbacks on a forest- and brush-covered slope to Flat Rock Junction, where you meet the trail from Redfish Lake. This trail is the source of all those white-shorts-and-tennis-shoe-wearing tourists you've been meeting, most of whom were dropped off by boat at the southwest end of the busy Redfish Lake.

You turn right and soon come to a flat, sloping rock shelf over which the creek slides—the origin of Flat Rock Junction's name. You cross the 25-foot-wide Redfish Lake Creek here. In early summer this can be a tricky ford, but there is usually a logjam about 100 yards downstream from the ford, where you can cross more safely. On the opposite side of the crossing is a good campsite.

The path goes gently upstream, generally staying close to the sparkling creek, which gives anglers many opportunities to pull out their trusty fly rods. After 0.5 mile, the trail works away from the water and goes up the hillside to the east. You gain about 800 feet in the next mile, and then level off and contour across a partly forested slope. A final short climb takes you to Lower Cramer Lake, the smallest of three beautiful alpine lakes tucked beneath the cliffs and talus slopes of Sevy Peak to the southeast and an unnamed pinnacle to the west. All three lakes have campsites and host lots of hungry brook trout. The best campsites are beside the two lower lakes, but Upper Cramer Lake is the largest and most scenic of the group.

Above Upper Cramer Lake the lightly used trail makes a sweeping ascent of a partly forested hillside, which provides ever-improving views of the Cramer Lakes and Redfish Lake Creek canyon. After about 0.5 mile, you hop across a little brook and walk uphill past a string of ponds and small lakes. The trail then steadily ascends an open, rocky slope to a high pass.

WARNING: Snow often lingers on this slope until midsummer.

From the pass, you go downhill across a talus slope above a narrow, rock-rimmed lake, and then reenter forest and make a moderately steep descent to a crossing of a small creek just above the west shore of Hidden Lake, which is large and narrow. The trail threads its way between the lake's water and steep slopes to the west all the way to the southern tip of Hidden Lake, where you'll find a couple of adequate campsites. Below the lake you pass a long, narrow pool on the outlet creek, and then switchback through forest down to a junction immediately after you hop over the splashing headwaters of the South Fork Payette River.

For the most direct route back to your car, turn right and walk 18 miles down the South Fork Payette River Trail to the trailhead. Having come this far, however, don't miss the string of beautiful high lakes along an alternate trail. This route adds 9 miles and 1,800 feet of elevation gain to your trip, but it compensates with lots of outstanding scenery. So, unless you are really pressed for time, turn left at the junction and slowly climb beside the river—which is really nothing more than a small creek at this point—to the kidney-shaped Virginia Lake. This forest-rimmed pool is backed by a rounded, granite butte and has good views to the north of the peaks around Hidden Lake.

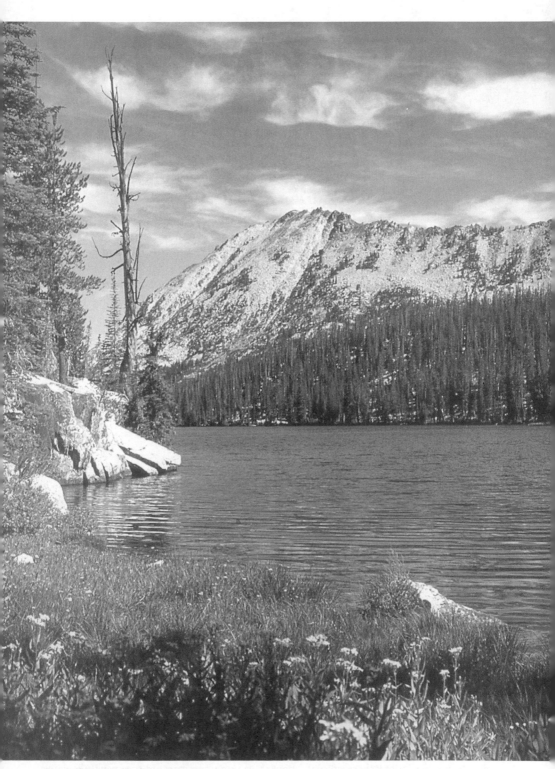

Payette Peak over Edna Lake

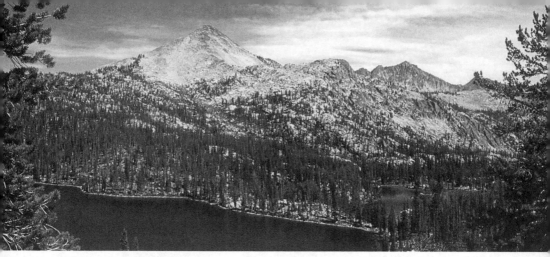

Glenns Peak over Spangle Lake

Beyond Virginia Lake you ascend six quick switchbacks to the 200-acre Edna Lake, which is surrounded by open, subalpine fir forests and has outstanding views of almost every nearby peak. The best campsites are near the south end of the lake, though they tend to be popular among equestrians, so expect dusty trails, horse apples, and the usual distinctive aroma. The trail follows the northeast shore of Edna Lake, and then switchbacks away from the water to a junction.

The trail to the left heads east over the view-packed Sand Mountain Pass and then drops to the popular Toxaway Lake (see Trip 15).

TIP: A side trip up this trail to either Sand Mountain Pass or the closer, off-trail goal of Lake 8,861 is well worth your time. Lake 8,861 is especially scenic, because it sits in a beautiful, grassy basin below the long ridge of Payette Peak. The few campsites at this lake are generally deserted and very scenic.

Back at the junction above Edna Lake, the main trail bears right, makes a few gentle ups and downs, passes a fine campsite at the south end of Edna Lake, and finally comes to the lovely Vernon Lake. This lake has good campsites along its gently sloping shores and stunning views of a triangle-shaped peak to the south.

TIP: For more solitude, try visiting the small, off-trail lake just southeast of Vernon Lake.

The trail crosses Vernon Lake's outlet creek, goes around the lake's northwest shore, and makes a series of nine uphill switchbacks. This climb takes you over a sparsely forested slope with lots of granite ledges, where you can enjoy a quick rest stop and fine views. Just before reaching a pass, you level off beside a small, island-dotted lake in a basin surrounded by subalpine firs, whitebark pines, and various alpine wildflowers.

TIP: Despite its relatively small size, this lake supports a population of brook trout. Because this lake gets less fishing pressure than nearby waters, you stand a better-than-average chance of catching dinner.

The best views at the pass are to the west over the forested Tenlake Basin, in the middle of which is the large Ardeth Lake. Dominating the skyline are the rocky heights and permanent snowfields of the 10,053-foot Glens Peak to the southwest. To reach Ardeth Lake, you descend 16 moderately steep switchbacks through open forest to the sparkling waters of this popular lake. Several large and exceptionally scenic camps are near the outlet and along the west shore, but be prepared to compete with horse parties for a spot.

The trail follows the northeast shore of Ardeth Lake, crosses its outlet creek, and goes another few hundred yards to a junction with a trail that goes down Tenlake Creek to the South Fork Payette River. If you want to cut the trip short, turn right at this junction and hike the 17 relatively easy miles back to your car.

WARNING: In early summer you may have to exit this way, because the trail over Tenlake Divide can remain snowbound until August. Ask other hikers for the latest information.

Assuming that snow is not a concern, bear left at the junction and walk to the southwest corner of Ardeth Lake, where the trail splits. The trail to the left goes down to a spacious horse camp beside the lake's inlet. You bear right (uphill) and gradually climb through lodgepole pine and subalpine fir woods to a spring-fed, marshy pond with a fine view of Glens Peak. You then make eight fairly long switchbacks up a talus slope to the 9,000-foot Tenlake Divide. Views from this windy location are superb, especially north over the Tenlake Basin to the colorful Payette Peak, Elk Peak, and Mount Cramer.

On the south side of the divide the gently graded trail snakes down three lazy switchbacks through open woods to the shores of the deep Spangle Lake. Camping here is limited, because the shoreline is quite steep and flat sites are hard to find, but a couple of good campsites are near the northeast shore. At the southeast end of the lake is a junction with a trail down the Middle Fork Boise River. You turn right and cross the narrow strip of rocky land between Spangle Lake and Little Spangle Lake, which is much shallower. The small stream connecting these two lakes is easily crossed on a logjam.

You climb six short switchbacks on the hillside west of Spangle Lake and come to a very attractive little lake tucked beneath a jagged line of cliffs. The trail just barely touches this gem, and then turns right and gradually ascends a few curving switchbacks to a high, flat ridgeline with exceptional views back to Spangle Lake and Glens Peak. Also of interest here, if you can pry your eyes away from the view, are several huge boulders that provide good, up close examples of the pink-tinted granite for which the Sawtooths are famous. A short distance past the viewpoint is Lake Ingeborg, which is deep, very scenic, and backed by a line of serrated peaks that are impressively streaked with snow in early summer. Several good campsites are at this lake, allowing you to spend an enjoyable evening snagging some of the lake's large brook and cutthroat trout. Sunsets are often spectacular at this lake.

The trail goes through an almost imperceptible pass west of Lake Ingeborg, and then descends a long switchback to a small marshy tarn. From here, you drop to the north shore of the very scenic Rock Slide Lake, which gets its name from a large rockslide that drops into the lake's south shore. The trail then descends seven switchbacks, crosses the lake's outlet stream below a small, sliding waterfall, and comes to a shallow, unnamed lake, which is little more than a marsh by late summer.

WARNING: Mosquitoes can be a problem here before mid-August.

At the north end of this lake–marsh is an unsigned junction with the 0.5-mile, dead-end trail to Three Island Lake, which sits in a lovely basin to the south and features three tiny, rocky islets that gave the lake its name.

The main trail goes straight (north), crosses Benedict Creek on a footlog, and gradually descends a couple of long switchbacks to the grassy shores of Benedict Lake, the last of the string of high lakes along this loop. The fine views up to an unnamed, rounded mountain to the northeast will make you sorry to leave the high country behind. But leave it behind you must, so reluctantly continue down Benedict Creek past a shallow pond. You then make a series of very gradual downhill switchbacks beside a sloping waterfall to a junction with a trail that heads left (southwest) to the Queens River drainage (See Trip 14).

TIP: Hikers who have not yet had their fill of beautiful mountain lakes can bear left, climb 1 mile to a junction, and then turn left to visit the remote Everly and Plummer Lakes. The farther of these two is only about 2 miles from the Benedict Creek Trail.

To continue on the loop, bear right at the junction and descend a short distance to log crossings of two forks of Benedict Creek. Over the next 3.5 miles the well-graded trail follows the relatively gentle canyon of Benedict Creek as that stream slowly curves northeast. The hiking is easy and pleasant as the trail passes through a series of avalanche meadows with fine views of numerous jagged peaks and plenty of wildflowers. About 0.9 mile from the Queens River junction is a nice creek-side campsite on the right. After this, the views are blocked by trees until you get near the bottom of the canyon, where the trail makes six irregularly spaced switchbacks to a small burn area and a junction with the shortcut trail down from Virginia and Ardeth Lakes.

You veer left, now on the dusty South Fork Payette River Trail, and soon pass the roaring Smith Falls, a sliding cascade that is well worth a lengthy visit or even an overnight stay at the campsite just upstream. Below this highlight, the trail follows the meandering stream for about 0.8 mile to a ford of the cold, 50-foot-wide river. A decent campsite is on the downstream side of this ford.

WARNING: In early summer this crossing can be dangerous. Wading shoes and a sturdy walking stick are recommended.

Below the ford it's a straightforward river walk all the way back to your car. The trail is never steep, so the miles are easy and go by quickly. The early miles are under the shade of stately Douglas-fir trees with an interesting mix of greenery in the understory. On your left, the river remains hidden in boggy areas bordered by nearly impenetrable tangles of willows and Engelmann spruces. These obstacles generally preclude access to the water, which is a shame, because the South Fork Payette River is one of Idaho's premier fly-fishing streams. The clear waters support both rainbow and brook trout, with opportunities for catching big fish improving as the stream gets larger down the canyon.

A little more than 1.5 miles from the ford, you reach the shallow and swampy Elk Lake. Except for around the campsite near its southeast end, this lake's shoreline is hidden by a tangle of spruce trees. About 1 mile past the lake you pass above a rocky gulch where the river tumbles through a narrow channel. This two-part cascade goes by the name of Fern Falls, though calling it a waterfall seems overly generous.

The trail descends a few gentle switchbacks, and then simply wanders down the widening canyon. There aren't any high peaks in view so the scenery is rather subdued, but woodsy ridges are visible on both sides of the canyon, and the nearby forests are continuously attractive. The trail is brushy in places, but the hiking is easy as you gradually descend through a mix of forests, avalanche chutes, and rockslides. The river is more accessible now, and anglers will be eager to avail themselves of every opportunity.

About 5 miles below Fern Falls the forest cover changes to lodgepole and ponderosa pines, with many of the open parklands and meadows so closely associated with the latter species. The temperatures can get uncomfortably warm at these lower elevations during the height of summer, especially because the ponderosas provide relatively little shade, but because the trail stays level or goes gradually downhill, the heat is tolerable.

The river slowly curves north and splits, with the various branches wandering in wide curves and eddies through increasingly large open areas that carry the rather uninspired name of Big Meadows. Near the largest of these you come to the site of Deadman Cabin, where you'll find several good campsites amid the pines with easy access to the river. Even hikers who aren't interested in casting a line should take the time to explore the meadow's fine views, wildflowers, and beaver activity.

Not far from Deadman Cabin the often-dusty trail passes the large Taylor Spring, and then travels through an area of dead and burned timber to a junction with a trail that heads west up the canyon of Mink Creek. You go straight, staying on the South Fork Payette River Trail, and continue another mile to the bridgeless crossing of Goat Creek. A good campsite is just north of the easy ford. After a refreshing rest stop here, you hike through burned forests for about 1.4 miles to a calf-deep ford of Baron Creek.

TIP: You can't see it from the ford, but a log goes across the creek about 50 yards upstream from the official crossing.

A short distance past this crossing is a junction with the Baron Creek Trail. To finish the hike, you go straight and make a gentle, 1.5-mile, up-and-down stroll back to the bridge over Trail Creek and the Grandjean trailhead.

POSSIBLE ITINERARY

	CAMP	MILES	ELEVATION GAIN
Day 1	Trail Creek Lake	5.0	3,100'
Day 2	North Fork Baron Creek	12.0	1,500'
Day 3	Baron Lake	7.0	2,700'
Day 4	Cramer Lake	7.0	1,900'
Day 5	Lake Ingeborg	12.0	2,800'
Day 6	Elk Lake	11.0	200'
Day 7	Out	11.0	500'

BEST SHORTER ALTERNATIVE ·

As mentioned above, consider making just the short loop up Trail Creek to Sawtooth Lake and back down North Fork Baron Creek to your car at Grandjean. With another day or two make the excellent side trip to the gorgeous Baron Lakes.

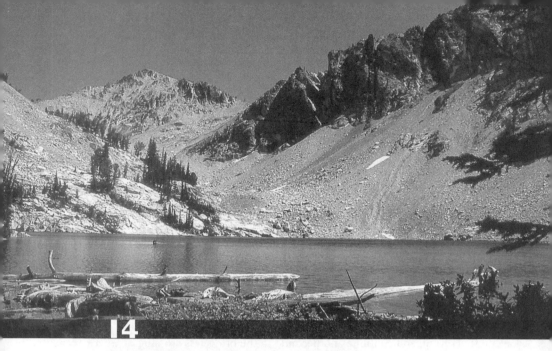

QUEENS RIVER LOOP

RATINGS: Scenery 9   Solitude 7   Difficulty 5
MILES: 37 (42)
ELEVATION GAIN: 8,100' (9,100')
DAYS: 3–4 (4–5)
MAP(S): Earthwalk Press *Hiking Map & Guide: Sawtooth Wilderness, ID*
USUALLY OPEN: July–mid-October
BEST: Mid-July–mid-August
PERMITS: Yes (free at the trailhead)
RULES: Maximum group size of 12 people and 14 stock animals; all fires must be in fire pans or on fire blankets; no fires allowed within 200 yards of Scenic Lake; dogs must be on leash July 1–Labor Day.
CONTACT: Sawtooth National Recreation Area, 208-727-5000

SPECIAL ATTRACTIONS ·

Fine mountain scenery; good lake and stream fishing; dramatic canyon scenery along the lower Queens River

CHALLENGES ·

Some burn areas with dense regrowing shrubbery; wear long pants

Above: Nahneke Mountain over Scenic Lake

HOW TO GET THERE •

From Boise, take exit 57 off I-84 and drive 12.9 miles northeast on the Ponderosa Pine Scenic Highway (ID 21) to a junction immediately after a large bridge over an arm of Lucky Peak Reservoir. Turn right, following signs to Atlanta and Arrowrock Dam, and drive 4 miles to the end of the pavement; then settle in for a long, rather tedious drive on a bumpy gravel road. Stay on this road, which becomes Forest Service Road 268, for 63.3 miles up the canyon of the Middle Fork Boise River to a junction directly across from Queens River Campground. Turn left onto the narrow FS 206 and follow it for 1.8 miles to a fork, where you veer left and drive a final 0.3 mile to the Queens River trailhead. A few campsites are at the trailhead, should you arrive late and want to spend the night before starting your hike.

INTRODUCTION •

The Sawtooth Mountains have an embarrassment of riches, including colorful fields of wildflowers, jagged granite peaks, and gorgeous, high-elevation lakes. This loop trip explores the southwest part of the range and includes a nice sampling of all these wonderful sights. In addition, it takes you through the impressive depths of the lower Queens River Canyon, a spectacular rocky chasm that features scenery not normally associated with a high mountain wilderness. Because this hike avoids the most famous attractions in the Sawtooth Wilderness, visitors here enjoy more solitude than in the better-known and more accessible parts of the range.

DESCRIPTION •

The trail drops briefly from the northwest end of the parking area to a sturdy bridge over the Queens River and a junction at the start of the loop.

For a clockwise tour, bear left and head up the canyon of the Little Queens River. The open forests at these lower elevations are a pleasant mix of ponderosa pines, lodgepole pines, Douglas-firs, and Englemann spruces. Beneath these trees, the forest floor is covered with a wealth of grasses and colorful wildflowers such as goldenrod, pearly everlasting, horsemint, and three flowers that grow up to 6 feet tall in this area—fireweed, coneflower, and larkspur. Apart from the flowers, the scenery is pleasant but unspectacular. You travel gradually uphill on a sometimes rocky tread for 0.6 mile, cross the river on a bridge, and come to a small meadow that holds an old wooden cabin and the rusted remains of an abandoned mine. The gentle trail then continues up to an easy crossing of Browns Creek and a slightly trickier, ankle-deep ford of the Little Queens River.

Another mile of gentle uphill takes you past a nice campsite and on to a broken-down miner's cabin, which is interesting to explore. The slope of your ascent picks up slightly after this—though it still isn't steep—as you go up three switchbacks, and then contour across a hillside well above the stream. Less than 1 mile from the cabin you hop over Scott Creek, and then wander through a mix of forests and meadows to a log crossing of Tripod Creek. About 0.5 mile later is a very good campsite just before a rock-hop crossing of the Little Queens River.

Beyond this crossing the trail goes through rolling, sagebrush-dotted meadows to a junction with the Neinmeyer Creek Trail, which heads northwest up to an obvious saddle.

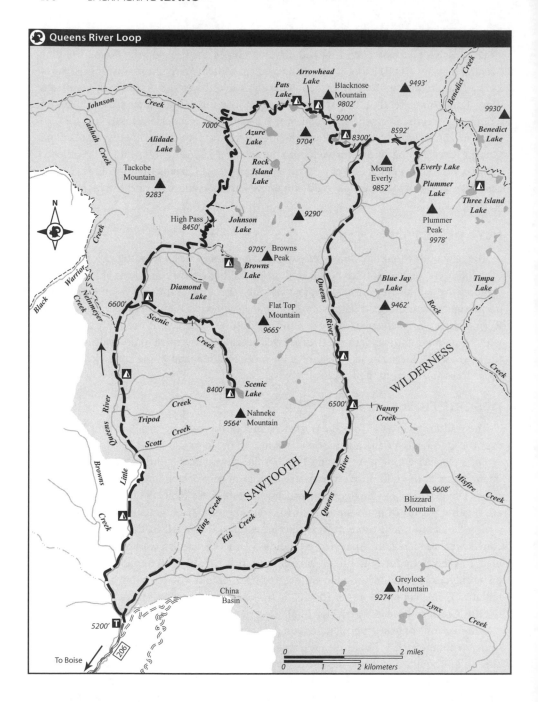

Queens River Loop

You bear right and soon pass a very large beaver pond about 200 yards before a tiny sign marking the junction with the Scenic Lake Trail.

If you want to make the side trip to this lake (and how could you not want to visit a place named Scenic Lake?), then bear right and travel down to an easy crossing of what's left of Little Queens River. A good campsite is on the right about 100 yards before this crossing, and another one is on the left just after the crossing. The trail climbs steadily away from the crossing through sloping meadows that in July are ablaze with the colorful blossoms of death camas, sulphur flower, paintbrush, and aster.

WARNING: Horseflies are common here and can be very bothersome on a warm afternoon.

At the end of the meadows you make six moderately graded switchbacks and then an uphill traverse to the base of a small, tumbling waterfall on Scenic Creek. Four more switchbacks lead to the top of the falls and just beyond to a sign stating HORSE TRAVEL NOT RECOMMENDED BEYOND THIS POINT. The reason for this sign soon becomes apparent as the trail winds very steeply up a rocky, almost shadeless hillside that is a challenge for two-legged visitors, not to mention livestock. The grade eases considerably at the top of the slope, where you go up and down through open, subalpine fir forests past a pair of small, marshy ponds.

WARNING: The trail is easy to lose in this area. Look carefully for blazes and a few cut logs that provide navigational clues.

In its final mile the trail goes through beautiful meadows beside the small Scenic Creek, crosses the creek once, and makes a short climb to a small but attractive lower lake, where the trail seems to stop. To reach the more spectacular upper lake, cross the outlet of the lower lake, follow its shoreline for about 150 yards, and then climb steeply for 0.2 mile to your final reward at Scenic Lake.

It's not easy to live up to a name like Scenic Lake, but this beautiful mountain pool manages to do so with ease. It is set in a dramatic cirque beneath Nahneke Mountain and is backed by tall cliffs and talus slopes. The best campsites are near the outlet, and for the pleasure of a night at this beautiful lake you'll be glad that you packed your heavy gear all the way up here. A bonus of camping here is that the lake has a good population of plump cutthroat trout and the fishing pressure is relatively light. Remember that fires are prohibited at Scenic Lake, so bring your cookstove.

After returning to the Little Queens River Trail, you turn right (upstream) and make a long, relentless climb at a moderate grade through spacious meadows on the rolling slopes above the river. Views improve as you climb, especially south down the valley of the Little Queens River and east up to the peaks around Browns Lake. You pass a cairn marking where the unmaintained trail to Diamond Lake comes in from the right, and then make two long, rounded switchbacks to a junction with the Browns Lake Trail. The 0.9-mile side trail to this lake gains about 500 feet of elevation, but it's worth the effort if you have the time.

The main trail goes left at the Browns Lake junction and steadily climbs 11 switchbacks through open forests to an 8,450-foot saddle with the rather unoriginal name of High Pass. The best views here are north over the drainage of Johnson Creek to Smoky Peak, and northeast to the tip of South Raker, a distinctive sharp pinnacle that peeks over the ridge west of Blacknose Mountain.

As the trail descends two well-graded switchbacks on the north side of High Pass it soon passes above a small pond. At about 0.2 mile from High Pass is an unsigned and easily missed junction with a blazed trail that goes 0.5 mile to the right to the very scenic

Johnson Lake. This is another worthy side trip if you can find the trail, though deadfall is often a problem on this unmaintained path.

The Little Queens River Trail makes a long, gentle traverse from the Johnson Lake junction into a sloping burn area. After this you make two more switchbacks and follow a small creek through flower-covered meadows with fine views of the nearby peaks. After following this creek for less than 0.5 mile, the trail gradually pulls away from the stream and passes through more of the burn area. A few final switchbacks take you down to a rock-hop crossing of Johnson Creek, a cascading stream that is bordered by lush riparian vegetation dominated by willows, monkshood, and Queen Anne's lace. About 200 yards after the crossing is a junction with the Johnson Creek Trail.

You turn right, following signs to Pats Lake, and climb a fire-scarred hillside, where fire-weed, ceanothus bushes, and young quaking aspen trees are quickly reclaiming the blackened landscape. The shadeless climb begins with four long switchbacks followed by an uphill traverse of a little less than 1 mile. At the end of the traverse, you ascend four short switchbacks to a log over the creek that drains this high valley, and then make a short, stiff climb to a second creek crossing near an intensely green meadow. The striking color of this meadow is in sharp contrast to the blackened snags all around. Only 200 yards later, you cross the creek a third time, just below a stair-step waterfall, and wind fairly steeply uphill to the top of the falls. Above the falls you make an uneven ascent to a final creek crossing a short distance below Pats Lake. The trail stays well to the north of this lake, so a short side trip is required for you to enjoy the excellent views across the water to Blacknose Mountain, northeast of the lake, and an unnamed, craggy ridgeline to the south. Some very good campsites are under a few unburned trees along the lake's northwest shore.

Above Pats Lake the rocky trail makes eight uphill switchbacks on a partly forested hillside to the lovely Arrowhead Lake. This deep gem is set in a beautiful alpine basin and has lots of hungry cutthroat trout, many of them large. The few campsites here are rather exposed (the ones at Pats Lake are better), but you'll find at least one good site on a little ledge above the north shore.

The trail ascends a series of moderately graded switchbacks above Arrowhead Lake to the highest point of this trip at a wide, 9,200-foot pass that sits just below timberline. The views from here are magnificent, especially southeast to the pointed Mount Everly and the upper basin of Queens River. Below the pass the trail winds down past a few weather-beaten trees and through alpine meadows, where high-elevation flowers such as Cusick's speedwell, owl's clover, pink heather, bistort, aster, and pussytoes add color to the magnificent mountain scenery. The trail then goes past three small- to medium-size lakes, all of which feature fine views of Peak 9,704 to the west. A good campsite is near the outlet of the second lake in this chain. A final nine switchbacks take you down to a junction with the Queens River Trail in a lovely meadow below the cliffs and snowfields of Mount Everly.

The return route of this loop goes right, but I recommend that you first take the opportunity for an outstanding side trip to Everly and Plummer Lakes, which are tucked in the high country on the east side of Mount Everly. To do this excursion, turn left, climb past a pair of lovely meadows to a low pass, and wind down a fairly steep and rocky trail past the crumbling cliffs on the north side of Mount Everly to a junction. You bear right, cross a boggy little basin with a great view of Mount Everly, and climb steeply up to the outlet of the rock-rimmed Everly Lake. To reach Plummer Lake, follow the trail around the east side of Everly Lake to where the path peters out in some meadows. From there, wander a few hundred yards south to an almost unnoticeable watershed divide, where you'll see Plummer Lake sitting in a dramatic basin beneath the dark summit of Plummer Peak.

TIP: Though very scenic, Everly and Plummer Lakes have only fair campsites, so it's better to visit them on a day hike.

Back at the Queens River junction, you turn south and begin the long descent of the dramatic Queens River Canyon. The first few hundred yards go through lovely meadows with scattered subalpine firs and views of several nearby granite cliffs and peaks. You then hop across the bubbling flow of the Queens River and make a moderately steep, 1-mile traverse of a mostly forested hillside to a second rock-hop crossing of the growing river. Still staying close to the water, the rocky trail winds steeply downhill through avalanche meadows that provide inspiring views of the tall peaks on either side of the canyon. At the bottom of this steep, 0.5-mile section, the trail becomes much gentler as it goes through or beside a series of grassy meadows to a tricky rock-hop or an easy, ankle-deep ford of the Queens River.

WARNING: Confusing game paths in the meadows near this ford falsely lead you to a point that is approximately 100 feet upstream from the official trail crossing.

Angler at Scenic Lake

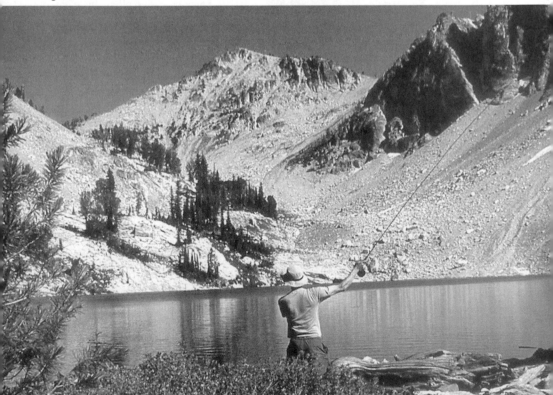

The next section of this very scenic trail goes through or just above some gorgeous meadows, which are bisected by the meandering Queens River and enclosed by towering granite walls and peaks that rise as much as 3,000 feet above the valley floor. About 1.5 miles below the last crossing, the trail makes a seemingly unnecessary uphill detour on a hillside to the east, and then goes steeply back down to river level and descends through a series of rocky avalanche meadows separated by strips of trees. These openings allow wildflowers to thrive and give hikers wonderful views of the high ridges on either side of the canyon. You pass a scenic riverside campsite in one of these strips of trees, and then continue the uneven descent to a very good campsite beside Nanny Creek just before the trail crosses the Queens River. This crossing can usually be accomplished on logs, but if these have been washed away, the ford is relatively easy and straightforward. The trail picks up again about 75 feet downstream from the crossing.

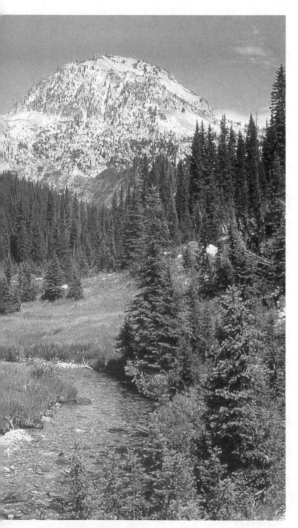

Along upper Queens River

About 0.5 mile after this crossing, you break out of the dense forest and enter large, brushy meadows, which provide unobstructed views of the dramatic canyon scenery. The topographic map shows lots of tightly packed contour lines here, and the landscape agrees, with tall pinnacles and towering ramparts, especially on the right (west) side of the canyon. On your left, the river cascades along in a narrow chasm, its flow augmented by small side creeks that trickle down from the heights on either side. The scenery in this canyon is far superior to that along the Little Queens River at the start of this trip, which means a clockwise loop is a good idea, so you can save the best for last. Not quite 3 miles from the last ford, you cross the river again, this time via a calf-deep ford.

TIP: Even though a few logs cross the stream here, they are all small and dangerously unstable, so you're better off with wet feet.

This crossing is necessary because for the next mile the northwest (right) side of the canyon rises in steep talus slopes and tall, dark-colored cliffs that are impressive to look at but would be very hard to push a trail through. Your much easier route goes up and down on the left side of the river through Douglas-fir woods and patches of succulent thimbleberries, which ripen in August. At the end of this section is another calf-deep ford of the river.

You can put the wading shoes away now, because for the rest of the hike you remain on the north side of the river, which now flows westward. Shortly after the last ford is a confusing area of brush and rocks, where you have to pick your way along the north bank until the trail becomes clear again. The canyon then widens and levels out as the trail leaves the river and goes through an old-growth, ponderosa pine forest with some Douglas-firs and lodgepole pines and an understory of grasses and manzanita bushes.

TIP: The Earthwalk Press map shows a junction here with a trail that goes left up to China Basin, but there is no trail sign and no tread is visible on the ground.

The last 2 miles of your hike are nearly level, through open forests of ponderosa pines where 4-foot-tall mullein plants bloom yellow in July and August. When you reach the Little Queens River junction, turn left, cross the bridge, and return to your car.

VARIATIONS

To extend this trip by two wonderfully scenic days, take the trail through the divide north of Mount Everly and make a loop past the high lakes at the headwaters of the South Fork Payette River. See Trip 13 for details on this route.

POSSIBLE ITINERARY

	CAMP	MILES	ELEVATION GAIN
Day 1	Scenic Lake	10.0	3,400'
Day 2	Pats Lake	11.0	3,400'
Day 3	Upper Queens River	8.0	1,000'
	Side trip to Everly and Plummer Lakes	5.0	1,000'
Day 4	Out	8.0	300'

BEST SHORTER ALTERNATIVE

For a fairly long weekend backpacking trip, make Scenic Lake your goal. Another fine alternative is a day hike up the lower Queens River Canyon for as long as your legs will carry you.

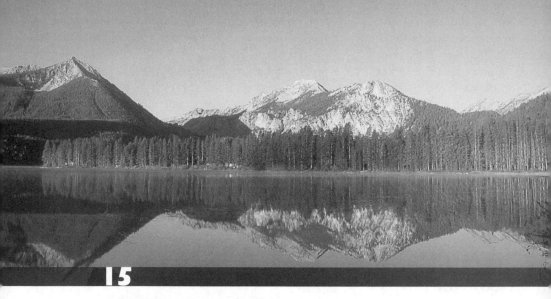

PETTIT LAKE:
HELL ROARING LOOP

RATINGS: Scenery 9   Solitude 3   Difficulty 5
MILES: 30.5 (35.5)
ELEVATION GAIN: 6,000' (7,200')
DAYS: 3–4 (4–5)
MAP(S): Earthwalk Press *Hiking Map & Guide: Sawtooth Wilderness, ID*
USUALLY OPEN: Mid-July–mid-October
BEST: Mid-July–August
PERMITS: Yes (free at the trailhead)
RULES: Maximum group size of 12 people and 14 stock animals; all fires must
be in a fire pan or on a fire blanket; no fires allowed in the Alice, Twin, or
Toxaway Lake basins; dogs must be on leash from July 1 to Labor Day.
CONTACT: Sawtooth National Recreation Area, 208-727-5000

SPECIAL ATTRACTIONS •

Beautiful mountain scenery; lots of large mountain lakes; wildflowers

CHALLENGES •

Rather crowded; mosquitoes in July

Above: Pettit Lake

HOW TO GET THERE •

From Stanley, drive 18.3 miles south on ID 75 to a junction just after the highway makes an angled turn to the left. (Coming from the south, this turnoff is 13.4 miles north of Galena Summit.) Turn right (west) on Pettit Lake Road (also known as Forest Service Road 208), and go 1.6 miles on this washboard-riddled gravel road to a T-junction. Turn right, and then drive 0.6 mile through a campground to the Tin Cup hiker's trailhead.

If you have two cars, you can shorten this trip by leaving a second car at the Hell Roaring trailhead. To reach it, return to ID 75 and drive 3.3 miles north to the junction with Fourth of July Road. Turn left (west) onto Decker Flat Road and drive 0.3 mile on this rough gravel road to a bridge over the Salmon River. Immediately after the bridge is a T-junction. Go left here and proceed about 0.4 mile to the signed trailhead, which has fairly limited parking.

INTRODUCTION •

This relatively short trip samples all of the attributes that make the Sawtooth Mountains the most popular hiking area in Idaho. The route wanders through attractive forests, goes past several beautiful mountain lakes, climbs over high passes with great views, and visits meadows with a wealth of wildflowers. Because of the excellent scenery and easy access, the trails here are some of the most popular in the state. It is, therefore, especially important that hikers be scrupulous in following all Leave No Trace principles.

DESCRIPTION •

A wide and well-used trail heads west through open forests of Douglas-firs and lodgepole pines on the slopes beside Pettit Lake. In the open areas above the trail are lots of sagebrush and early-summer wildflowers such as lupine, fireweed, groundsel, balsamroot, and sulphur flower. Numerous short side paths lead down to the lakeshore, which is especially appealing on calm mornings when the still waters reflect McDonald and Parks Peaks to the southwest.

About 200 yards from the trailhead is a four-way junction. A horse trail goes sharply right, while the path to Yellow Belly Lake angles slightly right. You will come back on the latter trail if you hike the full loop. For now, bear slightly left and stick with the rolling trail along the lakeshore. In about 1 mile you reach the end of Pettit Lake, enter Sawtooth Wilderness, and pass a registration box from which you are required to obtain a free permit.

For the next 1.5 miles you gradually gain elevation through relatively dense forests that in addition to the pines and Douglas-firs now include Engelmann spruces. The drier slopes in this area feature flowers like yarrow, paintbrush, and a particularly fetching variety of mariposa lily. The boggy areas, which are often crossed by wooden plank bridges, host thimbleberry and monkshood.

The trail passes beneath a long, craggy rock formation as it slowly ascends beside an unnamed, cascading creek. Along the way you cross the creek twice. Neither of these crossings offer a bridge, and the first is fairly deep and may present a hazard in early summer. The second crossing often has a log, but even if this is unavailable, the ford is easier than the first crossing. After the second crossing, you leave the stream and make 10 well-graded switchbacks up an open slope above a marshy little lake. This slope often has lots of fireweed in bloom during July. The switchbacks take you to an attractive upper valley, where you twice rock-hop across a small creek and gradually ascend through rocky

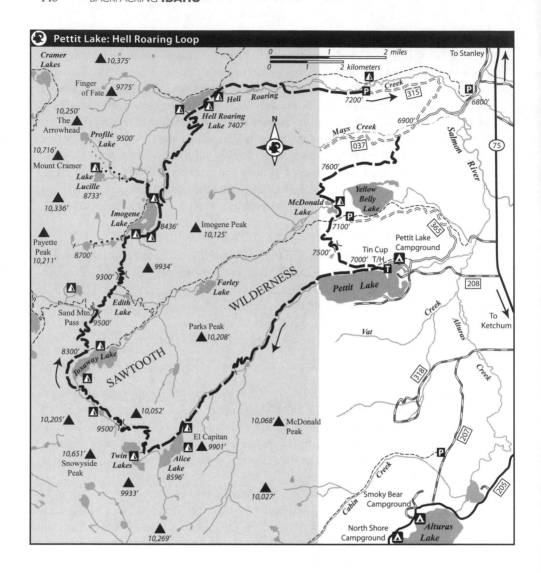

Pettit Lake: Hell Roaring Loop

meadows and open forests. After about 0.5 mile, you climb 300 feet in lazy switchbacks and cross the creek again, this time on a bridge not far above a small waterfall.

The next mile is easy and lovely as you slowly climb through open, subalpine fir woods with good views of the many granite summits on either side of the valley. At your feet are a wealth of wildflowers, especially aster, arnica, lousewort, pussytoes, and a deep-magenta paintbrush. After a final rock-hop crossing of the creek, you pass two lovely tarns and come to the large and very scenic Alice Lake. This gorgeous lake has numerous good campsites and outstanding views west to a craggy group of unnamed summits. The most attractive campsites are near the outlet.

TIP: Alice Lake is very popular, so if you plan to camp here it is better to visit on a weekday. For a less crowded alternative, look for the nice camps on the northeast (off-trail) side of Alice Lake or continue to the campsites at Twin Lakes, just ahead.

The trail follows the shore of Alice Lake for a short distance and winds uphill on gentle switchbacks for 0.5 mile to a poorly signed fork. The trail to the left goes about 200 yards down to the strip of land between the heather-rimmed Twin Lakes. These lakes both have good campsites and feature excellent views across their tranquil waters to Snowyside Peak.

The main trail bears right at the fork and gradually climbs in long traverses and short switchbacks up an open slope. Alpine wildflowers abound here, especially Cusick's speedwell, bistort, cinquefoil, paintbrush, Douglas's knotweed, stonecrop, Rocky Mountain goldenrod, and blue beardtongue. Views of the sparkling Twin Lakes and a group of nearby serrated peaks improve with every step. *Note:* The trail above Twin Lakes has been rerouted and now is very different from what is shown on older contour maps. You top out at a narrow, 9,500-foot pass on the northeast shoulder of Snowyside Peak.

WARNING: Snowfields often block the trail on the north side of this pass well into July.

From the pass, you descend 19 switchbacks to a pair of small, scenic lakes with a good campsite between them, and then go gradually downhill for about 1.5 miles on a sometimes rocky tread beside a small creek. The trail crosses the creek on logs just below a sloping waterfall and comes to the basin holding the mile-long Toxaway Lake. Though the trail stays well above this large lake, you can follow any of several boot paths down to good campsites and fishing spots on the shore.

You hop over several small creeks feeding Toxaway Lake and, about halfway down the north shore, come to a junction. For a short, easy loop back to Pettit Lake, go straight and walk 6 miles downhill on the popular trail that goes past Farley Lake to a junction just before Yellow Belly Lake. From there, you turn right and hike over a woodsy ridge to the trailhead.

For a longer and more scenic loop, turn left at Toxaway Lake and begin a long, 1,200-foot climb. The very rocky and moderately steep route uses dozens of switchbacks and longer traverses to ascend a partly forested slope with fine views back to Toxaway Lake and Snowyside Peak. You top out at a small notch in a side ridge, go around a knoll beside an orange-tinted peak, and drop a bit to a junction at Sand Mountain Pass.

WARNING: Sand Mountain Pass can be snowbound until late July or even, occasionally, early August. Ask about current conditions before you leave on this trip.

Your trail bears right at the pass, climbs about 200 feet, and switchbacks down into the next basin to the north. You'll see Edith Lake below you on the right just before you come to a tiny, wet meadow with a trickling creek. Hop over the creek, and walk a short distance beneath a rocky slope to a junction beside a small pond. You go left and climb a dozen moderate switchbacks on a talus slope to a 9,300-foot pass with fine views northeast to the basin holding the large Imogene Lake, and north to the crags around Mount Cramer and The Arrowhead.

The trail now descends a series of short switchbacks, first down a long talus slope and then through rolling meadows.

WARNING: Snow typically blocks this section of trail until mid-July. At the bottom of the switchbacks you follow a seasonal creek to its confluence with a larger stream, which flows down from a string of unnamed and trailless lakes on the slopes of Payette Peak to the west.

RECOMMENDED DAY HIKES FROM IMOGENE LAKE

Having reached Imogene Lake, it would be a shame not to spend a layover day exploring some of the outstanding possibilities for day hikes to this area's exceptionally scenic, off-trail lakes. One easy and especially superior outing goes to a string of beautiful, unnamed lakes along Imogene Lake's inlet creek to the southwest. A second, somewhat more challenging trip visits the drop-dead gorgeous Lake Lucille and, if you are up for a tough climb, Profile Lake, which is also stunning and sits high on the slopes of Mount Cramer to the northwest.

To take the first day hike, begin by making your way on the old trail around the west side of Imogene Lake to its unbridged crossing of the inlet creek. Cross the inlet, and then leave the trail and climb briefly up a granite ledge beside a waterfall on the creek. After a little more than 0.2 mile you will reach the first lake. This beautiful, irregularly shaped body of water offers excellent views up to an unnamed peak to the south and Payette Peak to the west. From here you pick up and follow an intermittent boot path that takes you around the right (northwest) side of this scenic lake and then follows the inlet creek for 0.1 mile to a second, smaller lake. This gorgeous oversize pond should whet your appetite for even more, so walk up the inlet creek past a lovely stair-step waterfall to a larger lake that sits at exactly 8,700 feet. This spectacular lake is in a wonderful setting beneath talus slopes and tall, pinkish peaks and ridges, and is extremely photogenic. For the adventurous, there is another smaller lake farther up the canyon above more waterfalls, but Lake 8,700 is the prettiest of this group and makes a logical turnaround point.

To make the second recommended day hike, walk the old trail around Imogene Lake until you cross to the north side of a logjam on the outlet creek at

Here there is an unsigned junction with an old and unmaintained trail that goes around the left (west and north) side of the lake. This trail is still easy to follow and passes numerous possible campsites. The newer and shorter trail goes to the right and skirts the lake's south and east shores. This trail also passes some very good, but popular, campsites. On either route are good views of the lake, its large island, and the peaks surrounding this basin.

TIP: Imogene Lake is less attractive in late summer because it often recedes several feet, especially during dry years.

The two trails reunite at the northeast end of the lake near several more good campsites. These sites are especially appealing, because they afford fine views across the water to the prominent Payette Peak. Anglers will be delighted to spend time here trying to hook some of the lake's abundant and quite large brook and cutthroat trout.

From Imogene Lake the newly rerouted trail descends gently from the northeast corner of the lake and crosses the outlet creek in the middle of a cascading waterfall. You then pass a marshy meadow and follow the creek downstream. You cross the creek again just above a small lake. From here the trail passes a couple of small tarns covered with water lilies and makes a long, nicely graded descent in several switchbacks. Occasional openings the northeast end of the lake. From there walk the trail another 0.1 mile or so to a point where the trail makes a turn to the left. Turn right (north) here on a very sketchy boot trail that goes up a little gully. This path soon leads you to a short but steep descent to a little, forest-rimmed lake. Here the way trail turns left and does several steep, little ups and downs for the next 0.4 mile until you reach an extremely scenic, little lake with a tall, sliding waterfall feeding in from the west. You cross this lake's inlet creek and then make your way steeply up the glacier-polished rock ledges well to the right of the waterfall. At the top is a shallow and narrow lake. Cross this lake's outlet and go left, gradually uphill, for about 0.15 mile to a large lake with no official name, but that locals typically refer to as Lake Lucille.

Lake Lucille is surely one of the most spectacular lakes in the Sawtooth Mountains. It is backed on three sides by tall spires and reddish-colored cliffs and is one of those spots that really has to be seen to be appreciated. If you want to spend the night, there is a campsite here. From this lake, ambitious and athletic hikers can make the steep and tiring 800-foot off-trail climb to Profile Lake at the base of Mount Cramer and The Arrowhead. The route is exhausting but does not require any technical climbing or scrambling skills. Those capable of the climb can pick out a route on the map and need no further instruction. The reward at the top is a deep, rock-bound alpine lake that is normally full of icebergs well into late July. The lake also has outstanding views of the steep granite ridges and peaks that enclose this stark basin. Mountain climbers often use Profile Lake as the jumping-off point to ascend Mount Cramer, the second-highest point in the Sawtooth Mountains.

in the tree cover along this section reward you with good views west to Mount Cramer and north to a group of extremely rugged ridges and granite outcrops that includes the ominously titled Finger of Fate. The final mile to Hell Roaring Lake uses numerous switch-backs to go down an old moraine that is still only lightly forested.

TIP: Just before the west end of Hell Roaring Lake, you pass an unsigned spur trail that drops to some good lakeside campsites.

The trail passes several fine and very popular campsites on its way to the northeast end of Hell Roaring Lake, where you will find several more excellent campsites and great views to craggy Finger of Fate on the western skyline. You cross the lake's outlet on a bridge and, about 50 yards later, come to a junction. Bear right on a heavily used trail and descend moderately for a short distance; then level off on an easy trail that travels through open forest in the lower valley of Hell Roaring Creek. Unfortunately, you rarely get close to the lovely creek, which remains out of sight on the right. About 1.1 miles from Hell Roaring Lake is a signed junction with the old Hell Roaring Trail.

If you left a car at the Hell Roaring trailhead, then go straight and continue down the wide valley. It's a pleasant stroll that passes an excellent creek-side campsite after about 2.5

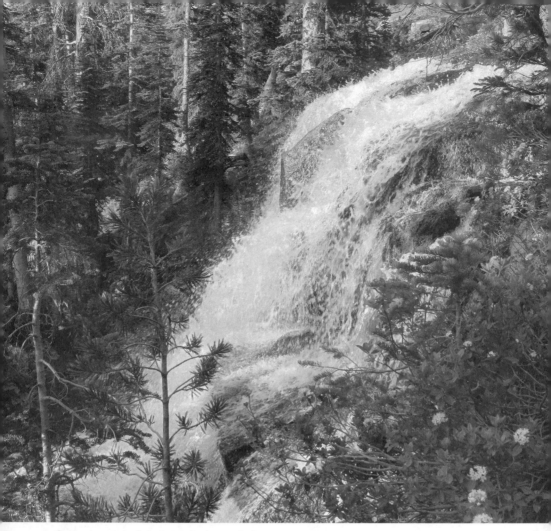

Stair-step waterfall above Imogene Lake

miles, and then goes up and down over old, rocky moraine that is sparsely forested with lodgepole pines. You'll reach the trailhead a little more than 5 miles from Hell Roaring Lake.

Those who are returning by trail to Pettit Lake will find the route is little used and a bit monotonous. Most of the way is on jeep roads or horse trails through a monoculture of lodgepole pines that are dense enough to block the views, but not thick enough to provide much shade. The route is also outside of the protected wilderness, so you must share the trail with motorbikes and mountain bikes. Still, for the most part it's a pleasant hike and certainly more interesting than walking back on ID 75.

To take this route, turn right at the junction with the old Hell Roaring Trail and cross Hell Roaring Creek on a log bridge. On the other side of the bridge the trail turns downstream and wanders through lodgepole pine forest, staying nearly level for 0.7 mile until you meet up with a long-abandoned jeep road. Follow this gently graded, old road for 0.1 mile to the wilderness boundary and then for another 0.9 mile to a developed trailhead. People with four-wheel drive vehicles sometimes use this trailhead, so you may encounter vehicles for the next few miles.

Continue walking on the dusty and rugged road for 2.4 miles as it curves right around a ridge, and then loses some elevation to a junction. You angle right on a dirt road and soon cross Mays Creek, which is usually dry for most of the summer. You then walk 0.4 mile along the road and bear left on a trail that is no longer shown on the U.S. Forest Service map, but which still exists and is easy to follow.

The narrow trail climbs fairly steeply to the top of a viewless ridge, and then turns to follow the ridgeline. After about 1 mile of undulating mostly uphill, the trail leaves the ridge and descends three switchbacks to the flat basin that holds both McDonald Lake, on your right, and the larger Yellow Belly Lake, hidden by trees on your left.

You soon make an easy, ankle-deep ford across the outlet of McDonald Lake, and then follow this lake's grassy shoreline, where there are good views to the west of the high peaks of the Sawtooth Range. No established campsites are at the lake, but there's plenty of flat ground and places to set up your tent. Shortly after McDonald Lake you bear right at a junction, and then walk 50 feet to a second junction, this time with the trail from Toxaway Lake.

To complete the loop, you bear left and gradually climb for almost 1 mile, gaining about 500 feet in three irregularly spaced switchbacks to the wide top of a woodsy ridge. From there, you make a gradual downhill traverse to a junction beside Pettit Lake, and then turn left and retrace the final 200 yards back to your car.

VARIATIONS •

If you want to extend the hike, consider a long side trip west from Sand Mountain Pass to Edna, Ardeth, and a string of other high lakes at the headwaters of the South Fork Payette River. See Trip 13 for details on this grand adventure.

POSSIBLE ITINERARY

	CAMP	MILES	ELEVATION GAIN
Day 1	Twin Lakes	7.0	2,000'
Day 2	Imogene Lake	10.5	2,400'
Day 3	Imogene Lake layover		
	Side trip to Lake 8,700	2.0	300'
	Side trip to Lake Lucille	3.0	900'
Day 4	Out	13.0*	1,600'*

* If you left a second car at the Hell Roaring trailhead, then these numbers are reduced by 3.5 miles and 1,300 feet of elevation gain.

BEST SHORTER ALTERNATIVE •

Perhaps the most popular loop hike in the Sawtooth Mountains is a shorter version of this trip. Starting from Pettit Lake, hike up to Alice Lake, go over the pass to Toxaway Lake, and return via Farley and Yellow Belly Lakes to your car. You should also strongly consider a weekend backpacking trip from the Hell Roaring Creek trailhead into Imogene Lake, perhaps with an extra day or two for the excellent side trips that are possible from a base camp at this lake.

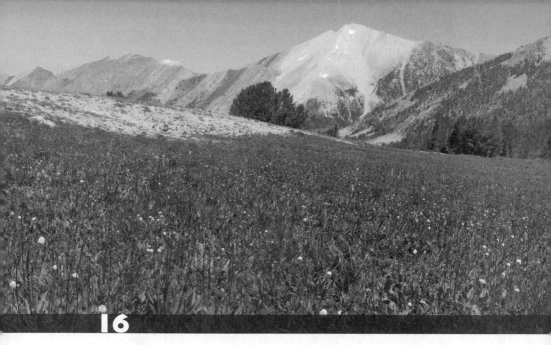

WHITE CLOUD PEAKS LOOP

RATINGS: Scenery 10   Solitude 5   Difficulty 8
MILES: 31 (32.5)
ELEVATION GAIN: 6,850' (7,100')
DAYS: 3–5 (3–5)
MAP(S): USGS *Boulder Chain Lakes*, USGS *Washington Peak*
USUALLY OPEN: Mid-July–October
BEST: Late July–September
PERMITS: None
RULES: Maximum group size of 20 people and 25 stock animals; fires are pro-
hibited within 200 yards of Scree, Shallow, Castle, and Upper Chamberlain
Lakes and in the Four Lakes Basin; fires are strongly discouraged in upper
Boulder Chain Lakes Basin; special rules apply to tethering, watering, and
feeding stock—call the Sawtooth National Recreation Area for details.
CONTACT: Sawtooth National Recreation Area, 208-727-5000

SPECIAL ATTRACTIONS ·

Spectacular mountain scenery; good fishing; wildlife, especially elk and mountain goats

CHALLENGES ·

Thin air at high altitudes; motorcycles allowed on part of the route; short but difficult
cross-country section

Above: White Cloud Peaks from Ants Basin

HOW TO GET THERE •

From Stanley, drive 15 miles south on ID 75 to a junction with Fourth of July Creek Road (also known as Forest Service Road 209). (Coming from the south this turnoff is 16.7 miles north of Galena Summit.) Turn left (east) and stay on this bumpy, gravel road for 10.2 miles through a large 2005 burn area to the developed Fourth of July Creek trailhead.

INTRODUCTION •

Though it would be difficult to pick a single favorite from among the dozens of mountain ranges that draw the admiration of Idaho hikers, you could make a strong case for the White Cloud Peaks as the best of the lot. All of the trails in this range take you through scenery that is so spectacular it simply defies description. This magnificent loop hits only a sampling of the best of these peaks. If you fall in love with this range's towering peaks and sparkling lakes, then you can expect to find yourself planning additional great adventures in the future. This loop trip requires a short, cross-country scramble over a steep, rocky pass followed by a longer off-trail romp past a series of lakes. Inexperienced hikers will find this challenging, but it isn't dangerous. Oxygen becomes noticeably scarce at the higher elevations along this trip, so it's not just the scenery that leaves lowlanders breathless. Take it slow until you get acclimated.

Many of the trails in this area have been rerouted in recent years. These changes were designed to make the trails less steep and to reduce erosion. Unfortunately, the new alignments are not shown on the U.S. Geological Survey (USGS) maps, and even the more up-to-date U.S. Forest Service maps do not include the changes. The new trail alignments have also changed the distances, so the mileages shown on trail signs are no longer correct.

DESCRIPTION •

The well-graded trail, which—to the chagrin of hikers—is open to motorbikes, starts in an open forest of lodgepole pines. In the first few hundred yards the path goes over Fourth of July Creek on a little wooden bridge, crosses a rough mining road, and begins a gradual ascent. The ensuing climb takes you through Engelmann spruce and subalpine fir forests on the edge of some very scenic meadows. These meadows border Fourth of July Creek, a small, cascading stream whose main stem and tributaries the trail crosses several times on flat-topped logs. About 1.3 miles from the trailhead the climb ends at a junction and the start of the loop.

> **TIP:** Hikers who get a late start will find a comfortable campsite above the north shore of the meadow-rimmed Fourth of July Lake, about 150 yards along the trail to the right.

To start the loop, you bear left at the junction on a trail that is thankfully closed to motor vehicles. The rocky footpath climbs fairly steeply to a small, scenic, rock-lined pond. The grade then eases as you make a gradual uphill traverse on a partly forested hillside to a windy pass with great views. To the south is an unnamed brownish-orange peak rising above Fourth of July Lake. To the southwest are several gray-colored summits near the distant Champion Lakes. Finally, to the north rise the aptly named White Cloud Peaks, a line of skyscraping mountains composed of striking whitish-yellow rock. Another prominent feature is Ants Basin, a large, green, relatively flat expanse directly below you to the north.

White Cloud Peaks Loop

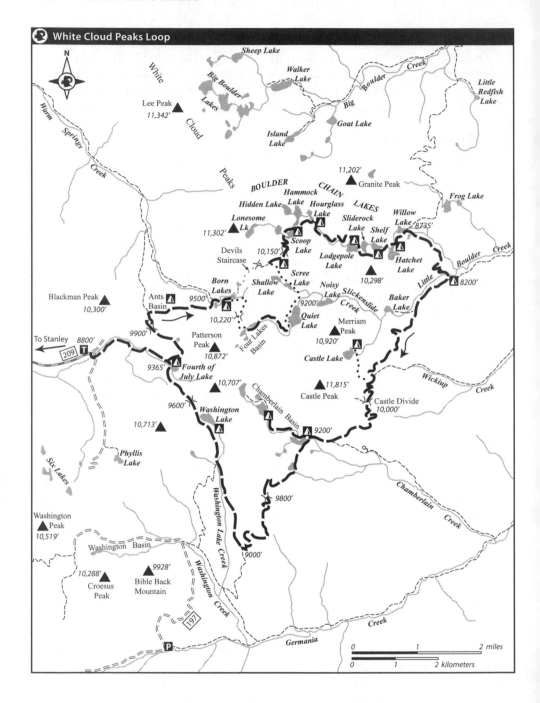

The trail briefly follows the ridge northwest of the pass, and then descends seven quick switchbacks across a talus slope to Ants Basin. This nearly flat, flower-covered meadow has great views, water from trickling springs and creeks, and some possible campsites beside a tiny pond about 300 yards left of where you reach the basin floor.

The old trail shown on the USGS maps goes across Ants Basin to the north. This path is now rarely used and very hard to find. Your route follows a more obvious maintained trail that goes east and heads more directly to your destination. From where you reach the basin floor, turn right and follow this good path across a meadow and over an insignificant rise. The path then goes steeply downhill, makes a rolling traverse across the lower end of a rock-slide, and climbs through open forest to an excellent campsite beside one of the lower Born Lakes. In a basin surrounded by brownish mountains and spires, this stunningly beautiful pool is a great location for a long lunch or a memorable night in the Idaho wilderness.

It will take some time to convince yourself to leave this idyllic spot, but once you do, follow the trail as it goes around the west shore of the lake; then travel gradually uphill through open forest to the largest and deepest Born Lake. Here there is a junction with a trail that goes northwest to Warm Springs Creek.

In a previous edition of this guidebook, I recommended a direct route over the ominous ridge northeast of the Born Lakes that was extremely steep and often dangerous for novice hikers. Fittingly, this route is locally referred to as the Devils Staircase and is best left for athletic and experienced scramblers. I now recommend a longer but much safer option that is still off-trail, but not nearly as steep, and includes visits to several previously missed lakes that offer truly outstanding scenery.

To follow this course, loop around the largest Born Lake and head generally south up a wide, rocky gully. This leads you to a steep and tiring climb up a rockslide to an obvious low point at the top of the gully. You may notice a few cairns and a sketchy boot path during this climb that offer guidance along the way. Even without these navigation aids, however, no expert skills are required to make this climb, just stamina. From the windswept pass you will have wonderful views, especially down to the stark cluster of rockbound lakes known as the Four Lakes Basin, just below you to the south.

Reaching the Four Lakes Basin requires a careful descent of a steep slope. At the top of this slope is a large snowfield with overhanging cornices that are often present well into August. It is usually possible, however, to work your way around this snowfield by going farther to the right. Once around the snowfield, the rest of the downhill isn't particularly dangerous, but it is very steep and does require steady nerves and maybe using your hands once or twice to balance yourself.

At the bottom of this steep descent is Emerald Lake, the largest of the four small lakes in this basin. Like all the others here, this is a wildly scenic spot set in a beautiful alpine setting beneath rugged peaks. Take some time to explore the other lakes in this cluster (Rock, Glacier, and Cornice), all of which are dramatically scenic. Do not camp in this area, however, because the terrain is rocky, exposed to the weather, and very fragile. Fires are prohibited in the basin, though there isn't anything to burn in any event.

To exit the Four Lakes Basin, pick up an obvious way trail on the slope above the south side of Cornice Lake, the lowest lake in the basin, and follow it east through a boulder-strewn drainage. This takes you to an overlook of the large and deep Quiet Lake, toward which you now steeply descend first over a rocky area, and then down a mostly forested slope. The sketchy boot path remains on the left (north) side of the creek, flowing steeply down from Four Lakes Basin all the way to Quiet Lake.

Once at Quiet Lake make your way around the western shore to the lake's north end and follow an intermittent boot route on the hillside above the west bank of the outlet stream, known, colorfully, as Slickenslide Creek. After about 0.3 mile you'll come to a significant tributary cascading down from the left. You turn up this tributary and follow it steeply upstream. This route will take you first to the green-tinged Scree Lake and then Shallow Lake. Both of these pools are very beautiful, though Shallow Lake has the slight edge in scenery. Fires are not allowed at either lake.

To complete the off-trail portion of this hike, climb the partly forested and relatively gentle slope just north of Shallow Lake to a wide, scenic bench that sits just below timberline. Here you will come across a well-worn maintained trail. Turn right and walk this trail to the northeast end of the bench, where there is a shallow tarn with a couple of wind-whipped campsites that tend to be rather bleak in bad weather. Just above the north side of the pond is a sketchy boot path that goes northeast. You follow this indistinct route as it goes over a low rise, cuts across a scree slope, and drops to a rocky saddle, where the tread becomes more obvious. The view from this saddle is stupendous, especially east to the distant White Knob Mountains and Lost River Range, and north to the nearby Boulder Chain Lakes Basin. This spectacular basin is backed by rugged, white-granite peaks and features a string of beautiful lakes, several of which are visible from this location.

The trail into this basin follows several well-graded switchbacks that take you down a rocky slope to lovely Scoop Lake, which has several good campsites above its northwest shore. After rounding Scoop Lake and crossing its outlet, you wind down to the deep Hammock Lake, which has a small island, excellent campsites, and a gorgeous setting. Next in the chain is Hourglass Lake, which is named for its distinctive shape.

After Hourglass Lake you descend, sometimes steeply, beside Boulder Chain Lakes Creek. The trail crosses the small creek three times during the mile-long, lakeless descent, and then levels off just before it reaches the very deep Lodgepole Lake. This scenic lake is the first in this basin's lower string of lakes and boasts very good campsites near both its inlet and its outlet.

The well-used trail now cuts across the narrow strip of land between Lodgepole Lake and Sliderock Lake, and then goes around Sliderock's scenic south shore. From there, you descend a bit to Shelf Lake, a deep pool with several excellent campsites and more good scenery. Next is Hatchett Lake, which has a good campsite and a great view of an unnamed, jagged pinnacle to the southwest. The trail barely touches Hatchett Lake, and then drops to Willow Lake, the last in the chain, and comes to a junction.

The most popular trail into the Boulder Chain Lakes comes in from the left, but your route goes right. This trail is open to motorbikes, so the tread is chewed up and rather dusty. The trail passes through a spacious, flowery meadow with a photogenic view of an unnamed peak to the north, and then descends gradually through dense forest. After it breaks out of the trees, the trail descends across an open slope of sagebrush and quaking aspens on three moderately long switchbacks. In early summer, this slope hosts a good variety of wildflowers, but the most spectacular color show is in late September, when the aspens turn yellow and orange and frame outstanding views of rugged Castle and Merriam Peaks to the southwest. At the bottom of the slope, the trail makes an easy ford of Little Boulder Creek and comes to a fair campsite on the south bank.

TIP: If you want to keep your feet dry, bushwhack upstream through some willows, where you can usually find a log across the creek.

About 50 yards beyond the campsite is a junction, where you turn right on a trail that is thankfully closed to motor vehicles. This path slowly climbs in forest for a little less than 1 mile to a fork that is not shown on most maps. The unsigned route to the right goes to the small Baker Lake, but your trail bears left and continues the long, woodsy ascent. Several level stretches along the way allow you to catch your breath and enjoy nice views through the trees. The best views feature the 11,815-foot Castle Peak, the highest point in the White Clouds, and neighboring Merriam Peak, which is not as lofty but is equally rugged.

The long climb takes you to a junction with the little-used Big Wickiup Trail, which goes straight where your trail switchbacks right. About 400 yards farther, it's time to drop your heavy pack and take an excellent cross-country side trip to Castle Lake, a dramatic pool tucked in a scenic cirque on the northeast side of Castle Peak. To reach it, work your way to the north end of a large, rolling basin west of the trail and look for two 3-foot-tall cairns. These mark the start of a sketchy trail that goes about 0.3 mile across a scree slope to Castle Lake. This deep, cold lake has some exposed campsites (fires are prohibited) and great views of the nearby cliffs of both Castle and Merriam Peaks. In addition to the occasional awe-inspired hiker, this area is a favorite hangout for a small band of mountain goats.

Back on the main trail, you climb eight long, lazy switchbacks on an exposed slope to the top of Castle Divide, a windy, above-timberline pass with inspiring views. The most impressive sight is the nearby Castle Peak, a towering mass of contorted white rock. An obvious boot path goes to even higher viewpoints on the ridge to the west.

To continue your loop, go fairly steeply down the gully south of Castle Divide; then descend at a gentler grade on a recently rerouted trail. The trail winds down a series of gentle curves and switchbacks through open whitebark pine and, later, subalpine fir forests, and then slowly curves around the south side of Castle Peak and comes to a junction with the Chamberlain Creek Trail. You go straight and soon reach a junction beside the outlet of lower Chamberlain Lake. This large, scenic lake is rimmed with meadows and has several fairly popular campsites along its east and southeast shores.

WARNING: The lake's water level recedes during the summer, so it may look rather pathetic by fall in dry years.

To visit the upper basin, take the trail along the north shore of the lower lake, climb beside a small creek, and go past a shallow pond to the large and very beautiful upper Chamberlain Lake. Fish often jump from the waters of this lake, disturbing the great reflections of the craggy Castle Peak, which rises directly from the lake's heather-lined shores.

TIP: Upper Chamberlain Lake has fewer campsites than the lower lake has, but its campsites are more scenic and less crowded.

After spending some time soaking in the view, consider taking the trail around the east side of upper Chamberlain Lake to another, unnamed lake, just a few feet higher in elevation.

To get back on the main loop, return to the junction beside lower Chamberlain Lake and turn south, following signs for Washington Lake. Your path wanders uphill through forests and small meadows for less than 0.5 mile to an unnamed lake. This lake can be rather unattractive by late summer in dry years because the water level may drop 30 feet or more. Above this lake you climb to a rolling, open basin and then make one switchback and a long, uphill traverse to the top of a high ridge. This grandstand not only provides your last good view north to the massive Castle Peak rising above Chamberlain Basin, but it also opens up an entirely new view south to the rugged peaks of the distant Boulder Mountains.

The trail descends two gentle switchbacks on the south side of the ridge and goes downhill at a gradual, then moderately steep, grade through viewless forest. The scenery improves as the trail curves right and passes openings in the trees that provide excellent views west to the multicolored peaks above Washington Basin. The trail then winds down a hillside to a junction with the trail to Germania Creek.

You turn right and go up and down (mostly down) across a steep slope to the pretty Washington Lake Creek, and then turn upstream and parallel this small creek through a pleasant mix of forests and meadows. At the prettiest of these meadows, you hop across the creek and immediately reach a trail junction. Your trail, which here is open to motorbikes, goes right and climbs steadily for another 0.5 mile to the meadow-rimmed Washington Lake.

> **TIP:** If you leave the trail and scout around a bit, you will find plenty of good campsites near the lake's southeast end. These campsites feature superb views across the water to the towering, tan slopes of an unnamed peak and ridge to the north.

The trail remains in the trees, far away from Washington Lake, and then angles right and touches the northwest shore. From here, you climb gradually through a low saddle with a seasonal pond and descend through forest to the scenic Fourth of July Lake. Your loop ends at the trail junction just past this lake, where you go straight and return to your car.

POSSIBLE ITINERARY

	CAMP	MILES	ELEVATION GAIN
Day 1	Born Lakes	4.5	1,500'
Day 2	Hatchett Lake	9.0	1,800'
Day 3	Upper Chamberlain Lake	7.5	2,050'
	Side trip to Castle Lake	1.5	250'
Day 4	Out	10.0	1,500'

BEST SHORTER ALTERNATIVE ·

Day hikes to either the Born Lakes or to Washington Lake are highly rewarding. For a one-night adventure, try hiking the southern part of this loop as far as the Chamberlain Basin.

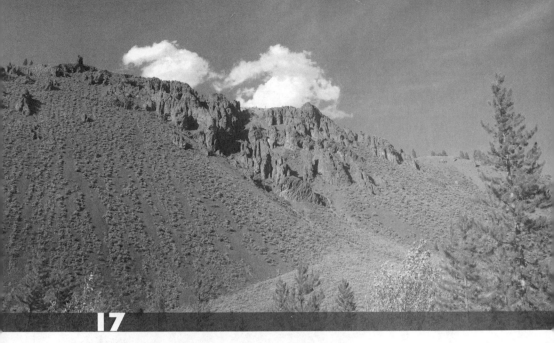

17

BIG BOULDER LAKES

RATINGS: Scenery 10   Solitude 3   Difficulty 6
MILES: 19 (including explorations up to the Big Boulder Lakes and Island Lake)
ELEVATION GAIN: 4,050'
DAYS: 3–5
MAP(S): USGS *Boulder Chain Lakes,* USGS *Livingston Creek*
USUALLY OPEN: Mid-July–early October
BEST: Anytime it's open
PERMITS: None, just sign the trail register
RULES: Maximum group size of 20 people and 25 stock animals. Fires are prohibited in the upper Big Boulder Lakes Basin (Cove, Sapphire, and Cirque Lakes and surroundings) and in the alpine basin around Slide and Sheep Lakes.
CONTACT: Sawtooth National Recreation Area, 208-727-5000

SPECIAL ATTRACTIONS ·

Some of the best high alpine lakes and scenery in Idaho; good fishing; excellent hike for those who like to backpack into a base camp and explore

CHALLENGES ·

The area is popular and the camps can be crowded. Mosquitoes are a problem in July. A portion of the lower trail is open to motorcycles.

Above: Railroad Ridge near Livingston Mill

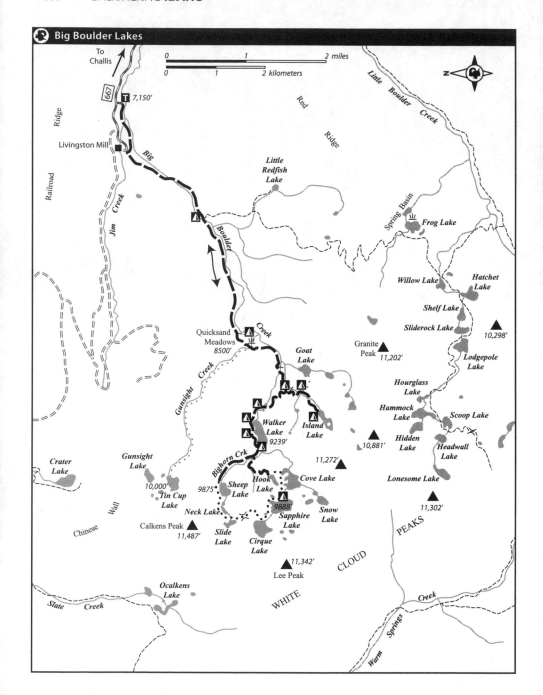

Big Boulder Lakes

To Challis

667   7,150'

Livingston Mill

Big Boulder Creek

Jim Creek

Railroad Ridge

Little Redfish Lake

Red Ridge

Little Boulder Creek

Spring Basin

Frog Lake

Willow Lake

Hatchet Lake

Shelf Lake

Sliderock Lake

10,298'

Lodgepole Lake

Quicksand Meadows 8500'

Goat Lake

Granite Peak 11,202'

Hourglass Lake

Hammock Lake

Scoop Lake

Gunsight Creek

Walker Lake 9239'

Island Lake

Hidden Lake

Headwall Lake

10,881'

Crater Lake

Gunsight Lake

Bighorn Crk

11,272'

Cove Lake

Lonesome Lake

11,302'

10,000'

Tin Cup Lake

Sheep Lake

Hook Lake

Wall

9875'

Neck Lake

9888'

Sapphire Lake

Snow Lake

Chinese

Calkens Peak 11,487'

Slide Lake

Cirque Lake

PEAKS

11,342'

Lee Peak

CLOUD

Ocalkens Lake

WHITE

State Creek

Creek

Warm Springs

HOW TO GET THERE ●

Drive ID 75 along the Salmon River either 19 miles west of Challis or about 37 miles east of Stanley; then turn south on East Fork Road immediately on the west side of a bridge over the East Fork Salmon River. Drive 16.7 miles to the end of pavement; then continue another 1.3 miles to a prominently signed junction. Turn right onto Forest Service Road

667, following signs to Big Boulder Creek, and go 4.2 miles on this narrow and somewhat rocky gravel road to a junction. Turn left at a sign for Big Boulder Trailhead and go 0.1 mile to the large trailhead parking area.

INTRODUCTION •

The White Cloud Mountains are full of wonderful hiking and outstanding scenery, so almost every trail is highly enjoyable and well worth hiking. Still, it would be impossible to write a book about the best backpacking in Idaho without including the outing to the Big Boulder Lakes.

Put simply, alpine scenery just doesn't get much (or, perhaps, *any*) better than what you will find in the upper basin of the Big Boulder Lakes. Here, there is the perfect mix of deep-blue alpine lakes, wildflower-covered meadows, small waterfalls, rock-garden wildflowers, and, most of all, dramatic peaks in every direction. Though no official trail reaches these wonders, a well-traveled boot route climbs from the end of the maintained route to Walker Lake, and from there the opportunities for relatively easy and exceptionally rewarding off-trail exploring are unlimited. The middle day of this three-day outing can be done as a short (but rugged) 5-mile day hike loop in just a few hours. However, you will surely want to spend many more hours and travel many more miles to check out all the lovely little nooks and crannies, visit the many ponds and small lakes, and just gawk at the scenery. Even scheduling an extra day to do it all again (or find some of the hidden corners you missed on the first day of exploring) would not be unreasonable and certainly would not be regretted.

DESCRIPTION •

The Livingston Mill–Castle Peak Trail departs from the south side of the parking area next to a large signboard. The heavily used route heads up the north side of Big Boulder Creek on a gentle course through sagebrush and scattered forests. To the north are nice views of Railroad Ridge, with its jagged, reddish pinnacles and steep slopes. Unfortunately this lower section of the trail is open to motorcycles, so don't be so distracted by the scenery that you end up with tire tracks running up your back. You can also expect the route to be rather dusty from all the spinning, knobby tires.

You cross the small Jim Creek and then at 0.3 mile pass the rusting equipment, tailings piles, and numerous wooden cabins of Livingston Mill, a historic mine. Just past this point the trail climbs onto the mostly forested hillside above Big Boulder Creek. The clear, rushing stream is soon beside you once again as you find yourself gently climbing through a mix of Douglas-fir and lodgepole pine forests and brushy little meadows that offer enticing views up to the peaks to the west. You cross the creek on a bridge at about 1.5 miles, and then at 1.9 miles reach a fair campsite next to an important junction.

You go straight on Big Boulder Trail, which is closed to motor vehicles (yeah!), and immediately cross the creek again on a flattened log about 15 yards upstream from the horse ford. You then make an intermittently steep climb on partly forested and partly sagebrush-covered slopes before coming to a pretty meadow on your left. A very photogenic view here looks west-southwest across the meadow to a reddish-brown mountain that forms the northern extension of Granite Peak. More climbing now offers even broader views of several pyramid-shaped peaks that tower over the lakes at the head of the Big Boulder Creek drainage.

At 3.9 miles a signed side trail angles down to the left to a stock camp beside Quicksand Meadows. You bear right here, following Big Boulder Lakes signs, and hike through forest to a log crossing of Gunsight Creek. A rather long, but very rewarding, off-trail route goes upstream along this creek for about 3 miles to very scenic Tin Cup Lake. Sticking with the maintained trail, you complete your wide loop around the north side of the large but mostly unseen Quicksand Meadows, and then resume going uphill beside the cascading Big Boulder Creek. You pass a loud, sliding waterfall about 0.5 mile above Quicksand Meadows, and then climb briefly to log crossings of two branches of the creek. About 0.25 mile above this point is a junction.

The trail to Walker Lake and eventually Big Boulder Lakes goes right. For a short and very worthwhile side trip, however, go left toward Island Lake. This path climbs rather steeply beside another sliding waterfall to a fair campsite just after a rock-hop crossing of the creek. An obvious cross-country route goes left here over a little ridge before dropping to the pretty Goat Lake. The official trail takes you to a second creek crossing, and then ascends a boulder-strewn landscape to reach Island Lake 0.8 mile from the junction. A very good and spacious campsite is right above the outlet. The lake is wildly scenic, with the towering, snow-streaked Peak 11,272 rising from its western shore.

Back on the main trail to Walker Lake, you go uphill on a winding trail that goes through thinning forest and past a large and interesting fluted boulder. The path then drops briefly to a log crossing of the creek between a pair of beautiful little tarns. You soon pass a good campsite and ascend gradually for another 0.4 mile to Walker Lake, which is incorrectly labeled as Walter Lake on the U.S. Geological Survey (USGS) map. This large and deep mountain lake has good fishing, fine scenery, a horse-tie location, a toilet, and many excellent (but popular) campsites. The best camps are near the outlet and scattered along the north shore. The lake makes a logical base camp for exploring the higher lakes in the basins above. Unfortunately, you should be prepared for lots of mosquitoes here in July.

Though Walker Lake is very attractive, the truly grand scenery lies in the basins above this lake. So to see the best of this country, follow an unofficial but very good trail that goes along the north shore of Walker Lake for 0.4 mile to the west end. From there continue on this steep and rocky path as it goes up the right side of Bighorn Creek, the main inlet stream for Walker Lake. After a little less than 0.3 mile look for a smaller creek, not depicted on the USGS map, that cascades down from the left.

To visit Big Boulder Lake, cross Bighorn Creek at this point and pick up an obvious and easy-to-follow boot path that steeply ascends initially along the left side of this tributary creek, though you'll cross it twice as you climb. The tread is hard to follow in a couple of marshy spots, but if you press on across these wet areas, the path becomes obvious once again on the other side. About 0.25 mile from Bighorn Creek you'll come to a lovely little flat basin set in a very scenic location below tall unnamed peaks and ridges.

The route goes to the left from the lower end of this basin and climbs very steeply on a winding course up a rocky slope. Near the top you skirt a couple of little ledges and voilà: You've reached the top of the headwall and much easier hiking. Ahead of you is one of the supreme alpine wonderlands in Idaho, and, in fact, it is probably the equal of any alpine area in the country—and I've been to most of them. The explorations are limited only by your imagination and the time available.

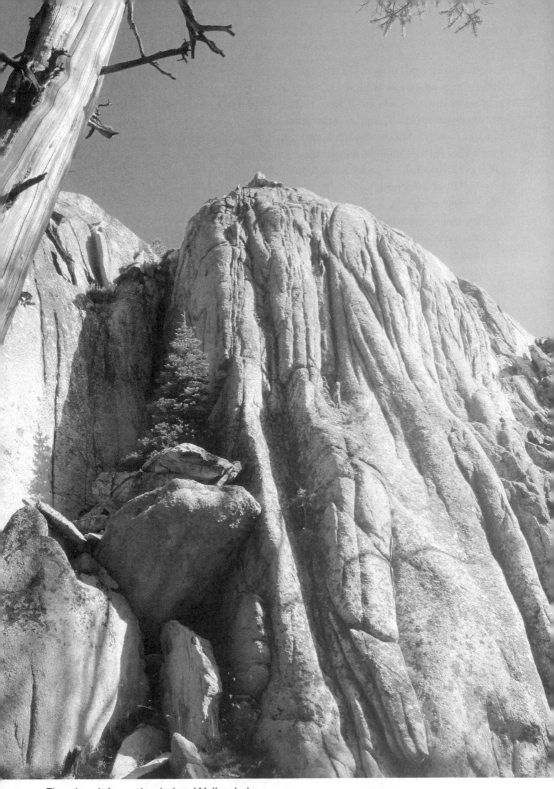

Fluted rock formation below Walker Lake

Directly in front of you lies the descriptively named Hook Lake, and numerous tiny ponds are scattered all around the large basin. The much larger Cove Lake is to your left, and Sapphire Lake and Cirque Lake, both outstandingly beautiful, lie farther up the basin to the northwest. Sheep and Gentian Lakes, tucked away in a side basin south-southwest of Cove Lake, are also well worth a visit. Every one of these bodies of water is tucked amid rocky shores, flower fields, and shimmering mountains of incredible beauty. The larger lakes even have fish. For added scenic interest, as if any were needed, the stream connecting the larger lakes tumbles over lovely little cascades and small waterfalls, and pink and white heather scattered all around provide color. Schedule as much time as possible to explore this high basin. You won't be disappointed.

Sketchy boot paths can be found in various places, but they really aren't necessary because the wandering is easy and spectacular no matter where you go. My recommended minimum itinerary is to first head down to Cove Lake, and then wander along the shore of this lake and up its inlet creek to Sapphire Lake, which offers the best potential campsites—no fires allowed. From there, scramble up to stark Cirque Lake and sit back and enjoy the view.

For hikers with the ability to do some easy scrambling, it is fairly simple to turn this day of exploring into a wonderful loop. To do so, simply climb the sloping, rocky ridge north-northeast of Cirque Lake, following a boot-beaten scramble trail up to an obvious low point. From there, drop down a steep scramble trail to Slide Lake, another spectacular alpine gem surrounded by rocks and bits of color from alpine wildflowers such as heather, moss campion, and alpine buttercups. The lake has a dramatic setting beneath unnamed bulky mountains. This lake is the source of Bighorn Creek.

From this lake you pick your way down rocky ledges on the left (north) side of Bighorn Creek. It is steep in places, but there are safe routes down if you search around a bit. The first part of the downhill leads to a flat area with a marshy pond called Neck Lake. From there you scramble down a second steep ledge to the very deep and scenic Sheep Lake. Camping is limited at both Slide and Sheep Lakes and fires are prohibited, so they are probably better visited in a day hike.

From Sheep Lake an established boot path descends beside the tumbling Bighorn Creek, staying on its left (northeast) side. This takes you steeply down to the unofficial junction with the trail that went up the side creek to the Big Boulder Lakes. Keep straight; soon find yourself back at Walker Lake, and from there return the way you came.

POSSIBLE ITINERARY

	CAMP	MILES	ELEVATION GAIN
Day 1	Walker Lake	6.0	2,250'
Day 2	Walker Lake	5.5	1,250'
	(day hike loop to Big Boulder Lakes and the basin holding Slide and Sheep Lakes)		
Day 3	Out, with side trip to Island Lake	7.5	550'

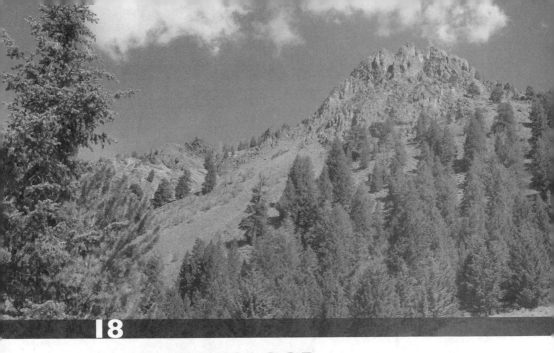

18

FALL CREEK LOOP: PIONEER MOUNTAINS

RATINGS: Scenery 9   Solitude 8   Difficulty 9
MILES: 18 (24)
ELEVATION GAIN: 4,200' (7,200')
DAYS: 3
MAP(S): USGS *Big Black Dome,* USGS *Standhope Peak*
USUALLY OPEN: Late June–October
BEST: July
PERMITS: None
RULES: The usual Leave No Trace principles apply.
CONTACT: Lost River Ranger District, Salmon-Challis National Forest,
208-588-3400

SPECIAL ATTRACTIONS ·

Dramatic alpine lakes and high basins set beneath towering peaks; excellent chance of seeing elk; plenty of solitude

CHALLENGES ·

A tough and very steep cross-country section is appropriate only for skilled off-trail scramblers. (Those without the needed cross-country experience can still do this hike as shorter trips on either end of the loop.)

Above: Rugged ridge above Left Fork Fall Creek

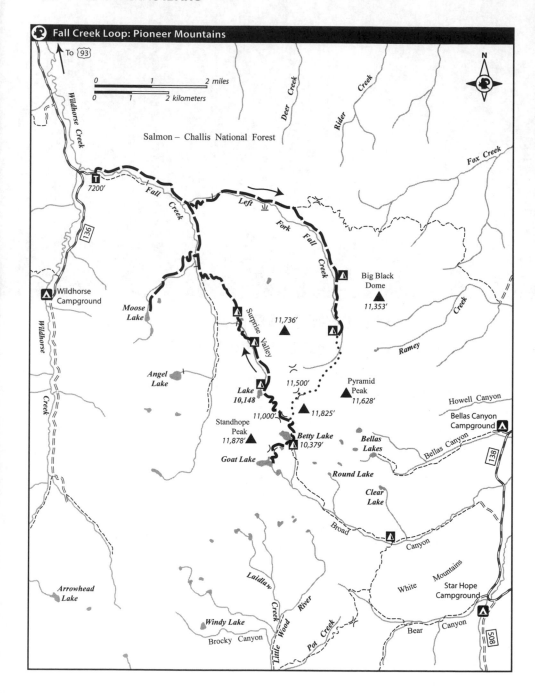

Fall Creek Loop: Pioneer Mountains

To 93

0   1   2 miles

0   1   2 kilometers

Salmon – Challis National Forest

Wildhorse Creek

Fall Creek

Deer Creek

Rider Creek

Fox Creek

7200'

936

Left

Fork

Fall

Creek

Big Black
Dome
11,353'

Wildhorse
Campground

Moose
Lake

Surprise Valley

11,736'

Ramey Creek

Angel
Lake

Wildhorse Creek

Lake
10,148

11,500'

Pyramid
Peak
11,628'

Howell Canyon

Bellas Canyon
Campground

11,000'

11,825'

Standhope
Peak
11,878'

Betty Lake
10,379'

Bellas
Lakes

Bellas Canyon

138

Goat Lake

Round Lake

Clear
Lake

Broad

Canyon

Arrowhead
Lake

Laidlaw Creek

Little Wood River

Pot Creek

White

Mountains

Star Hope
Campground

508

Windy Lake

Brocky Canyon

Bear Canyon

HOW TO GET THERE •

Drive US 93 about 39 miles south of Challis or 41 miles north of Arco to a junction where you turn southwest onto Trail Creek Road. Go 11.8 miles to the end of pavement; then continue another 6.6 miles on very good gravel to a sign marking the boundary of national forest land. Exactly 0.4 mile later you go left on Forest Service Road 135, following signs for Wildhorse and Copper Basin. Proceed 2.1 miles, and then go straight at a junction, now on FS 136 heading toward Wildhorse Guard Station. After 3.5 miles you turn left at a junction immediately after a bridge over Wildhorse Creek and drive 0.5 mile to the road-end Fall Creek Trailhead. Another parking and picnic area is just above the main trailhead, but overnight hikers are asked to park in the lower lot.

INTRODUCTION

I specifically included this outstanding and fun excursion for more experienced hikers who are looking for a little adventure. Most of this trip is on trails, though some are rather faint, but a section in the middle of the loop requires a little extra skill and ability. No technical climbing or even advanced scrambling skills are needed, but you will need steady nerves and experience in steep, off-trail hiking to safely complete the climb over the ridge between Left Fork Fall Creek and Betty Lake. That said, if the off-trail portion doesn't dissuade you, this is a great trip that travels through some of the best of what the outstandingly beautiful, but often overlooked, Pioneer Mountains have to offer. The relatively short trip is packed full of enough high mountain lakes (including what is purported to be the highest named lake in Idaho), broad alpine meadows, jagged peaks, large herds of elk, colorful wildflower fields, and splashing waterfalls to warm the heart of any mountain-loving backpacker. It is a cornucopia of delights that you are likely to have nearly all to yourself. Those without the desire or necessary off-trail skills to complete the middle section can still see almost all of the best of this hike by doing this as two separate, shorter trips—one up Left Fork Fall Creek and the other to Betty Lake through Surprise Valley. So, the magnificent scenery of the Pioneers is available to anyone willing to seek out this little-visited wonderland.

DESCRIPTION

Though a shorter trail leads up the west side of Fall Creek from the picnic area and upper parking lot, the trail you want starts from the lower lot and goes directly down to a wooden bridge that takes you over to the east side of Fall Creek. Shortly thereafter the trail goes through a gate in a fence and heads upstream. The surrounding landscape is an attractive mix of open sagebrush-covered flats, willows and cottonwoods lining the creek on your right, and Douglas-fir forests on the nearby hillsides. The views of some nicely rounded ridges and a few craggy nearby mountains are good throughout.

Following the remains of a long-abandoned jeep road, the trail climbs past an unseen waterfall at 0.75 mile, and then descends to a pair of large, open flats. In the second of these flats, Left Fork of Fall Creek tumbles down through a canyon on your left. At 1.6 miles, immediately after you make a log crossing of this side stream, is a signed junction and the start of the potential loop.

Go left on Highline Trail #059 and settle in for a steady climb. It starts with three switchbacks that ascend a partly forested hillside with nice views back down the canyon of Fall Creek and to the southwest of the peak-backed cirque of Moose Lake. At the top of the switchbacks the grade eases off and you come to a rock-hop crossing of the creek at about 2.7 miles. Continuing to go slowly uphill, you pass through lovely aspen groves and then above a large, wet, willow-choked meadow and several beaver dams on the creek. Once past this meadow, and just as you approach the top of a hill, you come to a fork in the trail. The official Highline Trail goes straight up a green little swale on its way toward the top of the ridge to the east.

You want to take the unofficial but very distinct livestock/boot trail to the right that begins with a gradual uphill on a sagebrush-covered slope. This route leads you up the wide, gentle, U-shaped valley of Left Fork Fall Creek. It's a relatively easy and very scenic walk with tall, multicolored ridges offering constant visual treats along the way. The tall, rugged peak you can see near the head of the valley is Pyramid Peak. The trail stays on the left side of the creek and passes a few potential camping areas as it slowly ascends the partly forested valley.

The tread remains distinct and easy to follow for about 2 miles, after which it becomes intermittent or simply disappears altogether. But you don't really need a trail anymore because the hiking remains relatively easy in this open and mostly gently terrain. The improving scenery will hold your interest, with ever-higher and more-colorful canyon walls and the abundance of wildlife. Elk are particularly common, and you could easily see dozens of animals. You will surely see their tracks, smell their musk, and walk over or around mountains of elk droppings. As you approach the middle of the canyon the route becomes somewhat steeper, taking you past rocky outcrops and drawing you closer to the cliffs, talus fields, and crags that enclose the upper basin. Though there are no established sites in this remote place, camping prospects are good in the upper basin, with abundant water from the creek and outstanding scenery.

From the headwaters of Left Fork Fall Creek it appears difficult or even impossible to exit this deep basin except by turning around and going back the way you came. And unless you are a fairly experienced off-trail scrambler, that is exactly what you should do, well satisfied with the rewards of your trip. However, for hikers with decent boulder-hopping skills and who don't mind a very steep downhill on a slope of dangerously loose rocks, there is a way to turn this into a challenging but enjoyable loop. To do this, make your way up game trails on the left side of the creek as that small stream curves to the right around the base of a large talus slope coming down off of a prominent ridge. You can see an obvious low pass at the head of the creek canyon on the right side of this ridge, but you do *not* want to go that way because the unseen cliffs on the other side of that pass require technical skills to safely descend.

Instead, when the tundra in the basin gives way to rocks, go left and make your way up the large talus slope on the prominent ridge that divides the upper basin. This requires a fair amount of tiring boulder-hopping but it is not overly difficult. Once on top of the ridge, things are pretty easy as you simply follow the top of this ridge as it climbs toward the left side of a peak with an obvious, dark layer of rock cutting diagonally across its face just below the top. Most of the ridgetop you are hiking on is solid tundra with embedded rocks and is not too steep, so the walking is relatively easy and perfectly safe. Just before the top of the climb you come to a small pinnacle of tan rock, which from a distance looks like a man-made cairn but turns out to be natural.

From the low point in the divide right beside the tan rock pinnacle is a wonderful view down to Surprise Valley, Angel Lake, and Lake 10,148 at the head of Surprise Valley. The gully leading straight down to Surprise Valley from this pass is too steep for safety, so veer left and climb another 50 feet or so to a rocky saddle. From there you contour across the top of a second steep gully on a mountain goat trail for 150 yards. Now you can see the tall pyramid of Standhope Peak and part of the shimmering Betty Lake in the next basin to the south. Your objective is to intersect a trail that travels through the rocky pass between you and Standhope Peak.

To reach that goal, you carefully angle to the left down a scree slope. The route is extremely steep, so it is important that you make sure you have good traction and solid footing with each step. Walking sticks will help you keep your balance. It actually turns out to be easier than it appears at the top, but care is still important. Occasional mountain goat tracks offer bits of tread to follow along the way. In general, try to take a course that leads nearly straight down toward Betty Lake. After rapidly, and cautiously, losing about 1,000 feet in elevation, you intersect a trail and are back on solid footing.

Once on the maintained trail, turning right (uphill) will take you over the pass and back to your car. First, however, you won't want to miss Betty Lake and the nearby Goat Lake, both spectacular alpine gems that are among the most impressive in Idaho. To visit them, turn left (downhill) on the trail, descend six switchbacks, and wind your way down through an area of impressive bus-size boulders to Betty Lake. Only a few scraggly whitebark pines survive near this lake, so camping, while very scenic, is quite exposed and often uncomfortable. The huge Standhope Peak towers impressively above the lake's northwest shore.

To visit equally gorgeous Goat Lake, take the signed but initially sketchy trail that crosses the outlet of Betty Lake. This path ascends an open slope to a smaller upper lake, and then climbs to a high pass on the side of Standhope Peak. From there the trail switchbacks steeply down to the shores of Goat Lake. This is said to be the highest named lake in Idaho and it's surely one of the most scenic.

To complete the loop, return to Betty Lake, climb back up to the point on the trail where you hit this route from the heights above, and go through the pass to the north. From

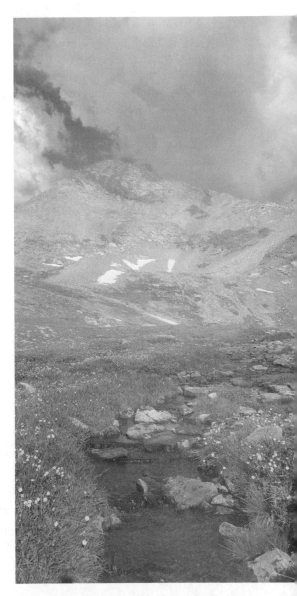

Standhope Peak over an outlet to Betty Lake

here you have a great view to the north of Surprise Valley and Lake 10,148. These land-marks are your next destination.

The trail descends some three dozen short and rather steep switchbacks to the base of a large boulder field where the tread temporarily disappears. The best plan is to angle to the left and descend relatively gentle slopes dotted with whitebark pines until you reach Lake 10,148. This incredibly beautiful gem sits right at the base of Standhope Peak and offers outstandingly scenic campsites.

The faint trail, marked with cairns, departs from the northeast shore of Lake 10,148, descends to cross a creek, and makes its way down the east side of nearly flat Surprise Valley. When the meadows of the valley give way to forest, about 1.5 miles below Lake 10,148, the trail grows faint once again. The easiest course is to cross to the west side of the creek and pick up a path that descends to cross the outlet of an unnamed but lovely little lake right where the creek drops over a waterfall to the west. Your trail goes around the west side of the unnamed lake, passes an excellent campsite, and heads north through the mostly forested north end of Surprise Valley. The rocky path descends to a small meadow and goes down a series of 18 very steep and rocky switchbacks to a junction just above the cascading Fall Creek.

Go right (downstream) at this junction and descend through forest at a much more reasonable grade for about 0.4 mile to a signed junction with the trail to Moose Lake. This is a good, but tiring, potential side trip that climbs fairly steeply for about 1.5 miles to the lake. This large, deep lake is set in a dramatic cirque beneath tall peaks and has good camps, though it's rather tiring hauling a heavy pack up that trail.

The main trail goes straight at the Moose Lake junction. An easy 0.7 mile later leads you back to the Highline Trail junction beside Left Fork Fall Creek. Go straight and retrace your route 1.6 miles to the trailhead.

POSSIBLE ITINERARY

	CAMP	MILES	ELEVATION GAIN
Day 1	Upper basin of Left Fork Fall Creek	6.0	1,700'
Day 2	Lake 10,148	6.0	2,400'
	Side trip to Betty and Goat Lakes	3.0	1,450'
Day 3	Out	6.0	100'
	Side trip to Moose Lake	3.0	1,550'

BEST SHORTER ALTERNATIVE ·

The best two-day hike options are to either Moose Lake or Surprise Valley. If you are backpacking but want to avoid the tough off-trail section in the middle of this loop, you can simply do either end of the described trip as separate one-night adventures to the upper canyon of Left Fork Fall Creek and to Betty Lake.

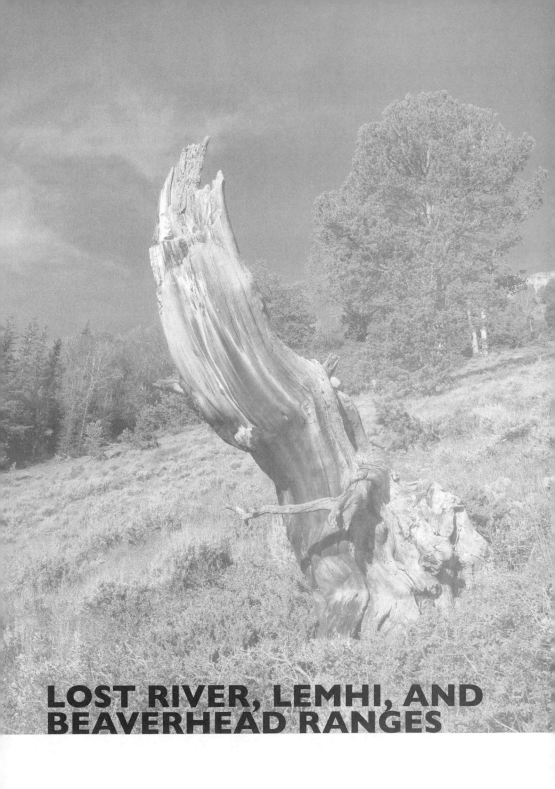

LOST RIVER, LEMHI, AND BEAVERHEAD RANGES

Snag along a trail south of Divide Creek Lake (Trip 21)

The highest mountains in the state of Idaho are in the east-central part of the state, about as far from major population centers as you can get in the Lower 48 United States. The Lost River, Lemhi, and Beaverhead Ranges run parallel to each other, rising from the canyon country along the Salmon River near Challis and petering out in the sagebrush plains near Arco about 100 miles southeast. The ranges are so rarely traveled that most of the highest peaks remain unnamed and are simply identified by their elevations.

The isolation ensures a high degree of solitude, even on holiday weekends. That solitude is enhanced by generally miserable road access and a scarcity of trails. A typical visit involves several miles of bouncing along at 5 miles per hour, preferably in a car you don't like very much, before you finally give up, pull off the "road," and walk the rest of the way to an unsigned trailhead. From there, you do your best to follow a sketchy path, but often give up on that as well, and continue your hike guided only by landmarks. Fortunately, the terrain is generally open, so navigation is easy.

Wildlife appreciates the isolation of these mountains, reveling in the quiet of a people-free landscape. So, if you make the effort to visit, you stand a good chance of seeing mountain goats, black bears, elk, moose, and even relatively elusive animals such as mountain lions.

Though tall, these mountains hide in the rain shadow of several mountain ranges to the west, so less snow falls here than on most Idaho mountains. The drier climate has some important consequences for hikers. First, trails open sooner in the year, with excellent hiking beginning in early to mid-June. Second, the open forests have relatively little ground cover, which makes cross-country travel a reasonable option for getting around in these mountains. Third, surface water is at a premium. Lakes are rare, and the smaller streams typically dry up by late in the season. Hikers should plan to visit early in the summer and take advantage of every available water source. Water problems are most severe in the southern parts of these ranges, due to slightly lower snowfall and an abundance of limestone rock, which allows water to percolate down from the surface. A big advantage of the water shortage is a relative lack of mosquitoes, at least in comparison to the wetter ranges in other parts of the state.

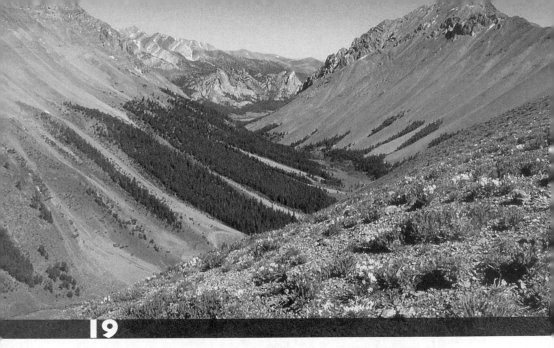

19

LOST RIVER RANGE TRAVERSE

RATINGS: Scenery 10   Solitude 9   Difficulty 8
MILES: 38 (48.5)
SHUTTLE MILEAGE: 33
ELEVATION GAIN: 11,200' (13,800')
DAYS: 4–5 (4–6)
MAP(S): USGS *Burnt Creek,* USGS *Leatherman Peak,* USGS *Massacre Mountain,* USGS *Warren Mountain*
USUALLY OPEN: Late June–October
BEST: Late June and July
PERMITS: None
RULES: The usual Leave No Trace principles apply. Call ahead about periodic fire restrictions.
CONTACT: Lost River Ranger District, 208-588-3400; Challis Ranger District, 208-879-4100

SPECIAL ATTRACTIONS ·

Solitude; outstanding mountain scenery; hiking amid the highest peaks in Idaho

CHALLENGES ·

Sketchy trail in places; motorbikes on some trails; thin air at high altitudes; in places the route is too dangerous for horses.

Above: East Fork Pahsimeroi Valley from Dry Creek Pass

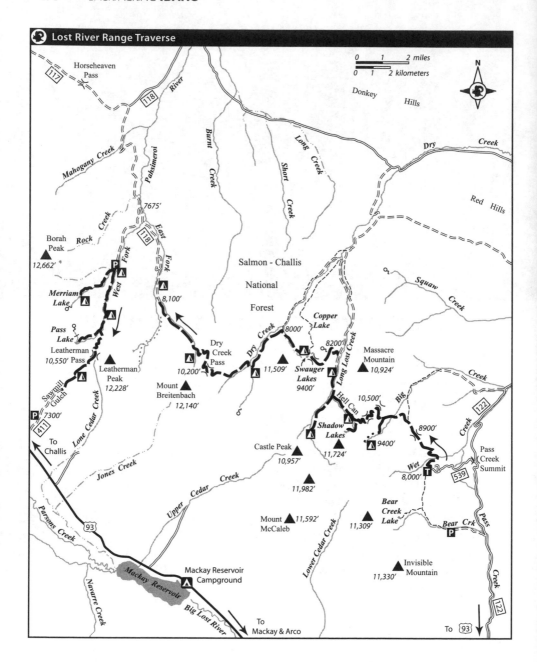

Lost River Range Traverse

HOW TO GET THERE

To reach the recommended ending point, drive about 13 miles north of MacKay on US 93 to a minor junction marked with a small sign saying SAWMILL GULCH. Turn right (northeast) here onto this rough dirt road, which immediately goes through a gate (please close the gate behind you). Drive this steep and very rocky track for as long as your nerves and your vehicle will allow. Most cars with decent ground clearance can get about 1.4

Despite being overlooked by the hiking public, the Lost River Range is both lofty and spectacular. Most of the state's tallest mountains are found in the Lost River Range. In addition to the 12,662-foot Borah Peak, the highest summit in Idaho, the range has eight other peaks higher than 12,000 feet in elevation (most of them unnamed), and a host of summits exceeding 11,000 feet. And there may be more to come, because the Lost River Range is a geologically young range that is still growing. Dramatic evidence of this came on October 28, 1983, with the Borah Peak earthquake, a 7.3-magnitude temblor that raised the mountains—or lowered the neighboring Thousand Springs Valley—by as much as 20 feet. The quake also started numerous landslides, left behind an interesting 21-mile-long crack in the ground, and was large enough to disrupt the geysers and hydrothermal activity in Yellowstone National Park, 150 miles away.

miles up the road to where Sawmill Gulch noticeably narrows. Beyond this point only tough four-wheel drive vehicles can continue.

To reach the starting point at the southeast trailhead drive 7.3 miles southeast of MacKay on US 93 to a junction with Pass Creek Road. (Coming from the south, this junction is 19 miles north of Arco.) Turn left (north) onto this gravel road and drive 1.2 miles to a junction. Angle slightly right and continue for 7.5 miles on this gravel then good dirt road, which becomes Forest Service Road 122, to a junction at Pass Creek Summit. Turn left (west) on FS 539, following signs to Loristica Group Campground, and drive 1.9 miles on this reasonably good dirt road to a junction. Keep straight and proceed another 0.3 mile; then park at a gate with a ROAD CLOSED sign.

INTRODUCTION •

The little-traveled Lost River Range is virtually unknown to hikers outside of Idaho, and even many residents of the Gem State have only a vague concept of where these mountains are. The most popular hike in the range is the route up Borah Peak, which isn't even an established trail. Elsewhere in the range only the occasional intrusion of a noisy motorbike gets in the way of complete solitude for hikers.

The best extended backpacking trip in the range is this rugged traverse that runs northwest from near Pass Creek Pass to the headwaters of the East Fork Pahsimeroi River, where you are smack in the middle of the highest peaks in the state. Along the way are countless open views, lots of wildflowers, and plenty of wildlife.

Though gloriously scenic, significant parts of this trail are so sketchy that much of the walking is effectively cross-country. In addition, junctions are almost never signed and many trails shown on the U.S. Forest Service maps either do not exist or are literally miles from where they are indicated. (The U.S. Geological Survey [USGS] maps show almost no trails at all.) Therefore, this trip is recommended only for experienced hikers who don't mind doing some bushwhacking to follow a poorly signed and rarely traveled route.

TIP: If the winter's snowpack was below or near normal, the best time to take this trip is in mid- to late June, before the local bovines have been released to graze the high meadows.

Note: This trip has been significantly changed from the first edition of this book by extending the outing to the Sawmill Gulch Road off US 93. While this adds 14 miles to the hike, it also adds some truly outstanding scenery around Leatherman Pass and offers easy access to two excellent, new side trips, to Merriam and Pass Lakes. This version of the trip also has a much shorter car shuttle and avoids the long and tortuous drive up the dirt roads on the eastern side of the Lost River Range.

DESCRIPTION ·

From the southeast trailhead, you are immediately faced with a confusing new sign saying simply TRAIL that points left (uphill) on a jeep road. This trail goes south toward Bear Creek and is *not* your route. Instead, you walk around the road-closure gate to the right and go 25 yards along a jeep road to an unadorned post marking the start of a trail that angles left. You turn onto this trail and follow it downhill through a selectively logged area to the lush, green meadow holding Wet Creek.

At this point, the USGS map shows no trail at all, while the Challis National Forest map shows the trail going left (southwest) up the canyon of Wet Creek. After hours of difficult bushwhacking, I discovered that this trail exists solely in the imagination of some U.S. Forest Service cartographer. The actual route goes about 200 yards down Wet Creek, and then crosses the creek on an unstable log (or you can make an easy ford). You then go downstream another 100 yards, curve left, and pick up an old jeep road that cuts across the base of a reddish rock outcrop. From here, the trail climbs the narrow jeep track up a hillside, makes two switchbacks, and heads up a side drainage that goes generally northwest. You turn left off the jeep track where a post has a small but helpful sign stating simply TRAIL.

The trail, which is now easy to follow despite being in the wrong place, according to the map, climbs at an uneven grade through forests and meadows with fine views of the surrounding mountains. Peak 11,309 to the southwest and another rounded mountain that tops out at more than 11,200 feet (there is no specific elevation because it hasn't even been accurately surveyed) dominate the scene. Like most peaks in this remote range, these summits have no names. If you shift your gaze downward to the lower and middle elevations of these peaks, you'll see a wide belt of attractive forests made up of Douglas-firs, Engelmann spruces, and lodgepole and limber pines. The magical scene is completed by the beauty at your feet, where several small meadows and rocky areas come alive in late June and early July with phlox, yarrow, valerian, bistort, wallflower, larkspur, lupine, skyrocket gilia, dandelion, alpine buttercup, forget-me-not, and many other wildflowers.

The trail crosses the seasonal flow of a tiny creek, climbs briefly to an intensely green little meadow, and ascends to a view-packed, grassy saddle just west of a jagged, reddish rock formation.

TIP: A side path goes to an excellent viewpoint at the top of this rock formation.

The trail disappears briefly here, but you can find it again if you go directly north through the saddle and descend to the bottom of an open meadow where the tread

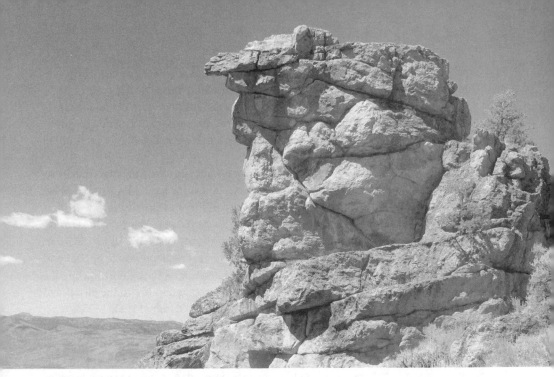

Rock formation in lower Sawmill Gulch

becomes more obvious. After losing about 350 feet, you bear left at an unsigned fork; cross a small, sagebrush-covered flat; and curve to the left.

The trail now makes a downhill traverse across a densely forested hillside and crosses the base of a large rockslide, where pikas squeak at passing hikers. Shortly after the rock-slide, the trail crosses Big Creek—which has reliable water, though the name greatly overstates the creek's size—and climbs very steeply away from the water up a little gully to the northwest. After quickly gaining about 250 feet, the gully splits and trails follow both branches. As usual in these mountains, there are no signs to help you determine the correct direction. However, you bear left and continue climbing steeply for 0.2 mile to another unsigned trail fork.

The main route goes to the right, but for a terrific (and difficult) side trip, keep straight. This trail soon levels out and gradually ascends through a low area, where the tread is often obscured by deadfall and cow paths. Following blazes, you climb left to a low point in the small spur ridge that separates you from Big Creek, and go steeply down the other side. The trail, which is now quite faint, makes its way back down to Big Creek, where the water disappears under the porous limestone rocks and the trail stops. Directly ahead of you is a towering cliff of tilted sedimentary rocks with a crumbly talus slope at its base.

TIP: Like many such places in the Lost River Range, this is a good area to look for fossils of shells, leaves, and other recognizable flora and fauna.

You follow the rubble-strewn creek bed upstream for about 0.5 mile, go around a rocky knoll, and come to a circular lake near the head of Big Creek. This small, deep lake is surrounded by spectacular, tan cliffs and rockslides, and is backed by an unnamed 11,724-foot mountain. Unfortunately, lack of flat ground near the lake precludes any comfortable camping. If you want to explore this area further, then scramble up the lake's cascading inlet creek to a stunning upper valley with a spring, flat ground where you can camp, and jaw-dropping views of the towering cliffs and peaks enclosing this little basin.

After this tough but very scenic side trip, return to the unsigned fork above Big Creek and follow the main trail. This path climbs through a rolling, sagebrush-covered meadow; ascends 12 short, steep switchbacks on a partly forested slope; and makes a long uphill traverse to a high saddle just above timberline.

North of this saddle, a gentle slope goes down to an undulating alpine meadow that looks very inviting. But the trail does not go that way. Instead, it turns left and goes up a steep, treeless slope that is covered with lichens, low grasses, and tundra wildflowers. The tread is very faint, but helpful cairns mark almost every turn in a series of switchbacks, which makes the trail easy to follow. You eventually end up just below the top of a nameless 10,535-foot summit. Alpine wildflowers sprinkle this tundra environment and invite you to lie back and enjoy the outstanding views. The rolling Massacre Mountain rises to the north, while the contorted crags of the Lost River Range spread out to the west and south. In the distance to the east is the Lemhi Range, dominated by Bell Mountain and Diamond Peak.

The tread completely disappears on the side of this 10,535-foot mountain. The correct route follows a string of low, strategically placed cairns that lead southwest down to a windy saddle, overlooking the rocky basin that holds the two very stark Shadow Lakes. From the low point at the southwest end of this saddle, the trail descends a talus slope via a series of very steep switchbacks, often across loose scree. The going is quite difficult, because time and lack of maintenance have obliterated many of the switchbacks. It's worth the effort to find them, however, because off the trail it is extremely easy to turn an ankle on the loose rocks. You reach the bottom at an unsigned junction in a lovely alpine basin near a wandering creek about 0.6 mile below the Shadow Lakes. The dead-end path to the left goes to the lakes (a terrific, must-do side trip), while the trail to the right descends along the outlet creek.

TIP: The best campsites are in the lower meadow, because those near the lakes are very exposed and rocky. Due to the rocky ground, a freestanding tent is a necessity.

To continue your trip, follow the sketchy trail along the lake's outlet creek, first through the undulating meadow, and then into the forests and down what the map labels as Hell Canyon. If you were coming up this increasingly steep trail, that name would probably seem appropriate, but going downhill it's not that bad. The trail can be easy to lose, but it generally stays close to the right side of the creek. Near the bottom you drop steeply through forest into the canyon of Long Lost Creek and reach an unsigned junction.

The main trail goes right, but if you have an extra hour or two, spend them on a side trip up the trail to the left. This path often has lots of deadfall, but it is easy to follow as it slowly climbs through forests for a little more than 1 mile to a lovely meadow in the upper reaches of Long Lost Creek. Wildflowers abound in this rarely visited basin, which is backed by the imposing limestone ramparts of Castle Peak and several unnamed mountains. Some wonderfully scenic campsites are in this area.

From the Hell Canyon junction, the main trail goes downstream, quickly dropping to an ankle-deep ford of Long Lost Creek, and then follows an undulating, sometimes rocky course a little above the creek for 0.4 mile to the end of a primitive jeep road. You follow this jeep road across a huge, nearly level meadow that has lots of sagebrush and wildflowers such as phlox, groundsel, owl's clover, and the tall spikes of monument plant. The acres of flat ground here make it possible for you to camp almost anywhere here and share an evening with the local coyotes, which hunt for ground squirrels in the daytime and howl during the night. About halfway across the meadow is a junction that, amazingly for these mountains, actually has a sign. The sign tells you that the Swauger Lakes, your next goal, are 2 miles away.

You turn left, leaving the jeep road for a trail that is often used by motorbikes, especially on weekends. One thing you'll immediately notice is that while hikers' trails in this range receive almost no maintenance (and aren't even accurately mapped), this motorbike trail has been very expensively built and is well maintained. The well-constructed route steadily climbs six moderately graded switchbacks over a partly forested hillside to a seasonal trickle of water in a little gully. You then make one more switchback to the base of a rolling, sagebrush-covered meadow and slowly ascend past a little spring to a wind-swept, 9,400-foot high point. From here, the trail curves right and loses about 350 feet of elevation to reach the two small but very scenic Swauger Lakes. A fair campsite is near the outlet of the upper lake, which gives anglers the chance to spend an evening trying to catch some of the plump cutthroat trout that live here.

A trail built specifically for motorbikes meets your route at Upper Swauger Lake and heads north toward Copper Lake, which is worth a visit if you have the time. Your less-traveled trail goes downhill to the left, passes lower Swauger Lake, and then follows a dry creek bed. For the next 2 miles you descend beside this dry creek, crossing its rocky bed several times and sometimes just picking your way along the bottom. A little before the bottom of the canyon, you cross the creek bed a last time and come to a signed junction with the Dry Creek Trail beside a small, marshy pond.

You turn left, walk past the marshy pond, and go up the canyon of the misnamed Dry Creek. The trail stays well away from the water for the first 0.5 mile and gets closer to the clear creek as the canyon gradually curves to the southwest.

TIP: A waterfall downstream leaves these upper reaches of Dry Creek with no fish, so anglers should not waste their time here.

Amid the marshes and willow thickets below the trail you can see many beaver dams along the creek. The views across these marshy meadows is stupendous, especially looking toward the head of the canyon, where a massive, snow-streaked wall of mountains is anchored by the 12,140-foot Mount Breitenbach on the right and a string of unnamed 11,000- and 12,000-foot peaks spread out to the left.

The trail crosses a rocky slope, and then wanders across a large, gently sloping meadow covered with sagebrush and a sprinkling of wildflowers. After the meadow, you go over a dry creek bed, and then splash across a fork of Dry Creek and enter a very green meadow, where the trail disappears. Angle slightly right and pick up the tread again near some good campsites just before an ankle-deep ford of the main branch of Dry Creek.

The sketchy trail turns left after the ford and, about 30 yards later, makes a short but very steep climb to the top of a little ridge bordering the creek. The trail follows the top of this ridge, gradually getting closer to the imposing wall of mountains ahead. The way through that wall is visible on your right at Dry Creek Pass on the northeast shoulder of Mount Breitenbach.

The way to Dry Creek Pass is indistinct (to say the least), so you will probably lose the trail several times. The pass is usually visible, however, and it's a straightforward scramble to make your way up. Once above timberline, you'll see several paths going up a very steep, rocky slope to the pass. Most of these are game paths, which are indistinguishable from the actual trail. The best advice is to follow whatever route looks to be the easiest.

The views from the 10,200-foot Dry Creek Pass make the considerable effort of getting there worthwhile. Tiny alpine wildflowers add color to the scene, but your attention is more likely to be drawn to the splendid views, especially down the U-shaped glacial valley of the East Fork Pahsimeroi River. Equally impressive is the awesome amphitheater created by the semicircle of 2,500-foot-high cliffs on the north wall of Mount Breitenbach. This is one of the most impressive scenes in all of Idaho.

To descend from Dry Creek Pass, follow the obvious trail to the right (north) as it goes gradually downhill for about 150 yards and then steeply descends a talus-and-scree slope. More game paths cross your route, but it's usually easy to determine which trail is intended for hikers. Eventually, you enter a whitebark pine woodland, where frequent blazes help you navigate.

> **TIP:** The switchbacks through this woodland are easy to miss. The best way to locate a switchback is to check behind you to see which direction the blazes are cut for uphill hikers to see.

The last of the steep downhill takes you through the forest just above the bottom of the amphitheater at the head of the East Fork Pahsimeroi River. You can leave the trail here and make an exceptionally scenic camp near the basin floor.

The trail then contours through the trees above the river's rocky gorge and drops to some lovely meadows along the creek. The tread often disappears in these meadows, but a few well-placed cairns help mark the route. About 200 yards after entering the first meadow, you hop over the river—really just a creek here—and follow the west bank downstream. Though the tread becomes increasingly obvious as you go down the valley, it's still easy to lose the trail, because you will probably be distracted by the excellent scenery.

You pass just above a marshy area with numerous beaver ponds and hike through a gap in an old, broken-down, wooden fence with a sign that almost laughingly says PLEASE CLOSE THE GATE. Shortly after this fence, you hike past a huge rockslide on the other side of the stream, and go downhill through forest for about 1 mile to a rolling, sagebrush-covered meadow. At the bottom of this meadow you cross a log over the East Fork Pahsimeroi River and immediately come to a remote trailhead at the end of a jeep road.

In the previous edition of this book, this was the trip's ending point—assuming you could coax your abused four-wheel drive vehicle to the end of this awful road. Now I recommend a better alternative, though it does involve an extra day or two of walking. The hike, however, is very scenic and saves your car from miles of abuse.

From the signed trailhead, walk down the jeep road, enjoying excellent views and scenery of the high peaks in this region. After about 0.4 mile you pass a nice potential campsite on your right at the edge of some woods; then it's another 0.5 mile to a knee-deep ford of the East Fork Pahsimeroi River. The road then climbs a short distance away from this ford and comes to a fork. Either route works here as the two forks both climb a hill and reunite after about 0.7 mile. At about 3.3 miles from where you started walking on the road is a second knee-deep ford, this time of the West Fork Pahsimeroi River. Past this point the road climbs for 0.6 mile to a major intersection.

Turn sharply left on the West Fork Pahsimeroi Road, another rugged jeep track, and walk through increasingly scenic terrain for not quite 3 miles to a road-end trailhead. A nice primitive camping area is located here in a grove of tall conifers.

From this campsite the wide trail crosses an intermittent stream, and then goes less than 0.1 mile to a possibly unmarked junction just before a ford of a branch of West Fork Pahsimeroi River. The trail to the right is a must-do side trip to Merriam Lake. It is approximately 2 miles up to this lake on a sometimes sketchy trail, with the last bit over impressive areas of white marble. The destination is a supremely scenic lake that is about as photogenic as a mountain lake can be. The beautiful, nearly white, and unnamed peak that rises above the lake's northwest shore is often mistakenly identified as Borah Peak, even though that lofty summit (the highest in Idaho) is actually hidden from view at this angle. Good campsites are near the lake, with the best ones along the north shore.

After returning to the junction near the end of the West Fork Pahsimeroi Road, you go south and immediately make a calf-deep ford of the side creek coming down from Merriam Lake. The trail now climbs gently along the West Fork Pahsimeroi River, staying mostly in an open forest of subalpine firs and lodgepole pines, but with frequent meadows that offer views up the canyon to Leatherman Peak and Pass. After about 1.7 miles the trail crosses the stream. If you search downstream a bit you can usually find some footlogs spanning the flow that allow you to keep your feet dry.

Now on the east side of the creek, you climb gradually in forest and through long meadows where the tread disappears from time to time (watch for cut logs and blazes to stay on course). You pass a nice campsite and then come to the upper end of the second of two especially large meadows, where an unsigned junction is so faint that it will be hard to notice. Directly ahead of you is a large talus slope up which the exit trail heads steeply uphill toward the obvious Leatherman Pass. If you look carefully, you will be able to pick out a faint tread going up the left side of this slope through some partially grass-covered areas.

Before heading that way, set aside a few hours for a terrific side trip to Pass Lake. To reach it, head generally south-southwest up to and through a narrow strip of trees that begins at the head of the meadow. Here you should pick up an initially sketchy trail that fords the creek and begins winding its way uphill at a moderately steep grade. This path becomes more obvious as it climbs, eventually reaching Pass Lake after about 1.2 miles. This scenic lake sits very near timberline and is situated immediately beneath a row of jagged tan, orange, and brown cliffs, peaks, and talus slopes. Icebergs typically remain in this lake well into July, though by late summer the lake usually recedes quite dramatically. A long, cascading waterfall graces the slope to the north, where the inlet creek emerges from a spring. The lake's shoreline is rocky and exposed, so camping, while possible, is not recommended.

To close out the trip, return to the elusive junction in the meadow 1.2 miles below Pass Lake and turn up toward Leatherman Pass. This steep, winding, and intermittent path is easy to lose, but your goal is always visible, so navigation is not really an issue. The steep climb eventually leads you up rolling alpine slopes to the narrow notch of the 10,550-foot Leatherman Pass. From the top, there are tremendous views of the tall Borah Peak to the north, the huge pyramid of Leatherman Peak immediately to the southeast, the Pahsimeroi Valley and Lemhi Range to the northeast, and the Big Lost Valley and White Knob Mountains to the southwest.

On the southwest side of the pass your trail makes a short but steep descent, and then traverses a steep slope below a jumble of rugged pinnacles. From there the trail is often faint, so you'll need to look for bits of tread and the occasional cairn to stay on course. The correct route stays to the right of a steep drop-off, making its way down a rocky meadow back toward timbered terrain. About 1 mile down from the pass you reach a relatively flat meadow area with fine views and good, but dry, campsites. Raucous Clark's nutcrackers are commonly found eating the nuts from the whitebark pine trees found here.

From the lower end of this flat meadow, look for a distinct trail that crosses the top of a large rockslide. Near the far end of this slide, the trail cuts to the left, steeply descends through forest, and then closely parallels the little creek in Sawmill Gulch as it goes very steeply downhill through brushy areas and groves of quaking aspens. About 2.2 miles down from Leatherman Pass you reach the end of the upper, four-wheel drive portion of the Sawmill Gulch Road. To reach your car, simply walk down this steep road as it eventually leaves the forest and crosses sagebrush-covered slopes. The distance you travel down the road depends on how far you were able to drive, but most people will walk between 1.5 and 2 miles to reach their waiting transports.

VARIATIONS ·

This hike presents several options for making rugged but highly worthwhile cross-country side trips. One of the best of these is the scramble over alpine ridges to the top of Massacre Mountain. You should also consider making the bushwhacks up to the high meadows and cirque lakes on the eastern branch of East Fork Pahsimeroi River and up the forks of Dry Creek.

POSSIBLE ITINERARY

	CAMP	MILES	ELEVATION GAIN
Day 1	Upper Big Creek Basin	6.0	2,600'
Day 2	Swauger Lakes	6.5	3,200'
	Side trip to Shadow Lakes	1.5	200'
	Side trip up Long Lost Creek	2.5	200'
Day 3	East Fork Pahsimeroi River along road	10.5	2,400'
Day 4	West Fork Pahsimeroi at Merriam Lake TH	6.5	500'
	Side trip to Merriam Lake	4.0	1,500'
Day 5	Out	8.5	2,500'
	Side trip to Pass Lake	2.5	700'

BEST SHORTER ALTERNATIVE ·

From the southern trailhead near Pass Creek Summit, try a weekend backpacking trip as far as either the upper basin of Big Creek or, for strong hikers, Shadow Lakes.

All other shorter options involve vehicular abuse that might get you sued by the People for the Ethical Treatment of Automobiles. If you are willing to risk it, then take your high-clearance vehicle to the end of the rough Dry Creek Road. From there, do a loop hike up Long Lost Creek, turn right and go past the Swauger Lakes, and return along Dry Creek. From the northern trailhead, a steep day hike is possible up to Leatherman Pass, or even as far as Pass Lake, if you are a really strong hiker.

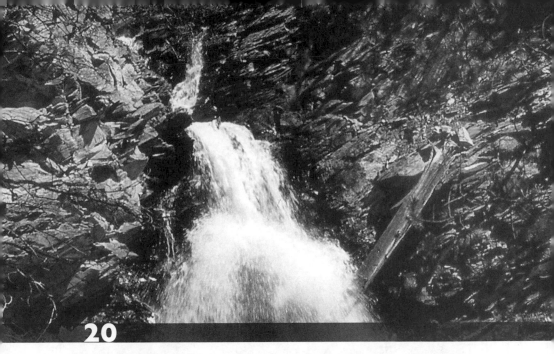

20

CENTRAL LEMHI RANGE LOOP

RATINGS: Scenery 8   Solitude 9   Difficulty 8
MILES: 45 (48)
ELEVATION GAIN: 10,300' (10,500')
DAYS: 4–6 (4–6)
MAP(S): USGS *Big Creek Peak*, USGS *Iron Creek Point*, USGS *Yellow Peak*
USUALLY OPEN: Late June–October
BEST: Late June and July
PERMITS: None
RULES: The usual Leave No Trace principles apply.
CONTACT: Challis Ranger District, 208-879-4100; Lost River Ranger District, 208-588-3400; Leadore Ranger District, 208-768-2500

SPECIAL ATTRACTIONS •

Solitude; outstanding mountain scenery; abundant wildlife

CHALLENGES •

Sketchy trail in places; motorcycles allowed on some trails; potentially difficult stream crossings; new and rerouted trails not shown on the U.S. Geological Survey (USGS) maps

Above: Falls on North Fork Big Creek

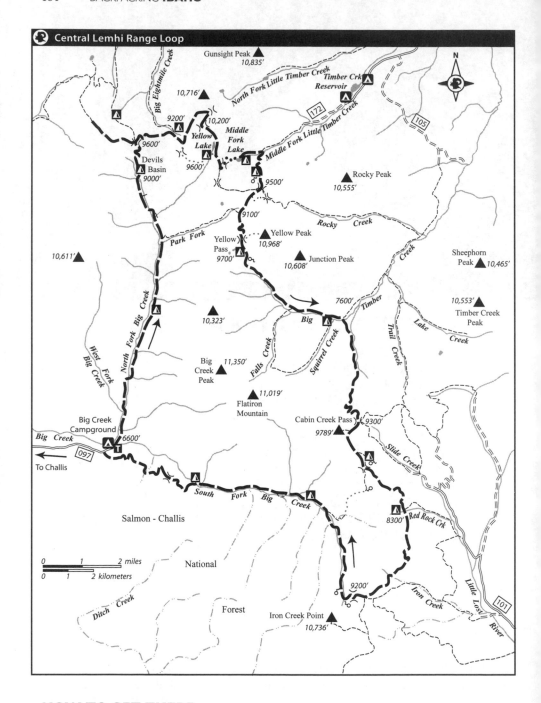

Central Lemhi Range Loop

Gunsight Peak ▲
10,835'

North Fork Little Timber Creek

Big Eightmile Creek

10,716' ▲

Timber Crk
Reservoir

172

105

9200'

10,200'

Yellow
Lake

Middle
Fork
Lake

Middle Fork Little Timber Creek

9600'

Rocky Peak ▲
10,555'

Devils
Basin
9000'

9600'

9500'

9100'

Rocky   Creek

Park Fork

Yellow
Pass
9700'

Yellow Peak ▲
10,968'

Junction Peak ▲
10,608'

Sheephorn
Peak ▲ 10,465'

10,611' ▲

Creek

10,553' ▲
Timber Creek
Peak

North Fork Big Creek

10,323' ▲

7600'

Big

Timber

Lake

Creek

Big
Creek
Peak

11,350' ▲

Falls   Creek

Squirrel Creek

Trail   Creek

West   Fork   Big Creek

11,019' ▲
Flatiron
Mountain

Cabin Creek Pass ▲ 9300'
9789'

Slide   Creek

Big Creek
Campground
6600'

Big   Creek

097

To Challis

South   Fork   Big   Creek

8300' Red Rock Crk

Salmon - Challis

9200'

0   1   2 miles
0   1   2 kilometers

National

Iron   Creek

Little   Lost   River

101

Ditch   Creek

Forest

Iron Creek Point ▲
10,736'

N

HOW TO GET THERE • • • • • • • • • • • • • • • • • • •

From Challis, drive 17.2 miles north on US 93 to a junction at the tiny crossroads community of Ellis. Turn right (southeast) onto a paved county road, following signs for the Pahsimeroi Fish Hatchery, and proceed 30.5 miles to a signed junction with Big Creek Road (also known as Forest Service Road 097). (Coming from the south, this turnoff is about 50 miles north of the tiny town of Howe.) Turn left (east) and slowly drive 3.6 miles on this rutted, dirt-and-gravel road to its end at primitive Big Creek Campground. The North Fork Big Creek Trail, signed simply Trail #075, starts at a T-junction just after a culvert over South Fork Big Creek. Because there is almost no long-term parking at the campground, it is usually better to park at the signed South Fork Big Creek trailhead at the top of the steep hill 0.2 mile before you reach the campground.

INTRODUCTION

To call the Lemhi Range remote is a little like saying that the weather in Siberia can get a bit nippy. Hidden behind the already isolated Lost River Range, the Lemhis may be the least known significant mountain range in the Lower 48. The nearest city is Idaho Falls, about 100 miles to the southeast, and the outdoor lovers of that town almost always head east to Grand Teton and Yellowstone National Parks rather than northwest to the Lemhis. So hikers in the Lemhi Range can expect plenty of solitude, even on holiday weekends. Because few people have even heard of this range, it might be difficult for you to convince potential hiking partners to come along. But persevere in your efforts, because the Lemhis are worth it.

This magnificent loop trip explores a spectacularly scenic part of this range, and does so from a trailhead with reasonably good road access, something of a rarity in these mountains. Wildlife is incredibly abundant in this area. In fact, at times the trail is turned into an obstacle course where it is virtually impossible to avoid stepping in the droppings of elk, deer, mountain goats, moose, and black bears. If you like this trip—and it would be hard not to—then you will probably find yourself joining that small group of devoted individuals who come back to these mountains time and again. You may also want to get involved in the effort to set aside this spectacular part of the Lemhi Range in the proposed Sacagawea Wilderness, a name chosen to honor the extraordinary young American Indian woman who helped guide Lewis and Clark across the continent, and whose branch of the Shoshone tribe lived in the adjacent Lemhi Valley.

TIP: I recommend doing this loop clockwise, especially early in the season, so you can get the most difficult stream crossings done at the start of the trip. This way you still have time to turn around if they look too intimidating.

DESCRIPTION

Shortly after the trailhead, you go through a gate and begin a gradual ascent that always stays close to the lush environment beside North Fork Big Creek. The vegetation is an interesting mix that fills a transition zone between the dry, sagebrush plains of the Pahsimeroi Valley and the wetter, coniferous forests of the Lemhi Mountains. On your left, the stream is crowded with riparian shrubs and trees such as willows and birches, while the open slopes on your right are dominated by grasses and sagebrush. In between are forests of quaking aspen, mountain mahogany, and Douglas-fir. There are also some lodgepole pines in this area, though many of these are dead, having been killed by a beetle infestation.

In late June wildflowers are abundant, creating a rainbow of colors, including the yellow of arnica, the red of paintbrush, the white of yarrow, the blue of lupine, and both red and yellow from columbine.

After about 1 mile, you pass a sign that identifies West Fork Big Creek, which comes down a side canyon on the left. A few yards later, you come to the first crossing of North Fork Big Creek. The ford where the trail crosses is cold, swift, and well over knee-deep in early summer, so you might try looking for a blazed route that goes upstream about 150 yards to a narrow log crossing of the creek. If the log has washed away or looks too narrow and unstable for safety, you'll have to return to the regular trail crossing and brave the cold water. Now on the west side of the creek, the trail gradually climbs across a series of boulder and talus slopes for 1.1 miles to the second ford, which is also cold and about knee-deep, but it's a bit easier than the first one. As with the first ford, a blazed trail goes upstream through willow thickets for about 130 yards to a possible log crossing that allows you to keep your feet dry.

Having passed these two potential obstacles, you now set out at a carefree pace, gradually gaining altitude through an increasingly dense forest that is dominated by lodgepole pines. The first good campsite comes at about the 4.5-mile point, just before you enter a pretty, creek-side meadow. Whether you camp here or not, this is a good spot to rest and try your luck at catching some of the hungry trout that live in North Fork Big Creek. The best fishing is usually in the ponds behind this creek's many beaver dams. Evidence of other wildlife comes in the form of large hoofprints and piles of pelletized droppings in the trail. Though elk are responsible for some of these signs, others are made by moose. On my trip, I was surprised to come face to face with a large, gangly bull moose, who stood for some time just staring at me, perhaps trying to figure out what I was since so few people hike these trails.

The trail crosses the base of a talus slope, and then, at about the 7-mile point, goes across several fairly small branches of Park Fork Big Creek and comes to a junction. If you want a somewhat shorter and easier loop, turn right and climb about 3.5 miles up the valley of Park Fork Big Creek to a junction below Yellow Pass. Hikers who are not accustomed to finding routes should take this trail, because the recommended route presents some navigation challenges. On the other hand, the trail up Park Fork Big Creek misses both Devils Basin and Yellow Lake, so I recommend that experienced hikers bear left and stick with the main branch of North Fork Big Creek.

Up to now the hike has been fairly easy, but after this junction the grade steepens. Also, the path is sketchy in places (keep an eye out for blazes) and in early summer numerous trickling tributaries cause the tread to be muddy in spots, which makes the going slow and messy. A little more than 0.8 mile from the Park Fork junction, you ford a tributary creek in the middle of a two-tiered sliding cascade, and then cross the main branch of North Fork Big Creek on a log. The forests at this elevation are more interesting than they were below, with some Engelmann spruces and subalpine firs added to the lodgepole pines and Douglas-firs. The scenery has become more interesting as well, because the forests are more open and provide occasional glimpses of the surrounding peaks.

About 0.9 mile from the last crossing, you pass an impressive waterfall on the main creek, which is worth a short, off-trail detour to fully appreciate. You cross the creek again above the falls, and then hop over numerous small creeks that comprise the headwaters of North Fork Big Creek. The last of these crossings comes at the edge of Devils Basin, a gorgeous mountain meadow that must have been named in error, because Satan would never want to be associated with such a heavenly place. The basin is bisected by a clear creek and carpeted with yellow buttercups and white marsh marigolds. The meadow also provides the first complete break in the tree cover, so you can appreciate unobstructed views of the surrounding mountains. A very nice campsite is on a little rise just after the creek crossing.

The trail disappears shortly after it enters Devils Basin. To relocate it, walk along the right side of the meadow for about 150 yards, and then turn onto an obvious path that goes into the trees on the right. This trail is gentle for a short while; then it steeply climbs a rocky slope where your pace is slowed by frequent stops to enjoy the ever-improving views, and by the thinner air at this relatively high elevation. The last 0.5 mile of the climb is over a boulder field where the route is marked by occasional cairns.

You top out at a wide, windy, 9,600-foot pass, where the harsh environment limits the tree cover to only scattered subalpine firs and whitebark pines. Wildflowers are limited as well, to stunted varieties of shooting star and alpine buttercup, mostly in wet areas.

WARNING: The trail is easy to lose here, so look carefully for cairns and blazes.

On the left side of this wide pass is a poorly signed junction. The trail that goes sharply left follows a wildly scenic ridgeline and is an excellent side trip, though it may be hard to know when to turn around. Another path, which is not shown on the U.S. Geological Survey (USGS) or U.S. Forest Service maps, goes straight, contours for a while, and then drops into a scenic basin with a shallow tarn and some decent campsites. This is a good side trip as well, if you don't mind making the steep climb back up to the pass.

Your trail, which is unsigned and the hardest one to locate, goes right and steeply descends a partly forested slope. If you can't find the trail, go downhill to the east over generally open terrain to where the tread becomes a little more obvious in the trees. The trail eventually turns right, levels, and crosses several small snowmelt creeks before intersecting an obvious trail at a junction marked by a cairn.

TIP: The USGS map incorrectly shows this junction about 400 feet lower in elevation.

You turn right on a good trail, and then walk gradually uphill for about 350 yards. Here you'll see a sign on a tree 50 yards to the right that points to Big Eightmile Creek in one direction and Timber Creek in the other. Several good campsites are in this area.

The old trail went south from this sign, climbed over a rocky pass, and then dropped to Yellow Lake. The somewhat longer new trail, which is not shown on the USGS maps, is much better graded and easier to hike. Stick with the well-built new trail as it curves up a wide, subalpine valley of meadows, rocks, and scattered trees. Directly ahead of you to the northeast is an unnamed, pyramid-shaped peak covered with loose, tan talus and boulders. The path slowly curves to the east around the base of this peak, and then climbs to a wide pass. From here, you can see Gunsight Peak to the northeast and look down the scenic valley of North Fork Little Timber Creek.

Instead of going through this pass, the trail turns right and gradually traverses uphill across a rocky slope to a 10,200-foot pass. From this above-timberline location, the trail curves gradually down to the east side of Yellow Lake, a sparkling gem in a grassy cirque surrounded by talus fields and the bare, tan slopes of several nearby ridges and peaks. The beautiful tan color of these mountains is from quartzite, a rock that makes up most of the Lemhi Range. The best campsites are in some clumps of trees near the outlet creek a few hundred yards below the lake.

TIP: In the evening and morning be sure to check the slopes around Yellow Lake for tiny, misplaced snow patches. If they move, they're mountain goats.

To exit the Yellow Lake basin, follow the well-maintained trail that gradually climbs the side of the sloping ridge southeast of the lake. After about 0.5 mile, this trail leaves a grove of stunted whitebark pines and presents you with a choice. If you want to stick with the official trail, then continue straight, climb to a high saddle, and descend gradually on a relatively new trail to a junction in the pass above Park Fork Big Creek. For a longer and more scenic alternative, leave the trail where it emerges from the trees and walk a short distance to the left over alpine grasses to an obvious wide pass. Below you to the northeast is the canyon of Middle Fork Little Timber Creek and, in the distance, the Lemhi Valley and the Beaverhead Mountains. Directly below you is the enticing Middle Fork Lake, which is your immediate goal.

The way to the lake follows the course of thousands of mountain goat hooves on an obvious track that goes down a very steep, rocky slope. Amazingly, the crafty goats have included a few steep switchbacks. The downhill grade lessens and the track disappears near a grassy spring, but a path is no longer necessary, because it's easy to make your way down from here past a small pond to Middle Fork Lake. On the north side of this scenic lake are a good trail and several excellent campsites.

The trail down from Middle Fork Lake, which is not shown on any map, follows the lake's cascading outlet stream for a little less than 1 mile to an unsigned junction with the Middle Fork Little Timber Creek Trail.

In the upper basin of Big Eightmile Creek

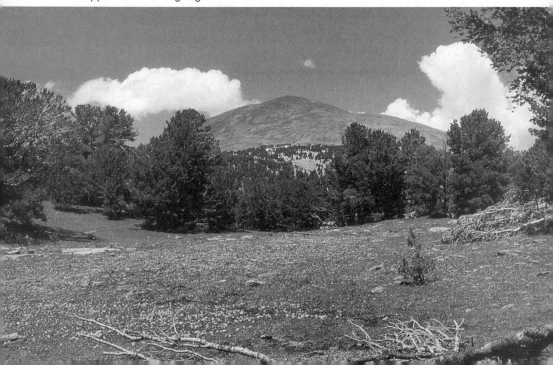

WARNING: This trail is open to motorbikes and all-terrain vehicles, so it's possible that your peace and quiet will be disturbed by machines.

You turn right, cross the creek on logs, and then steeply climb the wide trail to a pretty little basin with a spring and possible campsites. Black bears and elk both frequent this area, so keep quiet and look for movement in the meadows and near the edge of the forest. The trail goes up a grassy slope above the basin to a 9,500-foot pass, where the view to the south is dominated by a striking, orange-yellow peak called, appropriately enough, Yellow Peak. Many other lesser summits are also visible from the pass, but they have no names.

There is a four-way junction at the pass, though the USGS map shows no junction at all. The path to the right is the trail from Yellow Lake. The trail to the left contours to a wide saddle with a scenic pond and drops down the canyon of Rocky Creek. Your route bears slightly right, following signs to North Fork Big Creek, and descends through lovely sloping meadows and strips of trees to an unsigned junction with the old trail to Rocky Creek. You go straight and descend to a junction with the trail down Park Fork Big Creek. This is where the alternate trail that skips Devils Basin and Yellow Lake rejoins your route. You bear left, climb through forest, and then skirt a small, rocky basin and steeply switchback seven times up a talus slope to the 9,700-foot Yellow Pass.

The view from Yellow Pass presents a whole new panorama of rugged peaks, dominated by Big Creek Peak and Flatiron Mountain to the south. Both of these summits top out above 11,000 feet, which makes them the highest in this part of the Lemhi Range.

TIP: It is relatively simple for ambitious hikers to make the scramble up open, rocky slopes east of the pass to the top of the 10,968-foot Yellow Peak. The commanding views from this summit stretch for hundreds of miles and encompass several nearby mountain ranges and valleys.

The trail now makes a long descent from Yellow Pass into the curving canyon of Big Timber Creek. Just below the pass is a shallow lakelet with a possible campsite above its northeast shore. The trail then gradually drops past a series of springs in a huge, sloping meadow that is home to a large herd of Rocky Mountain elk throughout the summer months. Observant hikers are almost certain to see some elk, or at least hear their distinctive grunts and high-pitched squeals.

At the bottom of this high meadow, the trail turns left and makes a lovely descent of Big Timber Creek's scenic canyon, generally staying on the slopes above the creek. In the lower canyon, these slopes are open, drier, and covered with sagebrush and a sprinkling of June-blooming wildflowers such as death camas, phlox, lupine, and dandelion. Views are superb from these slopes, especially of Flatiron Mountain and its surrounding ridges. In a particularly large sloping meadow is a signed junction with the upper end of the little-used Flatiron Mountain Trail. You go straight and continue gradually downhill, now mostly in lodgepole pine forests with a few meadows and aspen glades. Almost 5 miles from Yellow Pass, the trail levels and goes through a large meadow to a junction with the lower end of the Flatiron Mountain Trail.

TIP: A comfortable and spacious campsite is about 100 yards down the Flatiron Mountain Trail in the trees at the meadow's border.

Just 200 yards past the Flatiron Mountain Trail is a junction with the Cabin Creek Trail, where you turn right and soon come to a ford of Big Timber Creek. You may be able to find a helpful log in this area, but, if not, the ford is only about 20 feet across and no more than calf-deep.

The Cabin Creek Trail goes upstream beside its namesake creek through attractive forests and small meadows. The ascent is fairly gradual for the first 1.5 miles; then the trail enters a side canyon and starts to climb more seriously. Things ease off again for the next mile as you go through a series of delightful, rolling meadows, where the trail has been rerouted to make the grade much gentler. The trail completes its ascent at a four-way junction in the 9,300-foot Cabin Creek Pass. Take a rest stop here to recharge your system, and to enjoy the excellent views looking northwest to Yellow Peak and southeast to an entirely new vista that stretches all the way to the towering Bell Mountain.

You turn right at the junction, following signs to Iron Creek, and make a short, steep climb up the shoulder of a hill to an unsigned junction. The trail to the right goes to the top of an unnamed 9,789-foot knoll. Your route bears left, traverses the east side of the knoll, and passes through some lovely ridgetop meadows.

TIP: The trail is easy to lose in these meadows. The correct route crosses the meadow with almost no change in elevation and picks up again in the woods.

The trail now gradually descends along the top of a ridge for about 1 mile to an unsigned fork, where you bear right. A few hundred yards past this fork, you travel above a meadow with a small spring and a possible campsite. Unfortunately, cattle often graze in this meadow, which reduces its appeal.

About 0.4 mile past this meadow the trail comes to a saddle and disappears. The only obvious route from here is a game path that angles downhill to the right (west) and goes 0.5 mile to a spring where it dead-ends. This trail is not shown on any map. The official trail, which is very hard to find, goes downhill to the left from the saddle.

For those who don't mind a couple of miles of moderate cross-country travel, consider this alternate route to complete the loop. Take the trail to the spring, and then turn right (west) and make your way steeply down through open, creek-side meadows and across sagebrush slopes. Whenever possible, try to follow game paths, because experience has taught the animals the best routes. At the bottom of the descent, you enter a steep and heavily wooded canyon where the route gets rugged and quite brushy. Eventually, you hit a switchbacking trail, not shown on the USGS or U.S. Forest Service maps, that takes you down to an unsigned junction with the trail along South Fork Big Creek. This cross-country section is all downhill and should only take you a little more than an hour to complete. Keep in mind, however, that this isolated area is no place to be stranded with a sprained ankle, so never travel alone and do this cross-country section only if you're confident, careful, and experienced.

If you prefer to take the longer, more scenic, official trail (assuming you can find it), then pick up the sketchy route at the saddle and go gradually downhill at an uneven grade across partly forested slopes. One immediately apparent feature of this area is the reddish rock, which here has replaced the tan quartzite and limestone that comprise most of the Lemhi Range. This colorful rock is part of the Challis Volcanic formations and adds greatly to the area's scenic appeal. In honor of this change in geology, the next landmark

If you're feeling ambitious, go straight at the junction below Iron Creek Point and hike 1 mile to a second junction. Turn right and climb steadily to the former lookout site atop the 10,736-foot Iron Creek Point. As with all lookout sites, the views from here are exceptional, including almost the entire southwest side of the Lemhi Range and the broad expanse of the Pahsimeroi Valley to the west. You can even pick out Borah Peak, the highest mountain in Idaho, in the Lost River Range to the southwest.

you come to is Red Rock Creek, where there is a junction with a trail that drops to the east. You'll find a possible campsite on the south side of the easy creek crossing.

Having lost about 1,300 feet from the knoll above Cabin Creek Pass, the trail now sets about regaining most of that elevation in an irregular ascent that mixes uphill sections with contours and even some downhills. Views are good throughout and keep the hiking interesting. About 0.5 mile beyond Red Rock Creek, you hop over an unnamed creek and go up and down for the next 3.5 miles to a four-way junction below the towering Iron Creek Point.

To complete the loop, turn right (west) at the four-way junction below Iron Creek Point and soon cross a trickling, seasonal creek. The trail then climbs fairly steeply through spacious meadows, gaining a little more than 400 feet to a wide saddle. After this, you descend a few switchbacks, pass some springs, and follow an unnamed creek that flows almost directly north on its way to meet South Fork Big Creek. Even though you must cross this creek, or various tributaries, numerous times, it's always easy to keep your feet dry at the crossings. After about 2.5 miles, you intersect an unsigned side trail (the cross-country alternative route) and come to the confluence of your creek with South Fork Big Creek.

Below this junction, the trail travels across a hillside, staying just above the creek for 1 mile to a spacious horse camp that is very comfortable but smells badly of equines. If you prefer the aroma of pines and wildflowers—who doesn't?—there are many smaller campsites under the trees near the creek.

Beyond the camp, you hop over a side creek and go around the base of a talus slope of colorful red and tan rocks. Less than 0.5 mile later, you ford or make a slippery rock-hop crossing of an unnamed tributary creek that comes out of a canyon to the north.

TIP: You may find a log across this creek hidden in the willows a bit downstream from the trail crossing.

Almost immediately after this crossing, the trail goes down to a horse ford of South Fork Big Creek. There is no need for hikers to make this ford. Instead, simply scramble a few yards to the right and pick up an obvious trail across a crumbly talus slope. Horses cannot safely negotiate this slope, but hikers should have no problem. After about 200 yards, the horse trail fords the creek again and rejoins your route.

Below these fords, the trail travels through a grove of willows and aspens, where you'll probably notice that many of the young trees have been chewed through and hauled away by beavers. You then go up and down through a mix of wet meadows and dense riparian shrubbery, and across rocky slopes covered with sagebrush and wildflowers. Though the landscape is very pleasant, it's not as wildly scenic as the high country earlier in the trip. Less than 0.5 mile after leaving the last large, sagebrush-covered slope, the trail drops to a nice campsite and a ford of South Fork Big Creek. The easy ford is only calf-deep and the cold water feels great on a hot afternoon.

After the ford, the trail climbs steeply beside a tiny tributary, the banks of which are crowded with 3-foot-tall bluebells, and then contours for 0.5 mile and steeply climbs to a sagebrush- and grass-covered saddle with good views.

TIP: For even better views, wander a short distance north to the top of a knoll directly overlooking the steep canyon of South Fork Big Creek.

You descend one long switchback to the bottom of the next side canyon, which contains a trickling creek, and then make a final, tough, sun-exposed climb. At the top of a spur ridge, you level off, travel through forest for a few hundred yards, and then leave the trees and enjoy a superb view of the Pahsimeroi Valley and the Lost River Range. The last 0.5 mile winds down open, view-packed slopes to the South Fork Big Creek trailhead.

POSSIBLE ITINERARY

	CAMP	MILES	ELEVATION GAIN
Day 1	Devils Basin	10.0	2,500'
Day 2	Yellow Lake (with side trip out ridge west of the pass above Devils Basin)	5.0	1,600'
	Side trip out ridge west of pass above Devils Basin	3.0	200'
Day 3	Lower meadow on Big Timber Creek	10.0	1,700'
Day 4	South Fork Big Creek Canyon	13.0	3,200'
Day 5	Out	7.0	1,200'

BEST SHORTER ALTERNATIVE •

For a shorter two- or three-day trip try a lollipop loop, starting from the Big Creek Campground, going up North Fork Big Creek, and then looping around via Devils Basin, Yellow Lake, and Yellow Peak before returning on the Park Fork Trail to North Fork Big Creek.

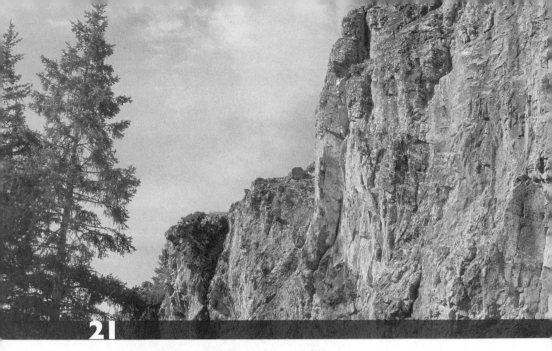

21

DIVIDE CREEK AND
WEBBER LAKES

RATINGS: Scenery 9   Solitude 7   Difficulty 6
MILES: 30 (including day hikes to Webber Lakes and Deadman Creek Basin)
ELEVATION GAIN: 5,800' (including day hikes)
DAYS: 3–4
MAP(S): USGS *Deadman Lake,* USGS *Scott Peak* (all in Montana)
USUALLY OPEN: Mid-June–October
BEST: Late June–mid-July
PERMITS: None
RULES: The usual Leave No Trace principles apply.
CONTACT: Dubois Ranger District, 208-374-5422

SPECIAL ATTRACTIONS ·

Dramatic alpine lakes set beneath towering peaks; very good opportunities to see moose, elk, mountain goats, and other wildlife; excellent hike for those who like to backpack into a base camp and explore

CHALLENGES ·

Most of the trail is open to motorcycles. Grizzly bears occasionally wander into this area, so camp and act accordingly.

Above: Cliffs lining Divide Creek Trail

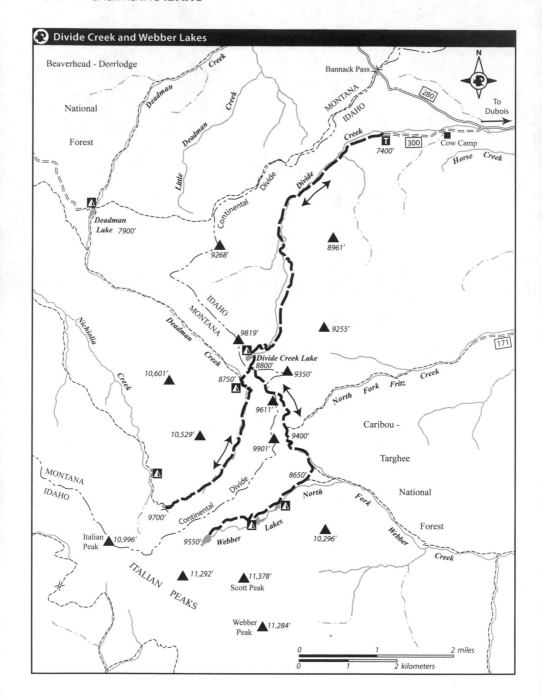

Divide Creek and Webber Lakes

HOW TO GET THERE

Take Dubois Exit 167 off I-15 north of Idaho Falls, go west on ID 22 for 6 miles, and then turn right (north) at a junction near milepost 62.8, following signs to Medicine Lodge. Stay on the paved county road through several turns and past the unincorporated town redundantly named Small, as the road heads up the canyon of Medicine Lodge Creek and toward the mountains beyond.

After 8.8 miles go left on Medicine Lodge Road at the junction with West Indian Creek Road; then continue another 12.6 miles to the end of pavement. About 1.5 miles later is a junction with a signed road going left toward Webber Creek Campground. Go straight on the main road and, 3.3 miles later at the junction with Irving Creek Road, continue straight. Your route continues to get narrower and a little rougher, but it remains generally good gravel and drivable in a passenger car. At 1.9 miles from the Irving Creek Road junction, bear left at a junction with Warm Creek Road and cross a bridge over Medicine Lodge Creek. Just past this bridge veer right at a junction with Fitz Creek Road and go 1.9 miles to the boundary of national forest land, where the route becomes Forest Service Road 280. From here the road deteriorates, and you will have to drive much more slowly and carefully, though passenger cars should still be fine. The road gets rougher after another 3.5 miles when you reach the junction with FS 300, where you want to go left. This road is quite rough and you will need a higher-clearance vehicle, though four-wheel drive is not necessary unless the road is wet. After about 0.3 mile you reach Cow Camp, a rancher's facility with a small cabin. Cars without good ground clearance should park here. The rough road continues another 1.1 miles to the road-end trailhead.

INTRODUCTION

A spear of Montana points south into Idaho in this remote section of the southern Beaverhead Mountains, creating something of a geographic oddity. Here the Continental Divide runs north–south, as usual, but, uniquely, the streams on the west side of this section of the divide curve around and eventually drain to the Atlantic Ocean, while water falling on the east side of the divide drains toward the Pacific Ocean. That fact, mildly interesting as it may be, has no effect on the scenery, however, which is great regardless of where the melting snow on these isolated peaks is flowing. Peaks topping 11,000 feet in elevation are clustered at the head of Webber Creek, where a string of absolutely spectacular lakes lie glistening in the sun. They are at least as impressive as any other alpine lakes in Idaho (which is saying something), but are familiar to only a tiny percentage of even fairly knowledgeable hikers in the Gem State. Now you are in on the secret, so enjoy. As an added bonus, you also stand a better than average chance of seeing big game animals (elk, moose, and mountain goats). For hikers who like to backpack into a base camp and do some exploring, this is a terrific option. Sadly, motorcycles are allowed to despoil this paradise and scare away the wildlife. The noisy machines are rare on weekdays, however, so if you can manage to visit midweek you will have a much more enjoyable trip.

DESCRIPTION

Whether you drove or chose to walk the last 1.1 miles of road, the official trail begins from the end of FS 300 next to a trailhead sign. Your immediate surroundings consist of rolling hills. The south-facing slopes across the canyon from you are covered with sagebrush, while the wetter hillsides hosting the trail that face north are cloaked with forests of Douglas-firs. On your immediate right is the small, marshy, willow-choked stream known as Divide Creek.

The rocky trail begins on the hillside a little above the tiny creek passing through a pretty mix of forests and open slopes. After a little less than 0.3 mile you drop to creek level and walk primarily in forest. In June and July wildflowers are very common in this area, with large numbers of paintbrush, yarrow, buckwheat, alumroot, phlox, yellow paintbrush, arnica, penstemon, stonecrop, and both red and white columbine. At about 0.75 mile the trail takes you through a gate in a fence line.

Don't be surprised if you hear elk bugling in this lower valley of Divide Creek. It is also common to see moose amid the willows and meadows nearby. Nesting songbirds find good habitat near the stream as well, and they will fill the forest with song in early summer. As always, hiking early in the morning generally allows you to see more wildlife, but that is especially true here because the trail is open to motorcycles and the first machine to pass through will scare away any animals.

Near 1.5 miles you cross the creek, which is dry at this point after early summer, and continue gently uphill in meadows beside the waterless creek. About 0.6 mile later the valley is constricted by low cliffs on either side where a wooden fence spans the narrow gap. Just above this point a bit of surface water returns to the creek and the valley forks.

Your trail follows the left (southern) fork of Divide Creek, and soon takes you above a short section of slot canyon on the stream. Above this short canyon you step over the creek's meager flow three times in quick succession and make a short, steep climb on a rocky section of trail.

Once this little climb is complete, the trail gradually ascends an open, sagebrush-covered hillside above the southwest side of the creek, slowly leading you into higher and more scenic terrain with tall ridges now flanking either side of the narrow valley. At a little more than 5 miles you step over the tiny creek again and make a moderately graded ascent in meadows and open forest, with two rounded switchbacks to Divide Creek Lake at 5.9 miles.

This beautiful, forest-rimmed lake has rugged buttes rising in three different directions, making it very photogenic, especially on a calm morning with nice reflections in the water. The low ridge to the west forms part of the Continental Divide and the border with Montana. Excellent campsites are on either side of the lake's bridged outlet, and you will even find a nice wood picnic table to make your evening meals more comfortable. The lake has so-so fishing, but is good for swimming, if you are so inclined. Best of all, though, is that the lake is an ideal location for a base camp to do some exploring. Climbing the nearby peaks for the wonderful views is an excellent option, but the two best and most highly recommended day hikes are the one to Webber Lakes, on the Idaho side of the border, and the romp up to the high basin at the head of Deadman Creek in next-door Montana. Both of those hikes are described below.

Webber Lakes: Pick up the trail that angles to the south (uphill) from the bridge over the outlet to Divide Creek Lake and ascend about 200 feet to just below the Continental Divide. Here you will see an unsigned but obvious trail forking to the right. This is the unofficial path that drops over the other side of the ridge into Montana, where it intersects with the trail along Deadman Creek.

To reach Webber Lakes, keep straight on the main trail, which soon takes you to the top of the divide where you can see a host of rugged and impressive peaks at the head of Deadman Creek. These are the Italian Peaks, which tower over not only Montana's Deadman Creek, but also your goal for the day, the Webber Lakes on the Idaho side of the divide.

As it hugs the Continental Divide, the trail temporarily changes residency, taking you into Montana as it traverses the open west side of the divide. After returning to the ridge-top in about 0.25 mile, you pass above a small pond on the Idaho (left) side of the trail and make a brief but steep climb to the base of a rocky and rounded knoll. From here you climb some more to a high point on the east shoulder of this knoll.

Now back in Idaho, the trail drops about 100 feet, passing a series of colorful limestone cliffs on your right, to a junction with Trail #112 to Fritz Creek Cabin. You go straight and soon regain the lost elevation to the top of a high, grassy ridge. From here you'll have breathtaking views of the extremely rugged Idaho side of the Italian Peaks. Your goal is a cluster of three lakes that lie in a deep canyon hidden amid these scenic mountains.

To reach that goal, the trail steeply descends a partly forested hillside for a little less than 0.7 mile to an unsigned but obvious junction. Bear right here and follow this cut-off trail as it curves into the upper canyon of North Fork Webber Creek. After just 0.25 mile you merge with a trail coming up North Fork Webber Creek, and the combined routes then go gradually uphill for a little less than 0.5 mile to the first Webber Lake.

This spectacular aquamarine body of water is rimmed with meadows and conifers and has tremendous views of the rugged peaks rimming this basin. If you have the understandable urge to stay awhile, very good camps are amid the trees near the outlet and at the upper end of the lake.

It's difficult to imagine that the scenery could get much better than this lake, but it actually does. So keep hiking and make a steep and rocky ascent of 0.3 mile to the second Webber Lake, which is even closer to the towering cliffs and is even more dramatic than the first lake. There is a good camp here on top of a little knoll near the lake's west end.

To reach the third and final lake, follow the motorcycle-eroded trail as it climbs fairly steeply away from Webber Creek and into the rocky areas at the base of the canyon's north wall. The third lake in this amazing chain is 1 mile from the second lake. This high alpine gem has almost no

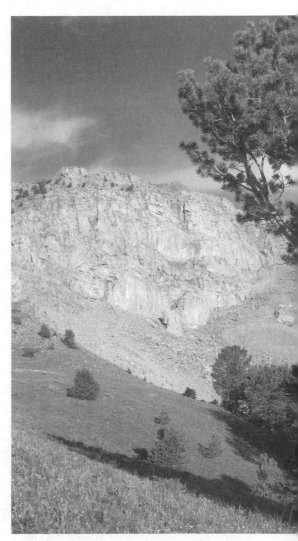

Limestone cliffs south of Divide Creek Lake

trees around it and is backed on three sides by snowfields and cliffs of twisted rock rising nearly 1,900 feet directly up to several imposing peaks, the highest of which is the 11,378-foot Scott Peak. The lake is completely surrounded by rocky shores, which makes camping effectively impossible. Budget as much time as possible for lots of gaping, before you reluctantly return to Divide Creek Lake the way you came.

Stark alpine cliffs above third Webber Lake

Deadman Creek Basin: After returning to your base camp at Divide Creek Lake, the other highly recommended day hike takes you over the border into Montana and up to a scenic basin with no lakes, but plenty of wildlife and virtually guaranteed solitude. To find it, start hiking from Divide Creek Lake as you did when going to the Webber Lakes. As before, you will reach the unsigned fork just below the Continental Divide after 0.25 mile.

Take the right fork this time and follow an unofficial but good trail that goes over the little ridge forming the Continental Divide and steeply down the other side to a meadow. Here you make an easy hop-over crossing of Deadman Creek and come to a junction with a trail along the creek's west side. Turn left (south) on this trail, which is supposed to be closed to motor vehicles, though this rule is all too frequently ignored, and climb through forest to a crossing of a small, dry lake bed. The creek is now dry as well, so except for snow patches that linger into early July, there is no water to be found in this drainage. From here the trail ascends steadily but never steeply through increasingly open terrain to the high basin at the head of Deadman Creek. Ringed by 11,000-foot peaks, this is an extremely scenic spot. Be sure to scan the steep slopes in this area because mountain goats and sometimes bighorn sheep are often seen here. The recommended turnaround point is the indistinct high point on the divide between the drainages of Deadman Creek and Nicholia Creek to the west. From here you have a jaw-dropping view of the towering cliffs on the northeast side of Italian Peak rising over the high basin at the head of Nicholia Creek. This spot is only about 4.5 miles from Divide Creek Lake and, despite the world-class scenery, is one you are very likely to have all to yourself.

Having filled your time (and your camera's memory card) with enough memorable images to last for years, return to your car the way you came.

POSSIBLE ITINERARY

	CAMP	MILES	ELEVATION GAIN
Day 1	Divide Creek Lake	6.0	1,700'
Day 2	Divide Creek Lake (day hike to Webber Lakes)	9.0	2,400'
Day 3	Divide Creek Lake (day hike to Deadman Creek Basin)	9.0	1,600'
Day 4	Out	6.0	100'

BEST SHORTER ALTERNATIVE

It is possible to do two of the principal highlights of this trip as day hikes. Unless you live in Idaho Falls and get an early start, however, you will probably have to car camp in the area to make this work. Divide Creek Lake is a reasonable day hike from the Cow Camp Trailhead as described above. To reach the Webber Lakes as a day hike, you should begin from the Webber Creek Trailhead near Webber Creek Campground. This trailhead is at the end of the rough (but drivable) FS 196, which you can reach directly off of Medicine Lodge Road on the drive up.

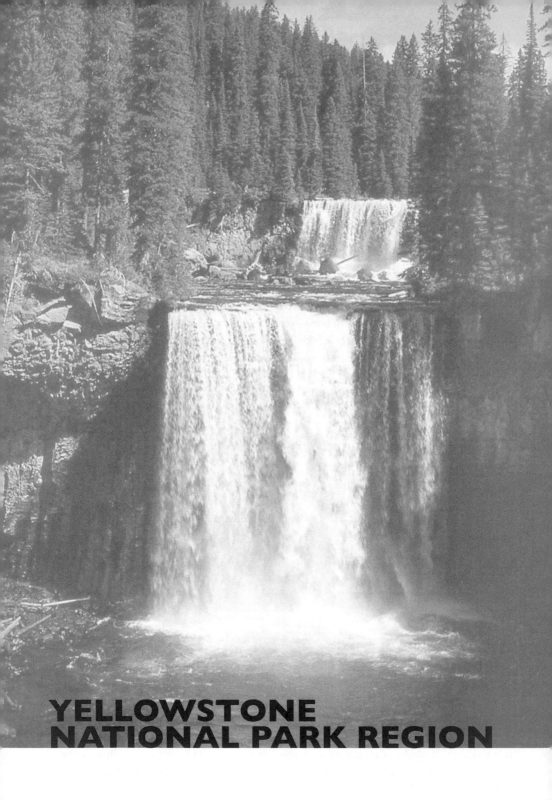

YELLOWSTONE
NATIONAL PARK REGION

Colonnade Falls (Trip 22)

W hile most of the world-famous Yellowstone National Park is in Wyoming, both Montana and Idaho proudly claim small parts of the magnificent preserve. Though the park's narrow western strip in Idaho has none of the geysers that made the park famous, in Yellowstone's southwest corner visitors will discover one of the highest concentrations of waterfalls in the Rocky Mountains. Trails along the Bechler River and its tributaries take visitors to waterfalls of every conceivable shape, size, and height.

This part of Yellowstone is accessible only by a gravel road from Idaho, so there are none of the crowds found in other parts of the park. And while wildlife may be less prevalent than it is in the more famous parts of Yellowstone, the animals here are less accustomed to people, so they are truly wild and therefore more natural.

Of course, one of the wildlife species for which Yellowstone is famous is the grizzly bear, and hikers may or may not be happy about the possibility of encountering this powerful denizen of the forest. The odds of seeing, much less being attacked by, a bear are extremely low, but backpackers are well advised to take extra precautions to avoid an encounter. Bear bells are not officially sanctioned, but they are not discouraged either. If you see a grizzly bear, give it a wide berth and consider turning around and staying out of its territory.

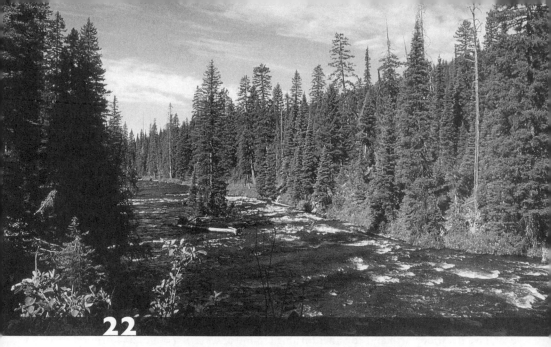

22

BECHLER RIVER TRAILS

RATINGS: Scenery 7 Solitude 3 Difficulty 3 (except for the fords, which can be very challenging)

MILES: 41

ELEVATION GAIN: 1,700'

DAYS: 3–5

MAP(S): Trails Illustrated *Old Faithful: Yellowstone National Park SW*

USUALLY OPEN: Mid-July–October

BEST: Late August–early October

PERMITS: Yes. Only a limited number of permits are available. The surest way to get the campsites you want is with a reservation. For a $25 fee (as of 2015), you can reserve a permit in advance by downloading a form from **nps.gov/yell/planyourvisit/backcountryhiking.htm.** Mail the form to Central Backcountry Office, Box 168, Yellowstone National Park, WY 82190, or fax it to 307-344-2166. All reservation requests received before April 1 will be processed and filled in random order.

RULES: Camping is allowed only at designated sites. Campfires are prohibited except in established fire pits at some campsites. For safety purposes, you are legally required to keep a clean camp; to properly hang all food, garbage, and other odorous items; and to report any aggressive bear activity. Anglers are required to have a special Yellowstone fishing license.

CONTACT: Yellowstone National Park, Backcountry Office, 307-344-2160. (Ask specifically for the informative brochure titled "Backcountry Trip Planner.")

Above: Bechler River in Bechler Canyon

SPECIAL ATTRACTIONS •

Waterfalls; wildlife

CHALLENGES •

Bears—both grizzly and black; several difficult stream crossings, especially before August; flooded areas in Bechler Meadows in early summer; clouds of mosquitoes June–early August

HOW TO GET THERE •

From Idaho Falls, drive 53 miles northeast on US 20 to a junction in the town of Ashton. Turn right (east) on ID 47, following signs to Mesa Falls Scenic Byway, and drive 1 mile to a junction just east of town. Go straight, staying on ID 47, and drive another 5.2 miles to a junction with Cave Falls Road. Turn right (east) on this paved road, which turns to gravel after 5.8 miles and becomes Forest Service Road 582. Exactly 16.6 miles from ID 47 is a junction immediately after the sign marking where you enter Wyoming. Turn left and drive 1.5 miles to the trailhead parking area beside the Bechler River Ranger Station. If you don't already have a reservation, you can pick up a back-country permit at this station, which opens at 8 a.m.

INTRODUCTION •

If you like the sight and sound of falling water, then you've hit the mother lode, because waterfalls are the prime attraction in this quiet corner of Yellowstone National Park. Sometimes called Cascade Corner, this compact area contains well over half of the park's waterfalls. The beauty and variety of the dozens of waterfalls here more than compensate for the lack of geysers, mud pots, and roadside bears, which have combined to make other parts of the park so famous. If the many trail-accessible waterfalls aren't enough, adventurous hikers can spend weeks happily bushwhacking to numerous cascades hidden in side canyons or on isolated sections of the main streams that the trails do not reach.

Though visitors to the Bechler (pronounced "Bek-ler") River country may be sorry to miss Yellowstone's famous geysers, they will be glad to be rid of the crowds, for which Yellowstone is also famous. Though the trails here certainly aren't deserted, the number of visitors is only a tiny fraction of what it is in other parts of the park.

WARNING: Both grizzly and black bears are present in this part of Yellowstone National Park. Though grizzly bears are uncommon here, you need to plan for their presence and act accordingly. See page 11 for more information on traveling in grizzly country. Black bears, though not as aggressive as their larger cousins, can be dangerous, and these smaller bruins are quite common in the Bechler River area. Park rangers strictly enforce the rules, which require that hikers properly hang their food and other odorous items from the wires provided at all designated campsites anytime they are away from camp, even for a few minutes.

The only road access to this area is from Idaho, so even though these trails are actually in the state of Wyoming, logic dictates that this trip is properly classified as an Idaho hike.

This hike is strictly for those who don't mind getting their feet, calves, knees, thighs, and maybe even waist wet. To enhance the area's wild character, the Park Service has

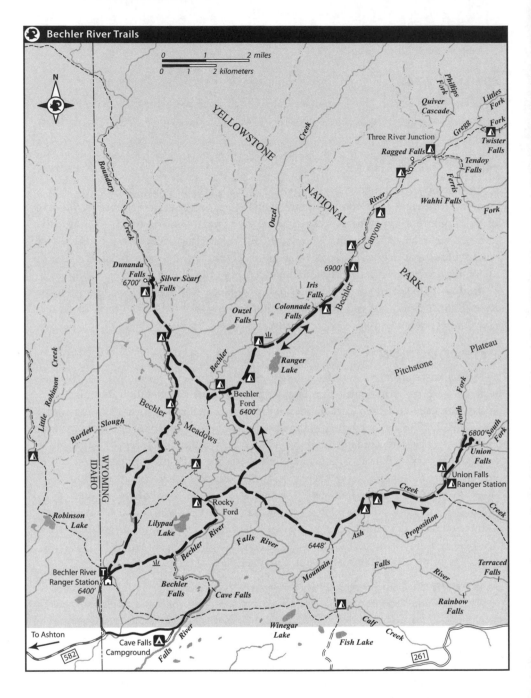

Bechler River Trails

0   1   2 miles
0   1   2 kilometers

YELLOWSTONE

NATIONAL

PARK

Phillips Fork
Quiver Cascade
Littles Fork
Gregg
Three River Junction
Ragged Falls
Twister Falls
Tendoy Falls
Ferris
Wahhi Falls
Fork

Creek

Ouzel

River
Canyon

6900'

Iris Falls
Colonnade Falls
Bechler

Ouzel Falls

Pitchstone   Plateau

Dunanda Falls
6700'
Silver Scarf Falls

Ranger Lake

Bechler

North Fork
South Fork
6800'
Union Falls

Bechler Ford
6400'

Bechler Meadows

Union Falls Ranger Station

Boundary   Creek

Little Robinson Creek
Robinson Creek

Bartlett Slough

WYOMING
IDAHO

Rocky Ford

Lilypad Lake

Bechler River
Falls River

Creek
Ash
Proposition
Creek

6448'

Robinson Lake

Falls

Terraced Falls

River

Bechler River Ranger Station
6400'

Bechler Falls

Cave Falls

Mountain

Falls

Rainbow Falls

To Ashton
582

Cave Falls Campground

Falls   River

Winegar Lake

Fish Lake

Calf   Creek

261

removed most of the trail bridges, which forces hikers to make numerous wet and potentially dangerous fords of the Bechler River and its tributaries. Bring a walking stick and
wading shoes for improved stability at the crossings, and save this trip for late summer,
when water levels are lower. Unfortunately, the waterfalls are marginally less impressive at
that time, but it beats drowning.

DESCRIPTION •

The Bechler Meadows Trail, which is marked only with a small metal sign, begins at the northeast end of the complex of historic buildings around the Bechler River Ranger Station. After 100 yards, the trail crosses a trickling creek on a log bridge and reaches a junction. If Union Falls is your first destination, then turn right and walk a nearly level trail through open forests of lodgepole pine with grasses, huckleberries, and various wildflowers on the forest floor. After 1 mile, you pass a large meadow with a shallow, lily pad–filled lake at its center, and then come to a junction beside the slow-moving waters of Bechler River.

You turn left, following signs for Rocky Ford, and closely follow the glassy river upstream. By late summer, which is the best season to take this hike, most of the wild-flowers in this area are long gone, but there should still be a few yellow goldenrod and blue harebells in bloom. Unlike the flowers, birds are common throughout the hiking season, especially woodpeckers and various small songbirds. As for larger birds, you are likely to see great blue herons and ospreys. If you are really lucky, you might even see a goshawk swoop down and catch an unlucky duck off the river.

> **TIP:** Plenty of rainbow and cutthroat trout are in the stream, but if you want to try to catch any of them, you'll need a special Yellowstone fishing permit and barbless hooks because the river is managed strictly for catch-and-release fishing.

The trail follows the Bechler River for 2 miles to a junction, where you turn right and immediately face the prospect of going across the 100-foot-wide Rocky Ford. In early summer this crossing can be extremely treacherous, but by late summer it's only a little over knee-deep. The water is always cold, however, and slippery rocks make the footing difficult, so be careful. The best place to ford is about 30 feet downstream from here.

The trail leaves the river at Rocky Ford and wanders across somewhat drier terrain covered with a nice mix of open forests and grassy meadows. Just less than 1 mile from the ford is a junction with the Mountain Ash Creek Trail, where you bear slightly right and walk 0.5 mile to a flat-topped log over a small creek at the edge of a beautiful, grassy meadow. The trail then goes through gently rolling terrain covered with lodgepole pine forests, a few quaking aspen trees, and dry meadows that are sparsely vegetated with scattered wildflowers and some sagebrush. Eventually, you come to a large meadow and a junction with a dusty, heavily used trail coming from the south.

You bear left, still following signs to Union Falls, and walk 1 mile to a junction with a short side trail to Camp 9U2. About 200 yards past this turnoff is the tricky, knee-deep ford of the swift-flowing Mountain Ash Creek. When I crossed, there was a rather precarious log over this creek a little upstream from the ford, but its future seemed pretty doubtful, so you should expect to get wet. Right after the crossing is Camp 9U3, a primitive, low-impact site, where fires are prohibited.

To continue on to Union Falls, walk gradually up Mountain Ash Creek through increasingly wet forests and meadows that now include more Engelmann spruces and Douglas-firs as well as wildflowers such as coneflower and monkshood. Though the flora has changed, the terrain remains nearly flat, so you may start to wonder how such a gentle landscape can have so many waterfalls. The answer lies a short distance to the north, where a line of rocky cliffs marks the edge of the Pitchstone Plateau. It is over these cliffs that the falls drop.

About 1.5 miles from the ford of Mountain Ash Creek is a junction. You bear slightly left and walk 0.4 mile to a junction with a side trail to the comfortable Camp 9U4 and a ford of South Fork Mountain Ash Creek.

TIP: To keep your feet dry, simply walk 60 yards up the side trail to the camp and then cross the creek on a flat-topped log.

After the crossing the trail goes 150 yards up the peninsula of land between the north and south forks of Mountain Ash Creek to the tiny, A-frame building at the Union Falls Ranger Station. The trail then passes the turnoff to Camp 9U5 and gradually climbs 1 mile on a sometimes-sandy tread to a trail fork.

Both forks of this dead-end trail are worth taking. For more subtle scenery, take the left fork, which leads 0.3 mile up North Fork Mountain Ash Creek to a small, cascading waterfall and a nice swimming hole. The more spectacular right fork climbs two switchbacks to an overlook of the 260-foot-high Union Falls, a broad veil of water that will take your breath away.

To see more of Yellowstone's waterfalls, return to the junction northeast of Rocky Ford and turn right (north) on the Bechler River Trail. This trail goes a few hundred yards through a meadow to a slow-moving creek, which you cross either on an unstable log or by a simple, knee-deep ford. A short walk through shady forest then takes you to a second creek crossing, this time on a larger, more stable log. After this, the trail climbs 200 feet up a small ridge, and then goes up and down on a mostly wooded hillside, where several small, splashing creeks provide water and nice places to rest. After 1 mile on this hillside, you lose a bit of elevation, and then walk beside the gently meandering Bechler River to a junction and your next choice of destinations.

To see Bechler Canyon, turn right at the junction and walk through a northeast extension of the grassy Bechler Meadows to Camp 9B3. The trail leaves the meadows here and wanders through forests for 0.5 mile back to the banks of Bechler River at very attractive Camp 9B4. If you look north through the trees here you can see the impressive, 235-foot-high Ouzel Falls, which drop over a cliff on the other side of the river. Unfortunately, a tricky river ford and a large marshy area prohibit easy access to the base of these falls.

The trail now follows the river upstream into beautiful, cliff-lined Bechler Canyon, which is a haven for some of Yellowstone's most charismatic wildlife. Don't be surprised to see black bears, which typically take a look at you, give a dismissive huff, and then go about their business. Or you could see moose, which are remarkably nonchalant and obligingly allow hikers to take their picture, as long as you don't get too close and make these large and potentially dangerous animals nervous.

In addition to wildlife and beautiful scenery, Bechler Canyon features unusually lush vegetation. The Bechler River area is the wettest part of Yellowstone National Park, because winter storms, which normally come from the southwest, dump their precipitation here first. The result of all this moisture is a dense forest of large Douglas-firs and Engelmann spruces with a thick understory of mountain ash, buffalo berry, horsetail, and gooseberry. The fern-lined trail also passes many wildflowers, including birchleaf spirea, coneflower, monkshood, Queen Anne's lace, grass-of-Parnassus, and a tall, white aster. In the latter half of August you can feast on both thimbleberries and huckleberries, though you'll be in competition with the bears for these tasty treats.

The trail closely follows the clear river upstream, often passing between the river and some large talus slopes where cute little pikas can often be seen and heard. Despite the rugged terrain on both sides of the narrow canyon, the trail manages to remain remarkably gentle as it stays in the shady forest beside the river. Not quite 2 miles from where it started up the canyon, the trail climbs more noticeably and you soon hear the thunderous roar of the canyon's first major cataract, Colonnade Falls. A 100-yard side trail descends to a dramatic overlook of this two-part falls, the lower half of which is a broad sheet of water that drops over a cliff into a basalt amphitheater. A short distance above Colonnade Falls is the very inviting Camp 9B5. This is an exceptionally nice place to spend the night, because not only is Colonnade Falls nearby, but just 400 yards upstream from this camp is Iris Falls. On sunny afternoons the wide drop of Iris Falls produces a lovely rainbow in its mist.

For the next mile above Iris Falls the river drops over a series of beautiful, gently sloping cascades. The trail provides lots of good views of these cascades as it gradually climbs to Camp 9B6 and, shortly thereafter, a knee-deep river ford over slippery rocks. This is far enough for most hikers because, in addition to this ford, you must make another one about 1 mile upstream and climb 2 more miles before you reach the next major highlight at Ragged Falls. If you are willing to make the hike, however, the rewards are great, including a series of hot springs, the impressive rock formation of Batchelder Column, and Three River Junction, where the three main forks of Bechler River all converge. If the sight of Ragged Falls inspires you to keep going, then continue fairly steeply uphill for 1.5

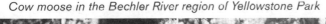

Cow moose in the Bechler River region of Yellowstone Park

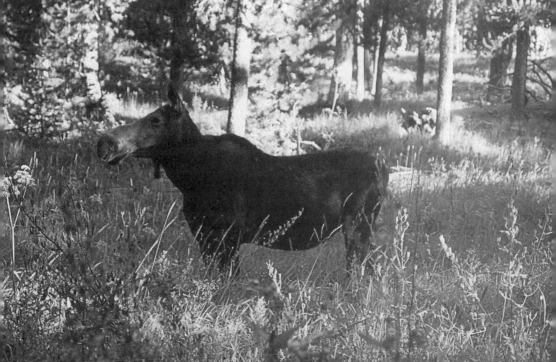

miles to the spinning drop of Twister Falls. Above these falls the trail gets gentler and you leave the lush canyon environment in favor of the drier, lodgepole pine forests that dominate most of Yellowstone National Park. Really ambitious hikers can keep going another 12 miles to Shoshone Geyser Basin and, from there, on to Old Faithful.

Having explored the wonders of Bechler Canyon, return to the junction at the edge of Bechler Meadows and bear right (west) toward your next major destination, Dunanda Falls. You soon go past a side trail to Camp 9B2 and, immediately thereafter, reach the thigh-deep Bechler Ford. This is one of the easiest major fords on this trip, because the water moves slowly and the sandy bottom provides good footing. The meadows near Bechler Ford are a good place to look for moose and sandhill cranes.

The trail immediately leaves the river and crosses part of the expansive Bechler Meadows, where you can look south across the waving fields of grass to the jagged spires of the distant Teton Range.

WARNING: In early summer, much of Bechler Meadows is flooded with a foot or more of water, which makes travel difficult and provides a breeding ground for an enormous population of voracious mosquitoes. The flying vampires don't completely disappear until sometime in September, so come prepared with bug repellent, long sleeves, and maybe even a head net.

About 0.4 mile from Bechler Ford is a junction, where you turn sharply right and walk 1.9 miles through meadows and forested terrain to a junction at the edge of a small meadow. Turn right and walk 600 yards through the meadow to a knee-deep ford of a branch of Boundary Creek. Immediately after the ford is the side trail to the designated backpacker area for Camp 9A2.

TIP: If you want to avoid the ford, walk about 75 yards downstream to a log across the creek, and return to the trail from the backpackers' camping area.

After the creek crossing, the trail goes gradually uphill for 1 mile through a 1995 burn area that is now covered with fields of bracken fern, sunflowers, and small lodgepole pines. You splash across several small creeks, and then reenter unburned forests and take a narrow log over a larger side creek. The trail soon passes a side trail to Camp 9A3; climbs steeply past the tall, flowing cascade of Silver Scarf Falls; and comes to a junction, where the Boundary Creek Trail goes steeply uphill and right.

To see Dunanda Falls, bear left and walk 200 yards to the top of this wide sheet of water, which drops into a scenic canyon of dark-gray rock. A very steep scramble route drops to the base of the falls, where you can soak in an idyllic hot-springs pool looking up at the spectacular, 110-foot falls and the rainbow they create on sunny days. Life just doesn't get much better than that!

To return to the Bechler River Ranger Station, go back to the junction just south of Camp 9A2 and bear right (south) on the Boundary Creek Trail. This nearly level route travels through forest, and then goes through the grassy, wildlife-rich area between the forest and the willow thickets beside the slow-moving Boundary Creek. Moose and beaver are common in this environment. After about 1 mile, you leave this life zone and cross the western part of Bechler Meadows to a calf-deep ford of Boundary Creek. Signs direct you to the best place to ford, which is about 100 yards downstream from here. Right after the ford is the scenic Camp 9A1 in a clump of trees near a lazy meander in the creek.

You go south from Camp 9A1 past a series of small tree islands amid the vast expanse of Bechler Meadows. You are likely to see at least a couple of pairs of tall sandhill cranes in this area, either feeding in the meadow or flying overhead and croaking their loud, guttural call. Less than 1 mile from the Boundary Creek crossing is a ford of Bartlett Slough, a stagnant backwater filled with lily pads. The slough can be up to 4 feet deep in early summer, but is usually only thigh-deep by August.

TIP: The bottom of Bartlett Slough is very muddy. Be sure that your wading shoes are securely tied, so they don't get sucked permanently into the goo.

After this crossing, the trail follows a gently rolling course through lodgepole pine woods, skirts a few small meadows, and passes a lily pond to a junction with the Bechler Meadows Trail. You bear slightly right and wander through open woods on a generally flat trail back to the junction just 100 yards east of the Bechler River Ranger Station.

VARIATIONS •

If you have some extra time and feel that a trip to Yellowstone just isn't complete unless you see a geyser, then continue up the Bechler Canyon Trail all the way to the Shoshone Geyser Basin. Because this area is too far away from the Bechler Canyon campsites for a comfortable day hike, you will need an overnight permit to stay at a nearby campsite, something that is nearly impossible without advance reservations.

POSSIBLE ITINERARY

	CAMP	MILES	ELEVATION GAIN
Day 1	Camp 9U4–below Union Falls (with side trip to Union Falls)	13.5	400'
Day 2	Camp 9B5–above Colonnade Falls (with side trip up Bechler Canyon)	12.0	600'
Day 3	Camp 9A3–below Dunanda Falls	7.5	500'
Day 4	Out	8.0	200'

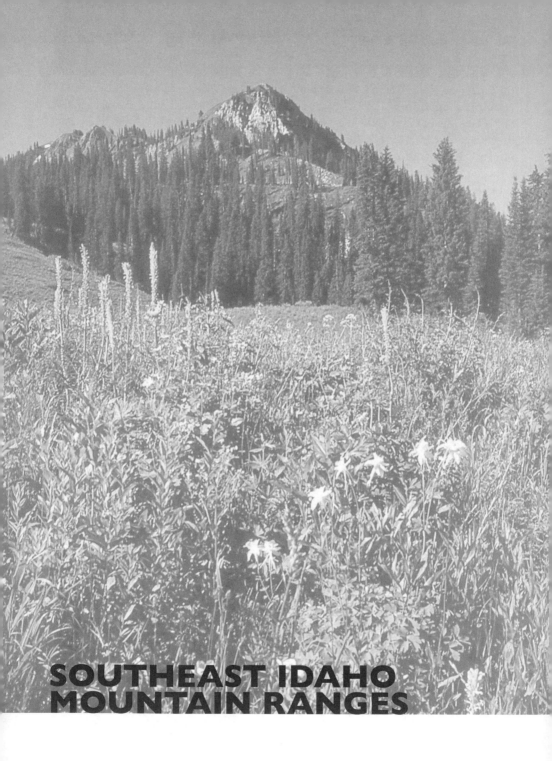

SOUTHEAST IDAHO
MOUNTAIN RANGES

Along the South Fork Indian Creek near Cabin Creek Canyon (Trip 23)

The southeast corner of Idaho is yet another scenic treasure in a state packed with glorious scenery. The landscape here is dominated by a series of relatively gentle mountain ranges separated by beautiful river valleys. The region has long been popular with vacationers, especially near Bear Lake, where people have built numerous summer homes and resorts. Despite this development, backpackers can still find solitude in the higher parts of the mountains, where the gentle, rolling hills become steeper and more rugged.

Winter snows are deep in these mountains, and when they melt, much of the water does something that is unique to this corner of Idaho. As part of the Great Basin, many of the streams here do not flow west toward the Columbia River and Pacific Ocean, as they do in the rest of the state, but travel south via the Bear River to Utah's Great Salt Lake, where the water simply evaporates and never reaches the ocean at all.

It's easy to get confused by the mountain ranges here because their names bear little relationship to any sort of logical geography. Often the name of what is clearly a single chain of mountains changes for no better reason than that a highway happens to cross the range. One continuous series of peaks, for example, goes by the name Big Hole Mountains in the north, is called the Snake River Range in the middle, and mysteriously changes again to become the Salt River Range in Wyoming.

Regardless of what you call them, these mountains are crucially important wildlife habitat, because they provide a corridor of wild land that connects the Greater Yellowstone Ecosystem to the north with the mountains of southern Wyoming and northern Utah. This corridor allows species such as moose and elk to extend their ranges and maintain the genetic diversity of their populations. In addition to these species, hikers stand a good chance of seeing mountain goats and black bears. There are even a few stray grizzly bears, though the species is so rare there is no need for hikers, even paranoid ones, to wear bear bells or lose sleep at night.

Fall is a particularly fetching time to visit this area, because the mountains support an abundance of quaking aspens, narrowleaf cottonwoods, and Rocky Mountain maples. In late September and early October these species combine to create some of the best fall-color displays in the state. The mid-elevation hillsides, especially above Palisades Reservoir, come alive with colorful splashes of vivid yellows, oranges, and reds that will dazzle the eye and keep photographers happy for days. Just keep an eye on the weather, because the first hard freeze or strong wind will quickly end the year's foliage display.

These mountains are part of the Overthrust Belt, which is at the center of a long-standing controversy. Oil and gas companies believe that this area holds significant energy reserves, and they strongly advocate drilling and exploration. Conservationists, concerned about the impact of drilling on the region's wildlife, scenery, and recreational values, are fighting these plans. Before making up your mind on this controversy, visit this magnificent region and see what is at stake.

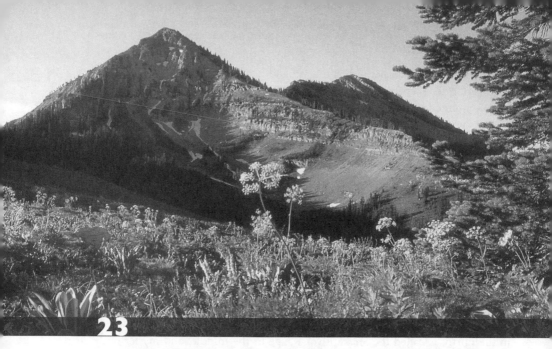

23

SNAKE RIVER RANGE TRAVERSE

RATINGS: Scenery 8   Solitude 6   Difficulty 8

MILES: 45

SHUTTLE MILEAGE: 19

ELEVATION GAIN: 9,800'

DAYS: 3–6

MAP(S): USGS *Alpine*, USGS *Ferry Peak*, USGS *Mount Baird*, USGS *Observation Peak*, USGS *Palisades Peak*, USGS *Teton Pass*, USGS *Thompson Peak* (all are wholly or partially in Wyoming except *Thompson Peak*)

USUALLY OPEN: Mid-June–mid-October

BEST: Mid-July, late September–early October

PERMITS: None

RULES: The usual Leave No Trace principles apply.

CONTACT: Palisades Ranger District, 208-523-1412

SPECIAL ATTRACTIONS •

Fall colors; great wildflower displays; wildlife

CHALLENGES •

Several moderately difficult stream crossings; mosquitoes in July; motorbikes allowed in the Indian Creek area; sketchy trail in places; several long, dry, steep climbs

Above: Mount Baird

HOW TO GET THERE •

Start by driving 50 miles southeast of Idaho Falls on US 26 to a signed junction with Palisades Creek Road (also known as Forest Service Road 255). To leave a car at the north trailhead, turn left (northeast) on this oiled gravel road, following signs for Palisades Creek Campground, and drive 2.1 miles to the campground and well-developed trailhead. Horse trailers and livestock facilities dominate the trailhead area, so the best parking for hikers is in a gravel lot just before the bridge over Palisades Creek.

To reach the recommended starting point, continue southeast on US 26 for 13.7 miles past the Palisades Creek turnoff; then turn left (east) onto FS 281 at the head of a large inlet in Palisades Reservoir. Proceed 1.9 miles on this narrow gravel road to a fork near the confluence of the North and South Forks of Indian Creek. Go straight, staying on the better road, and drive 1.6 miles to the South Fork Indian Creek trailhead, where a fence line marks the border with Wyoming.

INTRODUCTION •

The Snake River Range contains the most jagged peaks, the prettiest lakes, and the best fishing streams of any mountains in southeast Idaho. The range is at its scenic best in mid-July, when the meadows are ablaze with colorful wildflowers, and again in late September and early October, when the hillsides are covered with the yellow, orange, and red of aspens, cottonwoods, and maples. Regardless of the season, wildlife is a common sight along the trails, including elk, moose, and black bear. There are even reports of an occasional stray grizzly bear, though they are so rare that hikers don't need to take any special precautions.

Though much of this hike is in Wyoming, it is categorized as an Idaho trip, because the road access and both trailheads are in that state.

It is better to start this hike from the south trailhead, especially if you begin on a weekend, because the popular north trailhead is often very busy. This also allows you to benefit from a net elevation loss of 600 feet. This hike includes several relentless uphills that have no water or shade. Avoid this trip during a spell of hot weather.

DESCRIPTION •

From the east end of the trailhead parking lot, you cross the fence at the state line, and walk along a jeep road for 100 yards to the start of the trail. This route is open to motorbikes, so the path is wide, dusty, and sometimes noisy. Apart from the motorbike problems, the hiking is very pleasant, as the trail goes upstream beside the lovely South Fork Indian Creek through a lush mix of grasses and tall wildflowers such as coneflower and cow parsnip. The tree cover includes both evergreen and deciduous species, especially Engelmann spruces, Douglas-firs, quaking aspens, and narrowleaf cottonwoods.

About 0.5 mile from the trailhead, you bear left at a junction with the Driveway Canyon Trail and, 200 yards later, come to a crossing of South Fork Indian Creek. On a hot afternoon during the June snowmelt this stream can be a raging torrent, but by mid-July it's no more than ankle-deep. There may even be a convenient log over the flow. Now on the north side of the creek, the trail goes gradually uphill, either traveling close to the creek's bank amid lush, riparian vegetation or crossing rocky slopes a little above the water. These drier slopes feature a different mix of colorful wildflowers, including skyrocket gilia, groundsel, yarrow, aster, pink geranium, birchleaf spirea, and harebells.

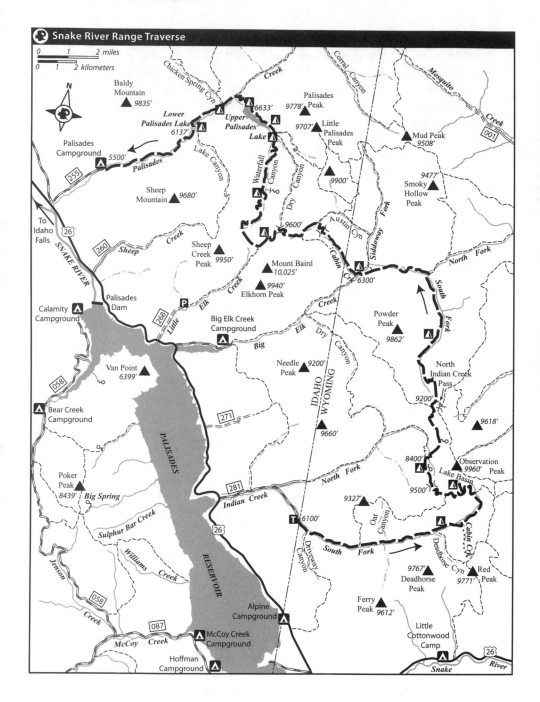

Snake River Range Traverse

With every added mile the scenery becomes more dramatic as you pass through increasingly large avalanche meadows that provide ever-improving views of the high peaks on either side of the canyon. In late September, the quaking aspens that rim these meadows put on an impressive display of color.

WARNING: The avalanche meadows encountered along this trip are often filled with stinging nettles. Wear long pants and be careful of what you brush up against.

At one of the largest of these meadows, about 3 miles from the trailhead, an easily overlooked sign marks a junction with the Little Oat Canyon Trail, a faint path that angles left. You continue straight and for the next 2 miles climb through brushy avalanche meadows crossed by a series of small side creeks that splash down from the high ridge to the north. In addition to wildflowers, the meadows are home to many deer and, in early summer, it is common to come across a small, spotted fawn squeaking out an alarm call at your arrival. The meadows are also excellent habitat for black bears, so keep an eye out for them.

About 5 miles from the trailhead the meadows are broken by strips of trees, which give you a chance to rest in the shade. This opportunity is welcome, because the grade of the climb picks up in this area and you'll really start to feel that heavy pack on your back. At the 6.5-mile point is a junction with an unsigned and little-used trail up Deadhorse Canyon, a grassy defile to the south that is worth exploring if you have the time. Just after this junction you enter a small strip of forest with a good campsite. About 200 yards beyond the campsite is the second crossing of South Fork Indian Creek.

WARNING: Though it looks like an easy rock-hop crossing, the rocks here are very slippery; it is much safer to make the ford.

The trail then makes a short climb away from the crossing and soon comes to a junction with the abandoned Cabin Creek Trail. This sketchy path ascends a beautiful sloping meadow that provides good views up to several nearby rocky peaks. In July, however, your attention is more likely to be drawn to the meadow's abundant wildflowers. Look for great displays of pink geranium, locoweed, giant hyssop (a member of the mint family), wild carrot, lousewort, and a large, white variety of columbine.

The main trail goes straight at the Cabin Creek junction and continues its moderately steep ascent, mostly through spacious, rolling meadows. Just before South Fork Indian Creek makes a sweeping curve to the north, you cross the now-small stream a final time, and then make a single switchback and resume the long, shadeless climb. The trail passes to the right of some low cliffs, and then makes an easy ascent to a junction with the Indian Peak Trail. You turn left and climb through a gently rolling meadowland to the delightful Lake Basin. This large, flowery expanse is backed by Observation Peak to the north and features two medium-size ponds set in grassy basins above the trail. Obvious boot paths lead to these ponds, and good campsites are found in the trees near each of them. The campsites near the larger pond to the north are better and more scenic.

TIP: From a base camp in this basin you can make a terrific day hike up the Indian Peak Trail to the high ridgeline of the Snake River Range. From there, you can follow view-packed routes to the tops of both Indian and Observation Peaks.

To exit Lake Basin, the trail turns west, switchbacks three times to the top of a small ridge, and makes a gradual downhill traverse to an obscure junction near a small pond in a scenic basin. You bear right and make a short, steep climb to a 9,500-foot pass. From this high vantage point you can not only look south to South Fork Indian Creek canyon, but also north to the rugged peaks and valleys that you'll be traversing for the rest of this trip.

The sometimes-obscure trail now makes an uneven descent across lovely, rolling meadows to a bubbling spring next to an elaborate hunter's camp. This camp is reserved for use by a commercial outfitter from late August to November, but at other times you are allowed to camp here.

WARNING: The camp has piles of horse manure and lots of flies, so backpackers probably won't want to stay here.

There are many confusing horse trails around this camp. The correct route stays below the main camp and follows a little creek through a sloping meadow for 300 yards to a signed junction with a trail to North Indian Creek Pass. If you only want to do a short loop, go straight and hike 7 miles down the North Indian Trail, back to the road fork 1.6 miles from your car.

For the full traverse, you turn right, hop over North Fork Indian Creek, and begin a series of little ups and downs. After climbing over a couple of low ridges, you pass a small spring, and then contour across a steeply sloping meadow just below some reddish cliffs. The trail then climbs eight irregularly spaced switchbacks, which steeply gain 600 feet on a sun-exposed slope that can be uncomfortably hot on a summer afternoon. Fortunately, the trail provides great views down the deep canyon of North Fork Indian Creek, so you have plenty of excuses for rest stops.

The trail tops out at a junction in the wide saddle a little west of North Indian Creek Pass. The trail to the left follows the top of a high, view-packed ridge for several miles before dropping to Big Elk Creek. The first few miles of this trail make a wonderfully scenic side trip. The main trail bears slightly right and winds steeply down into the little basin at the head of South Fork Big Elk Creek. Near the top of this basin is a junction with a trail that switchbacks up to North Indian Creek Pass on the ridge to the east. This trail is a worthwhile side trip for those who want a nice view into the vastness of Wyoming.

Your trail goes straight at the junction and traverses the steep slopes above the ever-deepening canyon of South Fork Big Elk Creek. After a little less than 1 mile, you bear left (downhill) at an unsigned fork and soon descend a set of eight well-graded switchbacks. These take you down to the meadows at the bottom of the canyon and an easy rock-hop crossing of the creek. The sketchy trail disappears just after the crossing. The correct route gains a little elevation, and then turns and closely follows the west bank of the creek. After a short while the trail enters the forest and the tread becomes more obvious. About 0.5 mile below the crossing is a decent campsite in the trees on the right.

The next 3.5 miles are an easy and very attractive walk that takes you gradually downhill through a series of large meadows beside the cascading waters of South Fork Big Elk Creek.

TIP: Be sure to look behind you from time to time to enjoy excellent views over the meadows to the jagged peaks at the creek's headwaters.

About 6 miles from North Indian Creek Pass is an easy, ankle-deep ford of the creek and a sign marking a junction with an obscure trail up North Fork Big Elk Creek. You bear slightly left on the more obvious trail and soon cross North Fork Big Elk Creek on a log.

The trail now follows Big Elk Creek downstream through meadows and open forests and past willow bogs with lots of beaver activity. Look for moose in these bogs feasting on the tasty, wet vegetation. Even if there aren't any moose around, you can usually count on seeing birds, which abound in this varied habitat. Mornings are particularly active, because the forest then is filled with the songs of western tanagers, American robins, white-crowned and chipping sparrows, red-breasted nuthatches, yellow-rumped warblers, various species of hummingbirds, and numerous others. After about 0.8 mile, you come to a ford of the creek. The water is cold and about knee-deep, but it isn't very swift, so the crossing is fairly easy. As I was preparing to make this ford, a large mountain lion came sauntering by on the other side of the creek. Once it caught sight of me, the lion slowly walked off into the trees and watched me cross.

TIP: Anglers might want to try their luck in Big Elk Creek because the stream has lots of trout.

You may as well leave the wading shoes on for a while, because you'll need them a few hundred yards later, when you have to ford the creek again, and 0.5 mile after that at a third crossing. After the third crossing you can put your boots back on, because the next ford is more than 1 mile away.

The trail climbs briefly from the third ford and makes an up-and-down traverse through the forests above the canyon of Big Elk Creek. You soon come to a small meadow and a junction with a connector to the Siddoway Fork Trail, which angles downhill to the right. You bear slightly left on the more heavily used trail and then descend six switchbacks to the final and most difficult crossing of Big Elk Creek. In early summer this ford is about thigh-deep and the water is quite swift, so you might want to scout around for a shallower crossing downstream. Unfortunately, no logs are nearby, so there is no alternative to getting wet.

Once on the other side of the creek, you reach a signed junction with the Siddoway Fork Trail. You go left and almost immediately come to a good campsite on the bench above the creek. Just 150 yards past this campsite is another junction, where you turn right on the very faint Cabin Canyon Trail. The junction is marked only with a small brown sign that faces toward hikers coming from the other direction, so look carefully for the sign.

WARNING: The rugged Cabin Canyon Trail receives little or no maintenance, so be prepared to climb over some deadfall and fight through overgrown areas. In addition to obscuring the trail, these overgrown areas have quite a few blackberries and stinging nettles, so you'll need to wear long pants. The trail's most difficult challenge comes near the head of the canyon, where the route diminishes to little more than a hypothetical dotted line on the map and forces hikers to travel cross-country to relocate the tread.

For a longer but less challenging alternate route, try the Austin Canyon Trail. To reach it, turn right on the Siddoway Fork Trail from the junction above the last ford of Big Elk Creek. After 1.5 miles, turn left on the Austin Canyon Trail and climb 4 miles to a junction with the Cabin Canyon Trail. This route is a little more than 2 miles longer than the more direct route up Cabin Canyon, but it is easier to follow.

On the Cabin Canyon Trail you face a minor navigation problem almost immediately, as the tread disappears in a narrow, flowery meadow. To relocate the trail, simply walk northwest through the meadow and look for old blazes when you get back to the trees. Once back in the forest, the now-more-obvious tread ascends beside the dry creek bed at the bottom of the canyon past a series of talus slopes that are home to a large population of pikas. Less than 1 mile into this climb, you cross the unsigned border and reenter Idaho.

For the next couple of miles the fairly steep climb becomes increasingly overgrown. Though the hiking is a bit tedious, you shouldn't lose the tread if you just stick to the right (northeast) side of the dry creek bed. About one third of the way up the canyon, an intermittent trickle of water flows at the bottom of the creek bed, allowing you to splash water over your head and cool off on a hot afternoon.

TIP: Fill up on water here because this is the last water source for several very tough miles.

From here on the climbing is almost entirely in meadows, either of tall grasses, which obscure the trail in the lower canyon, or of shorter wildflowers that dominate the upper canyon slopes. In both places shade is nonexistent, so on a hot day you'll sweat gallons.

About halfway up the canyon the trail pulls its disappearing act. The overgrown tread fades away completely in the grasses and, adding to the confusion, sketchy game paths head up almost every side canyon. The newly rerouted trail shown on the U.S. Forest Service map, which is extremely difficult to locate on the ground, turns left *somewhere,* goes up one of several side canyons, and then climbs around the left (west) side of an unnamed high point to a junction with the Austin Canyon Trail. Because you probably won't be able to find this trail, your best bet is to go cross-country straight through the upper canyon's grassy meadows, and then climb the very steep slopes on the canyon's headwall to a low notch in the ridge just to the right of a high, unnamed peak.

Once you reach the pass, the trail becomes obvious as it goes down several extremely steep switchbacks to the meadow at the bottom of Austin Canyon. You cross a small creek in this canyon, which has much-needed water, and come to a cairn marking the junction with the Austin Canyon Trail, where you join the alternate route from the Siddoway Fork.

You turn left (west) and climb at a moderately steep grade for 0.5 mile to where the creek goes under a small but interesting stone arch. More climbing takes you through steep, view-packed meadows; then the trail flattens out, goes over the now-dry creek bed, and crosses to the left side of a large meadow. On the south side of the meadow is a waterless camp and a signed junction with the newly rerouted but faint Cabin Canyon Trail.

You turn right at the junction and gradually climb through meadows and past a few groves of subalpine firs toward the impressive, tan cliffs at the head of Austin Canyon. The trail disappears in these upper meadows, but you can find it again if you angle right and look for an obvious trail that goes up the steep slopes on the north headwall. The last 0.5 mile climbs very steeply up a shadeless slope of loose rocks to a junction in a pass with a good view north down Dry Canyon. The trail to the right follows Dry Canyon to Upper Palisades Lake and is a pleasant shortcut, especially if the weather is bad. If you take that trail, however, you will miss Waterfall Canyon, one of the highlights of the trip, so I recommend that you turn left.

After the long climb to the pass, you were probably looking forward to some downhill. But you'll have to put those hopes on hold for a little while longer, because first the trail climbs steeply along the top of a ridge. After gaining another 300 feet, the trail finally tops out on a side ridge and makes a long downhill traverse. At the bottom of this traverse are two switchbacks just before you enter a basin directly beneath an unnamed, pyramid-shaped mountain. In early summer a tiny snowmelt creek flows out of this basin, providing water for a scenic campsite.

The faint trail goes several hundred yards across the basin and then steeply ascends the ridge to the southwest. It is possible, and fairly easy, to avoid this climb by leaving the trail and rambling to the west across rolling meadows for about 1 mile until you hit the Waterfall Canyon Trail. But if you do that, you will miss perhaps the best views of the trip. So take the sketchy trail to the top of the ridge, and then drop your pack and gawk. The high peak to the south is Mount Baird, the tallest summit in this area at 10,025 feet. To the southwest you can see a part of the large Palisades Reservoir, while to the northwest is a rolling, grassy basin at the head of Waterfall Canyon. On a really clear day you can even see the jagged Teton Range in the distance to the northeast. The flowers on this high ridge are also outstanding. The peak bloom, in mid-July, features a colorful collage of blue larkspur, pink vetch and geranium, white wild carrot, red paintbrush, and yellow balsamroot.

The official trail descends a short distance, and then turns right and climbs back up the south side of the ridge. But there's no need for you to lose this elevation, because it's just as easy, and more scenic, to simply turn right and walk along the open, view-packed ridgeline for several hundred yards until you meet the official trail angling up from the left. Shortly after this, you go straight at a signed junction with the Little Elk Trail and make a moderately graded downhill traverse to the rolling basin at the head of Waterfall Canyon.

The trail wanders down through this delightful basin, which has lots of flowers and excellent views of the surrounding peaks and ridges. You soon pass an easily overlooked junction with an abandoned trail, and then exit the basin via six gently graded switchbacks through a pleasant mix of forest and small meadows.

TIP: Quiet hikers stand a good chance of seeing deer and elk in this area.

After these switchbacks, you follow a dry creek bed (the water flows underground) past a pair of seasonal waterfalls, and then make seven more downhill switchbacks. When the trail levels out, you cross the rocky creek bed twice and enter a large meadow that holds a small lake. The highlight of the scenery here is a tall waterfall that emerges from a cave high on the canyon's east wall and drops several hundred feet in a series of cascades to the lake. It's quite impressive and dramatically demonstrates how Waterfall Canyon got its name. Some very good campsites are at the north end of the lake, though they tend to be quite buggy.

Immediately below the lake, the water goes back underground, so you are left to follow a dry creek bed once again as you gradually descend through meadows and forested areas. Things get steeper when you come to the edge of an old glacial basin and descend eight well-graded switchbacks past an unseen spring on your left. At the bottom of the switchbacks the trail lazily descends through a forested area with lots of huckleberries to a horse camp and a log over the clear creek that drains the misnamed Dry Canyon. About 100 yards later is a junction with the Dry Canyon Trail.

You bear left, walk past some silvery snags in an old burn area, and make your way around the northeast shore of Upper Palisades Lake. This long, deep subalpine lake was created when a large landslide blocked the canyon and streams filled the basin behind the slide. The lake is a fairly popular goal for both hikers and equestrians, in part because it has good fishing for cutthroat trout (though it can be hard to get to the fish without a boat). Several camps are above the lake's inlet and near the outlet, but elsewhere the lakeside slopes are too steep for camping. Unfortunately, all the best campsites smell badly of horses. When you get to the lake's landslide dam, you will undoubtedly note that no outlet flows over the dam. Instead, the water emerges from a large spring partway down the ancient landslide.

From Upper Palisades Lake, you lose almost 400 feet in lazy switchbacks and come to a junction just before an unstable log bridge over Palisades Creek. You turn left, cross the bridge, and then climb about 100 feet up the opposite bank and turn to the left (downstream). About 0.5 mile from the bridge is a small log cabin and a junction at the mouth of Chicken Spring Canyon. To reach the spacious designated camping area at Chicken Spring, walk 100 yards downstream from the cabin and cross Palisades Creek on a log bridge to the camp.

If you are not going to the camping area, continue straight beside the creek. There are several little ups and downs along the way, as the trail follows the lazy stream for 1 mile to the willow-lined Lower Palisades Lake, which is a good place to fish and watch for moose. At the southwest end of this lake is a sturdy bridge over the lake's rushing outlet creek and a camp area near a junction with the Lake Canyon Trail.

You can expect crowds from here on, because the trail from Lower Palisades Lake to Palisades Creek Campground is very popular with day hikers, weekend backpackers, and equestrians. Though the people are almost always friendly, the horses leave behind smelly souvenirs in the form of an entire orchard's worth of horse apples in the middle of the trail. Surprisingly, despite all the pounding it receives, the trail has very little of the dust and erosion commonly associated with popular horse trails.

From the Lake Canyon junction, you descend a half dozen gentle switchbacks, and then make three bridged crossings of the cascading Palisades Creek as it snakes through a scenic, steep-walled gorge. After the third bridge the trail stays in the trees above the creek's north bank and travels past a series of scenic cliffs and rock outcrops in a narrow canyon. Near the bottom of the canyon you enter a noticeably drier vegetation zone, where scattered Douglas-firs, bushy Rocky Mountain maples, and twisted Rocky Mountain junipers are added to the mix of trees. About 1 mile after a final bridged crossing of the creek, the trail skirts the left side of Palisades Creek Campground to the spacious trailhead.

POSSIBLE ITINERARY

	CAMP	MILES	ELEVATION GAIN
Day 1	Lake Basin	9.0	3,300'
Day 2	Upper Canyon of South Fork Big Elk Creek	9.0	1,900'
Day 3	Big Elk Creek (at last ford)	8.0	400'
Day 4	Lake in Waterfall Canyon	10.0	3,900'
Day 5	Out	9.0	300'

BEST SHORTER ALTERNATIVE •

For an excellent weekend backpacking trip, start from the southern trailhead and make the scenic loop that goes up South Fork Indian Creek and returns via North Fork Indian Creek. Lake Basin makes a good place to spend the night. From the north trailhead the popular trail as far as Upper Palisades Lake makes a good goal. For grander scenery and fewer people, extend your hike on the trail above the lake into Waterfall Canyon.

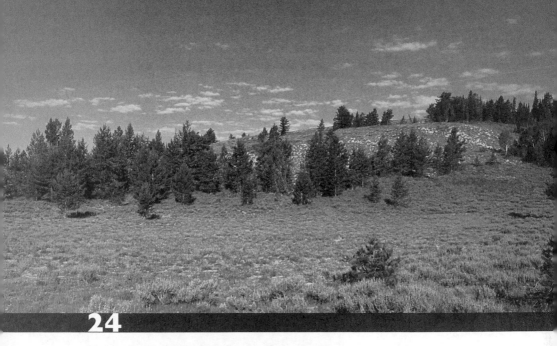

24

BEAR RIVER RANGE HIGHLINE TRAIL

> **RATINGS:** Scenery 8   Solitude 7   Difficulty 5
> **MILES:** 25 (The distance may be slightly longer for the hike, and shorter for the car shuttle, depending on how far you can drive on the access road to the north trailhead.)
> **SHUTTLE MILEAGE:** 37
> **ELEVATION GAIN:** 2,800'
> **DAYS:** 3–4
> **MAP(S):** USGS *Egan Basin*, USGS *Midnight Mountain*, USGS *Paris Peak*
> **USUALLY OPEN:** Late June–October
> **BEST:** Late June–mid-July for flowers; late September and early October for fall colors
> **PERMITS:** None
> **RULES:** The usual Leave No Trace principles apply.
> **CONTACT:** Montpelier Ranger District, 208-847-0375

SPECIAL ATTRACTIONS •

Fine views; exceptional wildflower displays late June–mid-July; fall colors

CHALLENGES •

Very limited water and campsites; mosquitoes in July; motorbikes along the entire trail

Above: Near Dry Basin

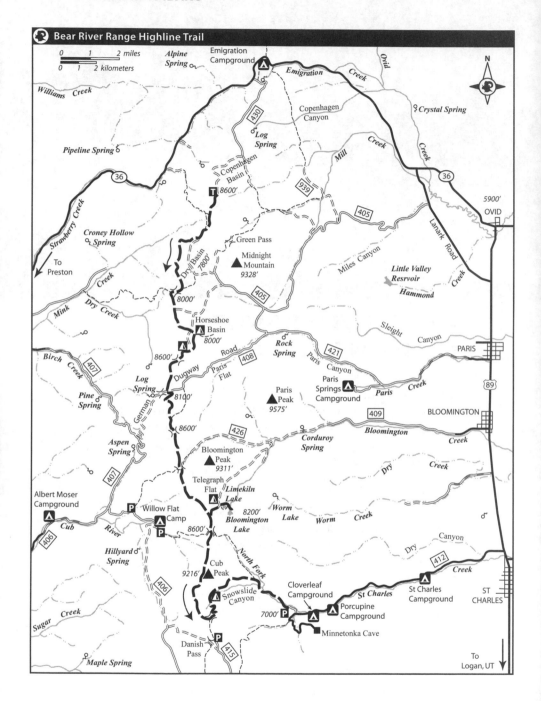

Bear River Range Highline Trail

HOW TO GET THERE •

From Montpelier, drive 6 miles southwest on US 89 to the tiny crossroads town of Ovid. To reach the exit point at the south trailhead, continue 11.3 miles south on US 89 to a well-signed junction with St. Charles Canyon Road. Turn right (west), following signs for Minnetonka Cave, and drive 8.2 miles on this paved road, which becomes Forest Service Road 412, to a junction 0.1 mile past Cloverleaf Campground. Turn right onto FS 716 and drive 0.2 mile on this narrow gravel road to the trailhead parking lot.

To reach the recommended starting point, return to Ovid and turn left (west) on ID 36. Drive 12.2 miles northwest to an unsigned junction 0.2 mile west of the pass at the summit of the Bear River Range. Turn left (south) on a paved road and proceed 200 yards toward a large snow park lot; then bear right on a dirt road (also known as FS 430). This bumpy road steeply climbs for 2 miles, and then levels off and gets increasingly rough. Unless you're driving a jeep or a high-clearance SUV, you should pull off the road and park in this area. About 3.5 miles from ID 36, you bear right at a fork and go through the huge meadow in Copenhagen Basin, which is covered with countless millions of white bistort blossoms in early July. About 1.5 extremely rough miles from the fork, the road ends at a trailhead sign. There is very limited parking here, but it doesn't really matter because you probably weren't able to drive this far anyway.

INTRODUCTION •

The Bear River Range, a northern extension of Utah's famous Wasatch Range, forms the western boundary of the popular Bear Lake Basin. Because the lower slopes of these mountains are crowded with lakeside resorts and recreation homes, it is surprising that so few people hike this range's scenic trails. After all, the Bear River Range has plenty of attractions, including view-packed ridges, open forests, and flowered-covered meadows. You'll find plenty of day hiking options, but for backpackers the best extended trip is the Highline Trail, which samples all of the diverse pleasures this range has to offer.

The most famous attraction in the Bear River Range is Minnetonka Cave. Caves like Minnetonka are typical of areas—the Bear River Range is one—with karst topography. The rock here is mostly limestone, which, unlike granite, allows water to filter down from the surface, slowly dissolving the rock as it goes. Once it gets to the cave, the dripping water deposits dissolved minerals to form stalactites and stalagmites. For hikers, the most important consequence of this geology is that when most of the water filters down from the surface, it leaves very little of that precious commodity above ground. As a result, there are very few lakes and streams to provide water to thirsty hikers. You should carry a minimum of 3 quarts from the trailhead and a lot more if you plan a dry camp for the first night—which is often a necessity.

TIP: The trail is best done from north to south, because that way you benefit from a net elevation loss of approximately 1,600 feet.

DESCRIPTION •

The Highline Trail starts as a jeep track amid lovely meadows that are framed with stands of lodgepole pines, Engelmann spruces, and white firs. The last species is found almost nowhere else in Idaho. After just 100 yards, you turn onto an obvious trail that leaves the jeep track and veers left into the trees. This trail soon enters a large, sloping meadow, which features a wide variety of colorful, July-blooming wildflowers. Of particular interest is a unique type of white columbine with unusually large blossoms that are both conspicuous and beautiful. This open meadow also has some excellent vistas, both south along the rolling Bear River Range and west to the farmlands around Preston.

WARNING: Strangely, even with so little surface water, in early July the mosquitoes can be fierce in these mountains.

Shortly after entering the meadow, ignore an unsigned motorbike track that angles in from the right and gradually descend across open slopes to a signed junction with the Snow Hollow Trail. The scenic ridgetop here is carpeted with wildflowers, especially blue lupine and yellow balsamroot, which make colorful foregrounds for some great photographs of the rolling Bear River Range. You go straight at the junction and descend about 400 feet on a wide and often dusty all-terrain vehicle track to the edge of the mostly forested Dry Basin and a junction with a jeep road.

You bear right, following a small, brown sign that says simply TRAIL, and travel mostly on the level past a delightful series of rock-garden meadows and a few less-appealing logging scars. The trail descends through a sloping meadow ringed by quaking aspens and goes up and down for 2 miles through forests and brushy meadows to a junction with the Dry Basin Trail. You bear slightly right and climb a short distance back to the scenic ridgetop.

At the top of the ridge is an unsigned junction with an obscure trail down Dry Creek. You turn left, gradually climb near the top of the ridge for 0.5 mile, and then contour across the west side of the divide on a partly forested slope, which is often covered with thousands of white columbines. At the end of the traverse you come to an open saddle, where an old jeep track crosses your trail. Go straight and hike gently up and down for 1 mile to a small, metal-roofed shack on the edge of an expansive meadow called Horseshoe Basin.

The trail crosses a primitive jeep road in this basin and goes 200 yards up a woodsy side canyon to a stagnant pond. This pond dries up by about late July, but it's the first water on the trip, and it is usually also the last water you'll see for another 7 miles. Before drinking the water, I strongly recommend that you treat it twice, first by either boiling or iodine, and then by filtering it to remove the silt and particulate matter. If you want to play it safe, carry enough water from the trailhead to make a dry camp. Some decent campsites are in the trees near the pond.

About 100 yards past the pond is a junction with a motorbike trail, which is not shown on either the U.S. Forest Service or the U.S. Geological Survey (USGS) maps. You veer right, climb over a minor ridge, and then go briefly downhill and curve to the left. Shortly after the trail starts to climb again, an unmarked, 100-yard side trail drops to the right to a lovely little meadow with a very pleasant campsite. In early summer there is sometimes a shallow, murky pond on the far side of this meadow (but don't count on it).

The Highline Trail makes a looping traverse up a forested hillside and passes two small, grassy basins, which in any other mountain range would almost certainly have water. Here they have only waving grasses and flowers. A short additional climb takes you up to a ridgeline.

The next mile is an especially appealing walk through flower-covered meadows near the top of a ridge with nice vistas to the southeast over the grassy expanse of Paris Flat. Halfway along this section is a saddle, where the trail angles left and makes a long downhill traverse. The descent is steep at first, but then it becomes quite gradual as you cross a sloping meadow liberally covered with picturesque quaking aspens. The trail splits near the bottom of the traverse under a set of power lines. Bear left and almost immediately come to the rough German Dugway Road.

You turn left, walk 20 yards along the road, and then turn right onto a dusty trail that is badly churned up by motorbikes. The trail makes one uphill switchback and gradually winds its way up through open forest and sloping meadows. As usual, there is absolutely no water on this climb, despite the fact that you will probably see a few lingering snow-fields on the ridge above the trail in July. A little more than 0.5 mile from the road you come to a pretty little basin where an unsigned motorbike trail joins from the left. You go straight, and then ascend steeply through forests to a high, grassy saddle just below the crest of the Bear River Range. This is a good spot to rest, have a snack, and enjoy the view southeast to the lofty Bloomington Peak.

TIP: For even better views, wander up the open slopes on either side of the pass to the windy summits of two small knolls.

For much of the remainder of the trip the trail goes along a beautiful open ridge, which features flowery meadows, stands of spire-shaped subalpine firs, and great views. The route stays close to the ridgecrest, so you can see not only up and down the Bear River Range, but also west to the relatively dry Bear River Valley and east to the shimmering, turquoise waters of Bear Lake. This easy, beautiful, and inspiring stroll is one of the best ridge walks in Idaho.

About 1.5 miles from the pass is a poorly signed, four-way junction in another saddle with fine views. The large meadow below you to the southeast is Telegraph Flat, but the more interesting view is southeast beyond Telegraph Flat to the rugged walls encircling the basin of Bloomington Lake. You go straight at the junction and hike 2 very scenic miles to a signed junction with the trail to Bloomington Lake.

Two factors will compel you to make the side trip to Bloomington Lake. The first is the impressive setting of the lake and a natural desire to see it up close. The second is that the lake is a permanent source of water and has good campsites nearby, both of which are extremely rare in these mountains. So turn sharply left, descend about 350 feet to a remote

MINNETONKA CAVE

Minnetonka Cave, a spectacular underground cavern filled with delicate stalactites and stalagmites, is visited by thousands of awestruck tourists every year. Discovered by a grouse hunter in 1907, the cave is now administered by the U.S. Forest Service. Because it's only a couple of miles from the south trailhead, interested hikers might want to take the 90-minute, half-mile tour after completing their hike. Guided tours run daily from June to September and they are well worth the relatively modest price. For more information call 435-245-4422.

trailhead at the end of a rough dirt road, and then walk 400 yards along this road to the signed Bloomington Lake trailhead on your right. This short trail makes a brief climb; splits to form a loop around a shallow, seasonal body of water called Limekiln Lake; and then passes a small pond and comes to Bloomington Lake.

The shimmering Bloomington Lake sits beneath a semicircle of craggy cliffs and is a great place to swim, fish, or just relax and enjoy the view. In recent years beavers have dammed the outlet creek, raising the lake's water level and flooding the angler's path around the shore. The U.S. Forest Service recently prohibited camping in the area immediately around the lake. Instead, they recommend that people camp southwest of the Bloomington Lake trailhead.

After returning to the Highline Trail, you continue south and resume the spectacular ridge walk along the crest of the Bear River Range. The trail traverses the west side of a high point and drops to a saddle where a large cairn marks a four-way junction. If you want to shorten the trip, turn left and descend 4 miles on the pleasant North St. Charles Trail to the south trailhead.

For the longer and more scenic route, go straight at the four-way junction and resume the gorgeous, up-and-down ridge hike. The remaining ridge walk is about 3.5 miles long, but the excellent scenery will make it seem like a lot less. The route never strays very far from the top of the divide, so the views in all directions are superb. The beauty at your feet is a match for the distant views, with an abundance of colorful early summer wildflowers. The most common varieties are cinquefoil, wild carrot, lupine, pink geranium, skyrocket gilia, and sulphur flower. Distracted by all this fine scenery, you will barely notice as the trail climbs high on the slopes of Cub Peak and then gradually descends to a low saddle and a signed junction with the Snowslide Trail.

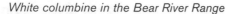

White columbine in the Bear River Range

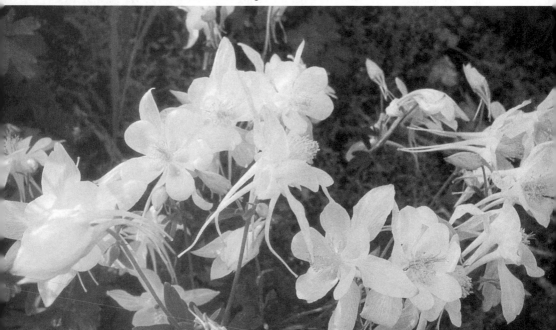

TIP: Quiet hikers may see both deer and elk in this area.

You turn left and descend four switchbacks to a partly forested basin at the head of Snowslide Canyon. Surprisingly, you'll find a creek in Snowslide Canyon, the first reliable running water on this entire trip. Just downstream from where you cross this trickling creek is a comfortable campsite at the edge of a small meadow choked with bluebells and false hellebore.

You briefly follow the tiny creek and then contour across a partly forested hillside through thickets of quaking aspen trees and ceanothus bushes. After splashing across the second of two spring-fed creeks, you make a gradual, 1-mile descent to a junction with the North St. Charles Trail. You bear slightly right and follow this wide, gently graded, and dusty trail to a bridge over Snowslide Creek and, shortly thereafter, a bridge across North Fork St. Charles Creek. You pass through a gate, and then, about 1 mile after the first crossing, come to a second bridge over North Fork St. Charles Creek. Just 300 yards later is the south trailhead and your car.

TIP: North Fork St. Charles Creek has good trout fishing.

VARIATIONS •

If you don't mind doing a fair amount of road walking, consider hiking all 55 miles of the Highline Trail from Beaver Creek, near the Utah border, to Soda Point, at the north end of the range. Unfortunately, the road access to these remote trailheads is long, rough, and complicated.

POSSIBLE ITINERARY

	CAMP	MILES	ELEVATION GAIN
Day 1	Upper Horseshoe Basin	8.0	500'
Day 2	Bloomington Lake	8.5	1,400'
Day 3	Out	8.5	900'

BEST SHORTER ALTERNATIVE •

The best short sampler here is a loop that starts from the southern trailhead. This route goes up Snowslide Canyon, follows the ridge north past Cub Peak, and returns via North Fork St. Charles Creek. Be sure to save enough energy on this loop for the excellent side trip to Bloomington Lake.

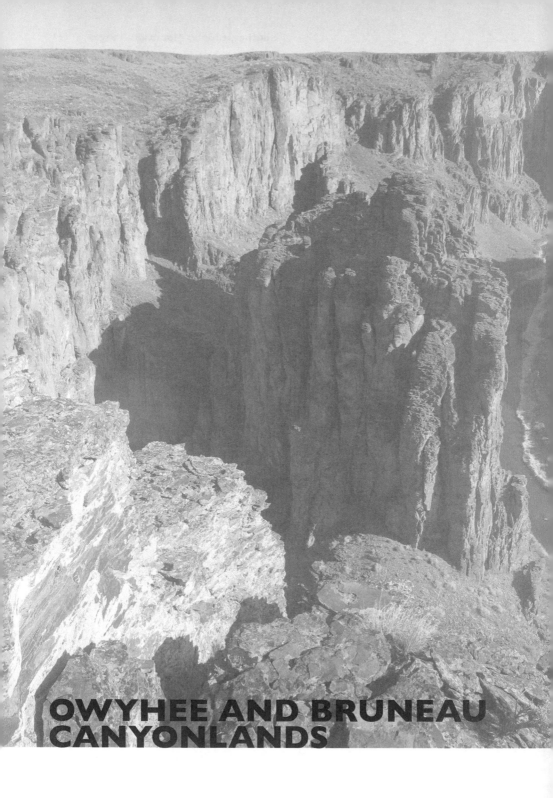

OWYHEE AND BRUNEAU CANYONLANDS

Rock tower in Owyhee River Canyon below Garat Crossing (Trip 25)

The vast deserts of southwest Idaho hide a rarely visited landscape of rolling sagebrush plains that are spectacularly broken by the deep, narrow canyons of two desert streams, the Owyhee and Bruneau Rivers. Extreme isolation and difficult access combine to ensure almost complete solitude for human visitors.

Hikers who do come here discover a harsh landscape that bears little resemblance to the scenery found in other parts of Idaho. First, unlike every other major hiking region in the state, there are no mountains here. Second, and most important, the weather is much drier.

The dry climate provides habitat for desert bighorn sheep, wild horses, badgers, sage grouse, and pronghorn, which are absent from the forested environments in the rest of the state. Birds of prey are abundant, because they find good nesting sites on the canyon rims and plenty of prey in the form of jackrabbits and desert rodents. Look for golden eagles, prairie falcons, and several species of hawks, all in greater numbers than almost anywhere else in North America. Reptile enthusiasts will discover that this desert environment is home to the highest concentration of lizards in the state. In addition, rattlesnakes, potentially dangerous reptiles, are common enough that visitors must watch their step, especially when traveling in grassy areas near water.

Water is rare in this desert realm. The occasional springs, ponds, and small streams shown on maps usually dry up by early summer and cannot be relied upon by thirsty hikers. The lack of available water forces hikers to stay in the canyons, close to major rivers. These main streams have water all year, but even that flow is highly variable. Though kayakers and rafters drool at the exciting whitewater possibilities, the rivers are runnable only in the high water of spring, and in some years there is never enough water for rafting.

Rattlesnakes and water shortages aren't the only problems posed by the desert environment. Unless you enjoy heat stroke, this is no place to hike in midsummer. Temperatures stay in the 90°–110°F range from about mid-June to early September and, except for the occasional western juniper or streamside willow, trees are nonexistent. The dominant plant species is sagebrush, which isn't exactly famous as a shade tree. Spring and fall are the most comfortable seasons for a visit.

While the absence of trees creates one problem, it is the presence of a different plant that creates another. Poison ivy is common in the stream canyons and can be hard to avoid. Hikers should consider carrying one of those new soaps or creams designed to block the plant's rash-producing toxin. A final concern is that the canyons are prone to flash floods. Thunderstorms, especially in the summer, occasionally bring large volumes of water down these narrow defiles.

A brewing environmental controversy in these canyon lands centers on the impact of military training flights. Air Force pilots routinely use this remote area for low-altitude training, often roaring by less than 100 feet above the ground. Environmentalists are concerned that the flights cause stress to the wildlife and make two-legged visitors feel like they are hiking in a war zone. The U.S. Air Force claims to do its best to minimize the impact on particularly sensitive wildlife, such as bighorn sheep, and they point out that their pilots have to practice *somewhere*. For now, the debate, and the flights, continue.

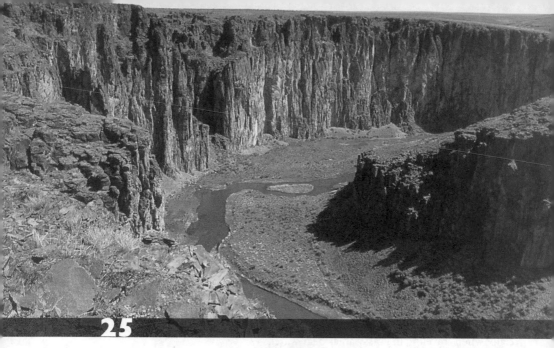

OWYHEE MEANDERS

RATINGS: Scenery 9   Solitude 10   Difficulty 8
MILES: 19+
ELEVATION GAIN: 3,400'
DAYS: 2–4
MAP(S): USGS *Jarvis Pasture,* USGS *Piute Basin East*
USUALLY OPEN: April–November
BEST: Mid-April–May, mid-September–October (Avoid the heat of midsummer.)
PERMITS: None
RULES: No specific regulations, though please follow the usual Leave No Trace principles.
CONTACT: Owyhee Field Office, Boise District, Bureau of Land Management, 208-896-5912

SPECIAL ATTRACTIONS ·

Dramatic desert canyons; excellent shoulder season hiking; almost complete isolation; abundant wildlife, especially birds

CHALLENGES ·

Rattlesnakes; extreme summer heat; limited water and campsites

Above: Meanders of Owyhee River Canyon below Garat Crossing

HOW TO GET THERE •

From Mountain Home, take ID 51 south for 92 miles to the Duck Valley Indian Reservation and the Nevada state line, where the road becomes NV 225. Continue south 0.8 mile from the sign at the state border, and then turn right (west) onto a paved road with a really tiny brown sign saying OWYHEE RIVER. This road soon curves to the north, taking you back into Idaho. After 5.3 miles the road turns to very good gravel and 0.8 mile later comes to a junction. Turn left here, following signs to OWYHEE RIVER onto a narrow but generally good gravel road that heads off into the seemingly endless sagebrush-covered desert. Follow this road for 11 miles to a signed junction. Go straight, following directions to East Owyhee River, and drive 9.8 miles to a fenced pipeline pumping station. The area immediately around the station is signed as private property, so do not park next to the station. Instead, park either a little back from the station off of the main road, or take the rough dirt road to the right (north-northeast) of the station that immediately reenters public land. If you drive carefully and the road is dry, most cars can continue for about 0.3 mile to where the road forks. Park amid the grasses and sagebrush on the side of the road here. There are no signs or amenities of any sort.

INTRODUCTION •

Don't be misled by the relatively short distances for this hike. Nearly the entire trip is off trail, and some of the route is rather rugged, so it will take you much longer to walk a mile here than on a well-maintained trail. In addition, the distance you actually cover will turn out to be much greater than the minimum distances listed here, both because you will have to walk around lots of rocks and sagebrush instead of going in a straight line, and because you will probably want to deviate from the shortest course in order to take in the superb views along the winding canyon rim. Finally, this country is so far removed from almost anywhere else in Idaho, it will take you a long time just to reach the starting point—I can't refer to it as the trailhead because there is no trail. Think of the drive as part of the adventure.

Now that those caveats are made clear, definitely take this hike. Navigating the cross-country route is relatively easy because the desert terrain is open and you can always see where you are going. More important, the scenery is tremendous, and completely different from any of the other hikes in this book. But even though it is different, you will soon discover that looking down into a steep-walled desert canyon is just as impressive as looking up at high mountains. Another bonus of hiking here is that this is one of the best early-season backpacking options in a state where most of the hiking is in mountain terrain that remains locked in the grip of heavy snows until months later than when this hike is at its best.

Note: There is some confusion about the name of the river carving the canyons on this hike. Signs along the road and most locals refer to this stream as the East Fork Owyhee River, while the U.S. Geological Survey (USGS) maps call it the main stem of the Owyhee River. For simplicity, I refer to it as the Owyhee River in this book.

WARNING: Rattlesnakes are common in this country. Be very careful where you step.

DESCRIPTION •

From the fork in the dirt road 0.3 mile north-northeast of the pumping station, take a few minutes to go straight to take in the view from the rim-top overlook into the canyon

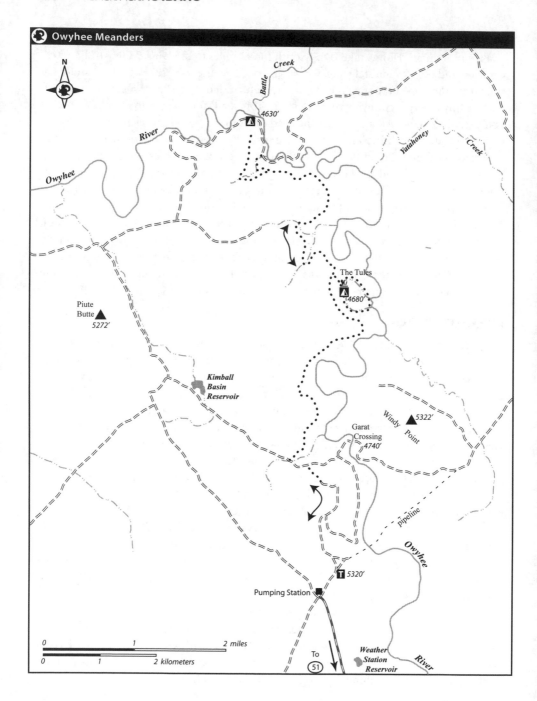

Owyhee Meanders

of the Owyhee River. It is a dramatic scene and a fine introduction to this region, even though the canyon walls here are neither as steep nor as impressive as those you will see later in the hike, and the wild character of the landscape is slightly marred by a pipeline bridge across the river below you.

The main route goes left from the road fork and follows a rough jeep road across the desert plateau. There are absolutely no trees in this dry landscape, so shade is only a distant rumor (bring a hat), but the lack of trees allows for unobstructed views. The best vistas are to the southeast of the distant snowy ramparts of Nevada's Jarbidge Mountains. Also vying for your attention, at least in early May, are the abundant desert wildflowers. Look especially for blue lupine, pink phlox, and yellow *Lomatium* and hawk's-beard.

The rough but nearly level jeep track begins, oddly, with four parallel ruts (what kind of vehicle are these people driving?) before narrowing to a more logical two ruts after 0.1 mile where another track joins in from the right. At just short of 0.7 mile a rough jeep trail angles off to the right (downhill) on its way to Garat Crossing and a very seldom used boat/kayak launch site on the Owyhee River. A sign at the junction says CAUTION: USE OF HIGH-CLEARANCE 4WD VEHICLES REQUIRED BEYOND THIS POINT (as if the rocky "road" you have been walking on up to this point was some kind of superhighway). The walk along the jeep trail down to Garat Crossing is well worth the time and effort: The launch site is in a very scenic location with reddish canyon walls and cliffs, making for a dramatic scene. It is 1.8 miles to Garat Crossing, and you will lose almost 550 feet along the way. If you go that way, you can make a shortcut back to the main route by taking a road that goes left about 0.3 mile before you get to Garat Crossing, and following it for 0.4 mile to a high point where those who take the shorter route meet this road.

For the shorter route to The Tules, go straight at the Garat Crossing turnoff, staying high on the canyon rim. A little more than 0.3 mile later the road you are following comes to a fine rim-top overlook of the Garat Crossing area. From here the route deteriorates to nothing but a wide, grassy track as it curves to the left and ends altogether after another 0.15 mile. From this location you can look down on a different jeep track that comes in from the west and that also leads to Garat Crossing. Your next objective is to make your way down to that jeep track, meeting it approximately where it tops an obvious rise. It is a fairly straightforward descent as you drop down through an obvious break in the rimrock right where the road you have been following ends. You then angle down the trailless and moderately steep slope of rock and shrubs for about 0.3 mile until you come to the road.

Turn left (west) on this rarely used "road" and follow it steeply downhill to the point where it crosses a generally dry creek bed. Leave the road here and angle a little to the right, climbing off-trail back up to the rolling top of the plateau. From here simply head north-northeast across the sagebrush-covered landscape until you reach the canyon rim where you are greeted with a jaw-dropping scene looking almost straight down to the snaking Owyhee River almost 500 feet below you. Broken cliffs and dramatic towers rise from the edge of the water, lining each side of the canyon. Across the defile you can see the long, tall rim of Windy Point, but it is straight down that will monopolize your attention. Don't be so distracted by the scenery, however, that you fail to look down at your feet. The canyon rim is very steep and a false step could be disastrous. In addition, rattlesnakes are common here. The sudden, heart-pounding sound of a reptilian rattle can make even the most hardened desert veteran jump back, with little thought for the drop-off behind them. (This very nearly happened to me, so I am not kidding here.)

Continue generally north (downstream), following the rim as the river meanders through its canyon far below. As you keep going cross-country you will have the option to save considerable mileage by crossing the gentle plateau and cutting off the wide meanders. Alternatively you can take the much more scenic route and stick with the view-packed, but wildly zigzagging canyon rim. It's your call, but if you're like me, you will find it very hard to stay away from the dramatic scenery at the edge of the drop-off. A bonus of hiking near the rim is the excellent bird-watching this provides. The desert canyons of southern Idaho have some of the highest concentrations of birds of prey in the world, and this stretch of the Owyhee River is no exception. Look for golden eagles, red-tailed hawks, turkey vultures, and prairie falcons, among many other species riding on the updrafts coming out of the canyon. Smaller birds you may see include violet-green swallows, white-throated swifts, and canyon wrens. If you stay on the plateau, you stand a good chance of seeing pronghorn antelope.

Eventually you'll come to a particularly grand overlook on the southern edge of an especially notable location in the deep canyon. Here a wide, looping meander in the river (called an oxbow) has been cut off from the main canyon where the river has carved through the canyon wall at the narrow part of the old oxbow. This has left behind a huge, cliff-edged tower that is now completely surrounded by the low area where the river either currently flows or used to go. The old course of the river in the wide oxbow is now a marshy, cattail-filled oasis called The Tules.

Though most of the canyon walls are sheer cliffs that are totally impassable to hikers, The Tules can be reached by a convenient break in the rim just to the west of the old oxbow. So to reach the fine scenery and possible campsites at The Tules, simply make your way around to the west side of the old meander and find a cairn near the top of the obvious break in the canyon rim. From here it is perfectly safe to make your way down the steep slope, losing about 400 feet to the relatively flat area beside the marsh in The Tules. There are several possible places to set up your tent in this area, all with stunning views up to the tall, multicolored walls of the canyon rising all around. You should expect a symphony of frogs and red-winged blackbirds coming from the marsh, and it is also worth spending some time to look for (but not disturb) the shy long-eared owls that often nest in the willows near the marsh.

Once your camp is comfortably established, you will undoubtedly want to do some exploring. The best itinerary is to spend a day or two from a base camp checking out the surroundings. One fairly easy option is to follow game trails around the base of the cliffs surrounding the old meander, making a loop down to the river and then back so that you completely encircle the huge tower in the middle of the old oxbow. You can fish in the river or maybe even see a whitewater rafter or kayaker go past on the way down the canyon. In most years there is enough water in the river for rafting only for a few weeks during the peak spring runoff, usually in April. Some years never see enough of a flow to support boats. If you are visiting in the fall, you can easily wade across the shallow river to explore the opposite bank.

For a much longer but even more enjoyable exploration, climb back up to the top of the rim and head north (downstream). After just a few hundred yards you will come to another excellent viewpoint of a huge meander. From there you'll have to make a wide loop around to the west to avoid the deep cut of a two-pronged side canyon before returning to the main canyon rim a little more than 1 mile as the crow flies (more than twice that as the hiker walks) north of The Tules.

The canyon continues to meander around from here, but now makes a general turn to the west, forcing you to follow suit. After about 0.7 mile of going west, another deeply incised side canyon cuts across your route. Here you have a choice. One option is to very carefully pick your way down this rocky and brushy little canyon to the flat bench beside the Owyhee River. At the bottom you can follow a jeep road to the north for about 0.4 mile to the confluence of Owyhee River and Battle Creek. This is a dramatic spot and it is possible to camp nearby, though there are parcels of private land here and it is not always easy to tell where the public land ends and the private land begins. Another option is to forgo the rough trip down the side canyon and to simply walk around the top of this side canyon to reach yet another excellent viewpoint, this time looking up the impressive canyon cut by Battle Creek as well as up and down the main canyon of the Owyhee River. Ambitious hikers can keep following the canyon rim downstream, enjoying a nearly constant string of tremendous rim-top viewpoints for as many miles and days as you desire. Most hikers, however, will likely choose to turn around at this point, having already enjoyed a superb sampling of what this remote desert region has to offer. So return to your camp at The Tules, and then back to your car the way you came.

POSSIBLE ITINERARY

	CAMP	MILES	ELEVATION GAIN
Day 1	The Tules (via Garat Crossing)	6.5	1,350'
Day 2	The Tules (day hike to Battle Creek)	8.0	1,000'
Day 3	Out (by shortest route)	4.5	1,050'

BEST SHORTER ALTERNATIVE •

It is possible to do the portion of this trip as far as The Tules as a day hike. You would need to get a pretty early start, however, which isn't easy with the long drive. A backpacking trip allows more time for exploring.

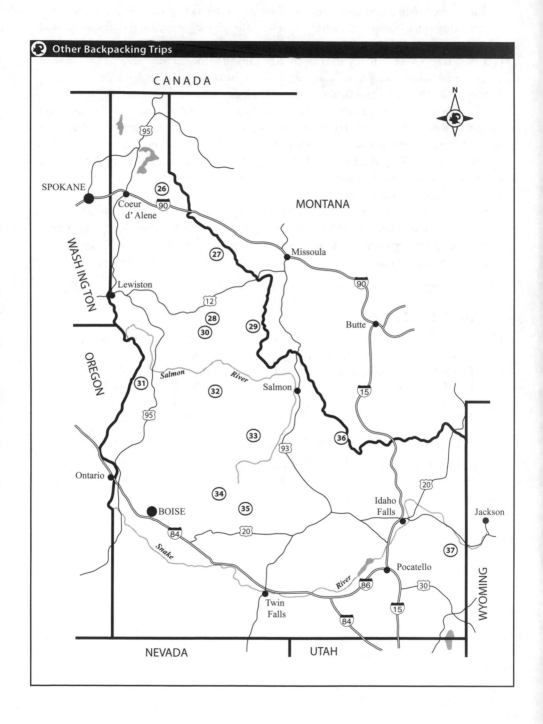

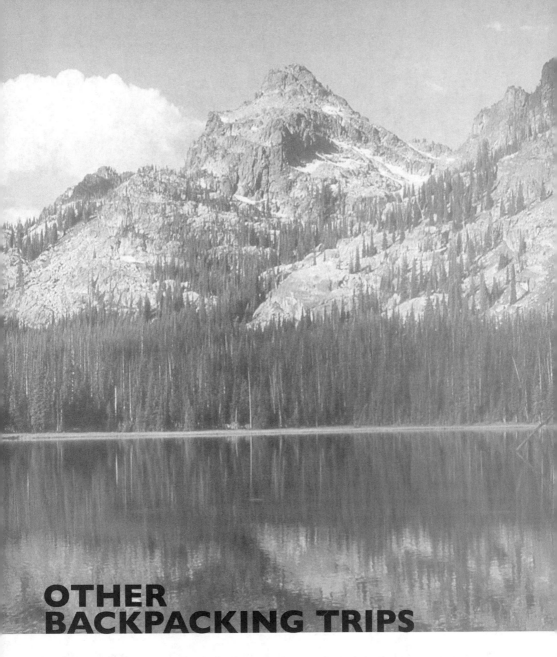

OTHER
BACKPACKING TRIPS

Though this book highlights my choices for the best longer backpacking trips in Idaho, there are many other options for the adventurous backpacker. With some creativity and a good set of topographic maps, a backpacker could spend a lifetime exploring the mountains, canyons, and deserts of this state.

What follows is an overview of some additional recommended trips, with just enough description to whet the appetite.

Above: Emerald Lake in the Southern Seven Devils Mountains (Trip 31)

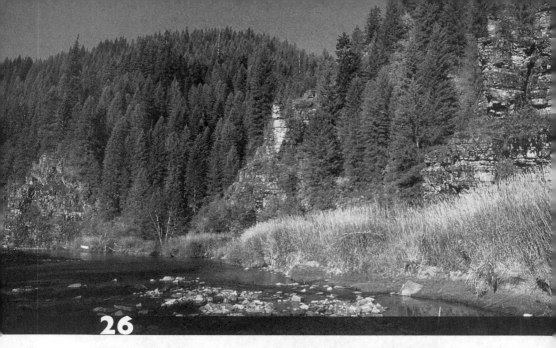

26

COEUR D'ALENE RIVER TRAIL

> **RATINGS:** Scenery 6   Solitude 5   Difficulty 3
> **MILES:** 14
> **DAYS:** 2–3
> **MAP(S):** USGS *Cathedral Peak,* USGS *Jordan Creek* (in Montana)
> **USUALLY OPEN:** May–October
> **BEST:** Mid-May–October

SPECIAL ATTRACTIONS •

Good fishing; early-season hiking

CHALLENGES •

The trail generally stays well above the river, so hikers must bushwhack to get to the water.

For most of its length, the Coeur d'Alene River is a tame stream that flows lazily through bottomlands where it is closely followed by roads. Near its headwaters, however, the river runs swift and wild through a scenic, forested canyon. A pleasant, 14-mile trail parallels this section of the river, with only one brief interruption by a logging road. The trail gives backpackers a wonderful introduction to one of the state's best fly-fishing streams, without the crowds found elsewhere on the river. But even if you aren't an angler, this relatively easy trail is worth hiking for the excellent canyon scenery. The stream is managed as a catch-and-release fishery; barbless hooks are required.

Above: Along the upper Coeur D'Alene River Trail

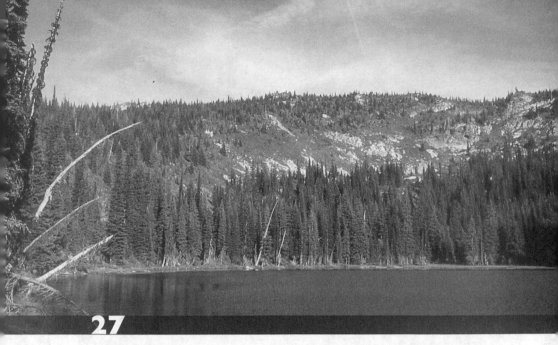

27

ST. JOE RIVER: BACON PEAK LOOP

RATINGS: Scenery 6   Solitude 7   Difficulty 6
MILES: 31
DAYS: 3–4
MAP(S): USGS *Bacon Peak,* USGS *Chamberlain Mountain,* USGS *Red Ives Peak*
USUALLY OPEN: July–mid-October
BEST: August and September

SPECIAL ATTRACTIONS ·

Huckleberries; excellent fishing

CHALLENGES ·

Two potentially difficult river fords in early summer

The strikingly beautiful and crystal-clear St. Joe River flows through a densely forested canyon and is considered one of the premier fly-fishing streams in the United States (barbless hooks and catch-and-release are both required). A wonderful trail parallels the river's upper reaches, and by adding a fun loop to the high lakes around Bacon Peak you gain wider views and better mountain scenery. The trip requires a couple of fords of the river, however, so save this trip for late summer or early fall. Conveniently, this is also when the huckleberries are ripe on the high ridges, adding pleasures for your palate to those for your eyes.

Above: Mud Lake in the upper St. Joe River area

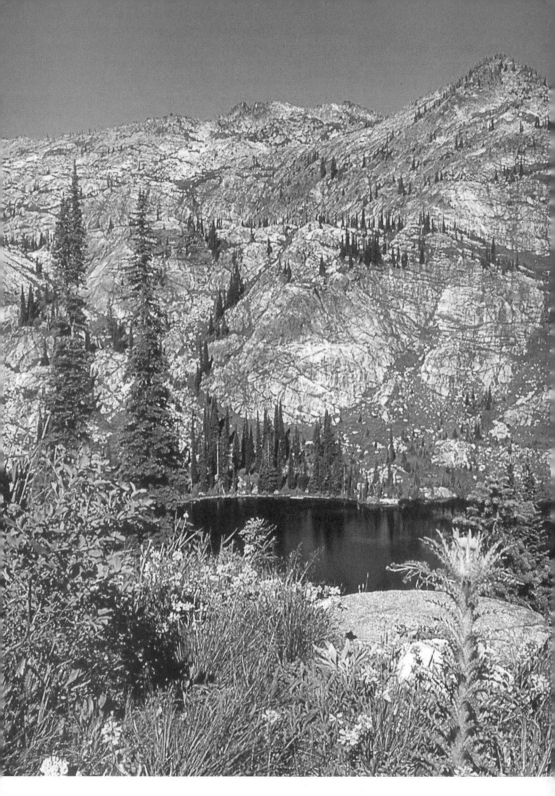

Lloyd Lake in the Selway Crags area

28

SELWAY CRAGS

RATINGS: Scenery 8   Solitude 5   Difficulty 4
MILES: Varies
DAYS: Varies
MAP(S): USFS *Selway-Bitterroot Wilderness: North Half*
USUALLY OPEN: July–mid-October
BEST: Mid- to late July

SPECIAL ATTRACTIONS •

High, craggy, granite peaks; cirque lakes

CHALLENGES •

Mosquitoes in July

This is a relatively popular hike into one of the most scenic parts of Selway-Bitterroot Wilderness. The Selway Crags feature classic mountain scenery with dozens of beautiful lakes tucked into glacial cirques amid a small group of granite peaks. There are two possible approaches to the area. The shorter and easier trail starts from Big Fog Saddle, at the end of a rugged, narrow, and steep dirt road that climbs from the Selway River Road near the Selway Falls Guard Station. The other trail is longer and much more tiring, but it starts from a good paved road, US 12, along the Lochsa River. Whichever route you choose, once you reach the Selway Crags, the best plan is to set up a base camp and spend several days exploring the area's many lakes and viewpoints. The Cove Lakes are the most popular choice for a base camp, but other nearby lakes, some off-trail, provide better scenery and more solitude. *Note:* The Crags are managed as a primitive region within the designated wilderness, so the U.S. Forest Service does not build or maintain any trails to most of the area. Over the years, however, people's boots have made numerous unofficial routes that visit most of the best lakes. These routes are not shown on any map, but they are generally easy to follow and make travel between locations relatively simple.

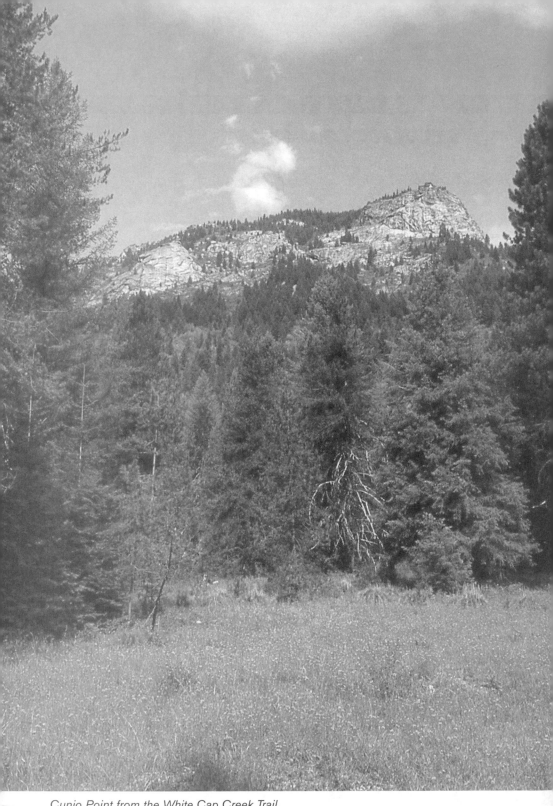

Cunio Point from the White Cap Creek Trail

29

WHITE CAP CREEK

RATINGS: Scenery 6   Solitude 8   Difficulty 5
MILES: 52
DAYS: 5–7
MAP(S): USFS *Selway-Bitterroot Wilderness: South Half*
USUALLY OPEN: July–mid-October
BEST: Mid-July–mid-August

SPECIAL ATTRACTIONS •

Solitude; wildlife

CHALLENGES •

A few rattlesnakes in the lower canyon of White Cap Creek; a very long drive from almost anywhere in Idaho

White Cap Creek is a major tributary of the Selway River and drains a significant area all the way up to the rugged Bitterroot Mountains along the Montana border. The long trail up this stream does not offer much in the way of outstanding scenery, but it does allow you to immerse yourself in the kind of solitude that just isn't possible in most of the Lower 48. The trip takes you all the way up to the creek's headwaters at a cluster of small lakes with good if not spectacular scenery. If you are looking for a place with excellent wildlife-viewing opportunities and lots of solitude, then this is the spot for you.

30

MEADOW CREEK

RATINGS: Scenery 5   Solitude 8   Difficulty 5
MILES: Varies
DAYS: Varies
MAP(S): USFS *Selway-Bitterroot Wilderness: South Half*
USUALLY OPEN: Late June–October
BEST: Late June–October

SPECIAL ATTRACTIONS •

Good fishing; wildlife

CHALLENGES •

Long car shuttle if done as a one-way hike

Meadow Creek flows out of an unprotected roadless area west of the Selway-Bitterroot Wilderness. The scenery is relatively subdued, with forested ridges on either side of the creek providing pleasant if not spectacular views. The main attractions are fishing, which is excellent, and abundant wildlife. A good trail starts near the Selway River and parallels Meadow Creek for about half the stream's length. Once the trail leaves the creek, you can either loop back to Indian Hill Lookout on view-packed ridge trails to the north and east, or make a one-way trip by going south to Red River Hot Springs. The latter exit gives you the chance to soak in the soothing hot water before making the dusty drive back to civilization.

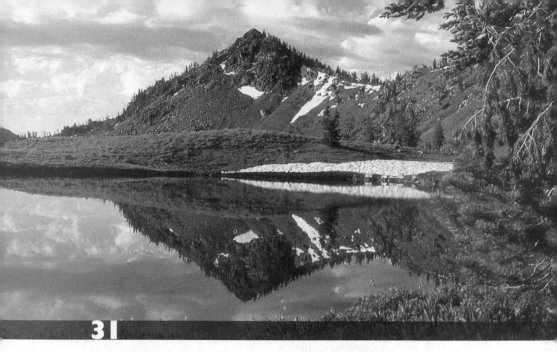

31

SOUTHERN SEVEN DEVILS MOUNTAINS

RATINGS: Scenery 7   Solitude 7   Difficulty 6
MILES: 24
DAYS: 3–5
MAP(S): USFS *Hells Canyon National Recreation Area and Wilderness*
USUALLY OPEN: July–October
BEST: July

SPECIAL ATTRACTIONS ·

High, craggy, peaks; cirque lakes; solitude

CHALLENGES ·

Mosquitoes in July; rough road access

Though not as well known as the loop through the northern Seven Devils Mountains (Trip 6), the Southern Seven Devils have a wonderful loop trail of their own with similarly grand scenery. This trip starts at the remote Black Lake Campground, at the end of a long, rough dirt road from the town of Council. From here, most hikers head west to Six Lake Basin, but to do the loop, you go north past the beautiful Emerald Lake, and then circle east around the craggy towers of Monument Peak and Black Imp. Excellent side trips lead to the spectacular Ruth Lake and the well-named Crystal Lake, the latter requiring a cross-county scramble.

Above: Pyramid Peak over a pond near Purgatory Saddle

32

BIG CREEK

RATINGS: Scenery 6   Solitude 5   Difficulty 3
MILES: 26
DAYS: 3–5 (one way)
MAP(S): USFS *Frank Church–River of No Return Wilderness: North Half*
USUALLY OPEN: April–October
BEST: Late June–October

SPECIAL ATTRACTIONS •

Excellent fishing; good canyon scenery

CHALLENGES •

Hot weather in midsummer; difficult transportation logistics

B eginning from the alternate trailhead for Trip 8, this is an easy, extended walk along the entire length of Big Creek, a first-class fishing stream that knifes through the heart of Frank Church–River of No Return Wilderness. In addition to fishing, hikers can gawk at the canyon scenery and watch the abundant wildlife. Snow usually blocks the road to the upper trailhead until late June or early July, so even though the lower parts of this trail are open as early as April, accessing the trail at that time requires either taking a long float trip down the Middle Fork Salmon River or hiring a bush plane to fly you into a remote airstrip.

After hiking downstream to the mouth of Big Creek, you face the prospect of either going back the way you came or finding another way out. Some people elect to make the long hike out on the relatively easy Middle Fork Salmon River Trail (see Trip 11). Others opt for the shorter but much more difficult Waterfall Trail, which makes a tortuous climb out of the canyon and exits through the Bighorn Crags to the east (see Trip 9). For a change of pace, you can also arrange to be picked up by a bush plane or float back to civilization on a raft. Both options are fun but rather expensive.

33

SLEEPING DEER MOUNTAIN: MIDDLE FORK SALMON LOOP

RATINGS: Scenery 7 Solitude 7 Difficulty 7
MILES: 32
DAYS: 3–4
MAP(S): USFS *Frank Church–River of No Return: South Half*
USUALLY OPEN: July–October
BEST: July–September

SPECIAL ATTRACTIONS ·

Solitude; dramatic fire lookout; fine canyon scenery; wildlife

CHALLENGES ·

Long drive on a narrow dirt road to reach the trailhead; lots of climbing to come back out of the canyon of Middle Fork Salmon River

S leeping Deer Mountain is a tall and impressive peak near the southeast corner of the enormous Frank Church–River of No Return Wilderness. A fire lookout sits at the top of this distinctive peak, and it's only a short walk from the end of a long dirt road. After such a tortuous drive to get to this area, however, it is much more satisfying to explore more of this remote and scenic region by taking a wonderful backpacking loop. The recommended route heads north on view-packed but little-used trails to Woodtick Summit and Grouse Lake before making a long, steep drop to the Middle Fork Salmon River near Tappan Falls. Loop back to your starting point via the trail up Cache Creek.

34

LEGGIT LAKE: MATTINGLY CREEK LOOP

RATINGS: Scenery 8   Solitude 6   Difficulty 8
MILES: 33
DAYS: 3–4
MAP(S): Earthwalk Press *Hiking & Map Guide: Sawtooth Wilderness, ID*
USUALLY OPEN: July–early October
BEST: Mid-July–September

SPECIAL ATTRACTIONS •

Excellent lake and canyon scenery; solitude

CHALLENGES •

Only experienced and confident hikers should attempt the difficult and challenging, 3-mile, off-trail section between Leggit Lake and the South Fork of Ross Fork River.

S tarting from a trailhead a little above the old gold-mining town of Atlanta in the upper reaches of the Middle Fork Boise River, this difficult but very scenic loop trip offers you a chance to explore a lesser-known part of the Sawtooth Mountains. The trip first follows a maintained trail to the beautiful Leggit Lake, and then forces you to climb off-trail over a couple of steep and rocky passes to the small but extremely scenic Ross Fork Lakes. From there you drop down to the little-used trail along Ross Fork River, climb over a pass to the north, and loop back along Mattingly Creek's deep and impressive canyon. There is a lot of fine scenery and variety for you to enjoy, but this trip should only be attempted by those who are skilled in cross-country travel.

35

SMOKY MOUNTAINS LOOP

RATINGS: Scenery 7   Solitude 8   Difficulty 6
MILES: Varies
DAYS: 4–6
MAP(S): USGS *Baker Peak*, USGS *Frenchman Creek*, USGS *Galena*,
   USGS *Paradise Peak*
USUALLY OPEN: Late June–October
BEST: July

SPECIAL ATTRACTIONS

Solitude; wildflowers

CHALLENGES

Motorcycles are allowed on some trails.

Though they are located relatively close to Idaho's largest population centers, the Smoky Mountains remain unknown to most Idaho outdoor lovers. In almost every way, these rolling, forested mountains are overshadowed by the neighboring Sawtooth Range. Unlike the Sawtooths, the Smokies have almost no lakes and few spectacular peaks. But even though they fall short in these important qualities, that doesn't mean they deserve to be ignored. Open forests, extensive views, colorful wildflowers, and solitude are more than enough to make a trip here worthwhile. For proof, try any of several possible loops that start from the Big Smoky Guard Station north of Fairfield. Probably the best trip goes up Smoky and Big Peak Creeks all the way to the scenic Baker Lake, which is about the only location in these mountains that sees many hikers. From there, you circle back to the north and west via Royal Gorge, West Fork Big Smoky Creek, and Skillern Creek to your starting point.

TIP: A side trip from Skillern Creek to the tiny Paradise Lake is well worth your time.

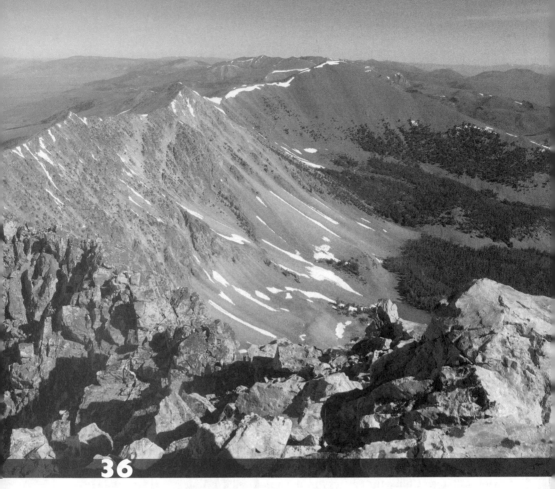

36

CONTINENTAL DIVIDE TRAIL

RATINGS: Scenery 7   Solitude 6   Difficulty 7

MILES: 57–85

DAYS: 5–9

MAP(S): USGS *Bannock Pass,* USGS *Deadman Lake,* USGS *Deadman Pass,* USGS *Eighteenmile Peak,* USGS *Morrison Lake,* USGS *Tepee Mountain* (all in Montana. Unfortunately, the recently completed trail sections are not shown on these USGS maps.)

USUALLY OPEN: Late June–October

BEST: Late June (to avoid the cows)

Above: The Continental Divide stretching north from Eighteenmile Peak

SPECIAL ATTRACTIONS •

Great views; lovely mountain scenery

CHALLENGES •

Some walking on primitive roads and incomplete trails; cows are allowed to graze in the high meadows in July.

O nce complete, the Continental Divide Trail will go 3,200 miles through America's Rocky Mountains from Mexico to Canada. Only a small section of this classic trail is in Idaho, where it travels through the Centennial and Bitterroot Mountains along the border with Montana. Some of the trail is still under construction, so hikers occasionally have to walk on primitive roads or travel cross-country. Construction is complete, however, on one particularly attractive section, where you can enjoy some great scenery.

Start at Bannack Pass, northwest of Dubois, and travel north through the Beaverhead Mountains to the recommended exit point at Bannock Pass (it's pronounced the same, but spelled differently). If you want more exercise, continue north from Bannock Pass to Lemhi Pass, where Lewis and Clark first crossed the Continental Divide. Don't miss the side trip into the ruggedly beautiful Italian Peaks, not far from the starting point.

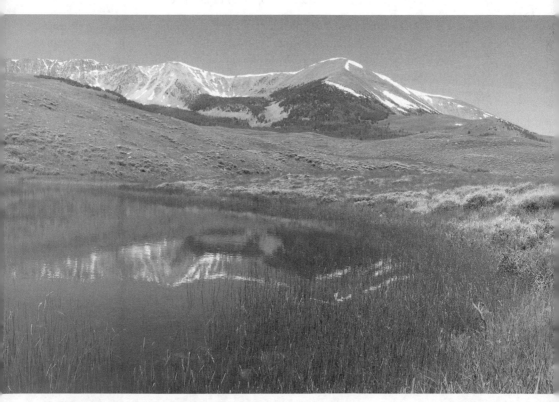

Cottonwood Peak over First Harkness Lake

3/

CARIBOU MOUNTAINS

RATINGS: Scenery 6   Solitude 7   Difficulty 6
MILES: Varies
DAYS: Varies
MAP(S): USGS *Commissary Ridge*, USGS *Palisades Dam*, USGS *Red Ridge*
USUALLY OPEN: Late June–October
BEST: July, late September, early October

SPECIAL ATTRACTIONS •

Excellent fall colors; solitude

CHALLENGES •

Lots of hunters in October; many trails are open to motorbikes.

There are many miles of interconnected trails in the Caribou Mountains southeast of Idaho Falls, and a hiker could spend several weeks happily traveling all of them. Those efforts would be especially rewarding in the fall, when the maples, willows, cottonwoods, and quaking aspens turn the hillsides into a colorful palette of yellow, red, and orange. The scenery is more subdued than in the nearby Snake River Range to the east, but wildlife is more abundant here and, except for hunters, people are few. No one trail is better than another, but most hikers start at the Bear Creek trailhead near Palisades Dam and select from any of several possible loops to viewpoints atop Red Peak and Deadhorse Ridge.

INDEX

ABOUT THE AUTHOR

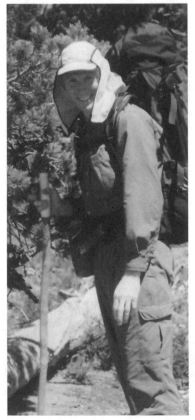

photographed by Becky Lovejoy

Douglas Lorain's family moved to the Northwest in 1969, and he has been obsessively hitting the trails of his home region ever since. Spurred by an unquenchable thirst for new trails to explore and a great enthusiasm for backpacking, he has now hiked more than 30,000 miles through every corner of the American Northwest and many thousands more in other western states and Canadian provinces. Despite a history that includes being charged by grizzly bears (twice!), being bitten by a rattlesnake, being shot at by a hunter, and donating gallons of blood to mosquitoes, Lorain claims that he wouldn't trade one moment of it because he has also been blessed to see some of the most beautiful scenery on Earth.

His other books for Wilderness Press include *Afoot & Afield Portland/Vancouver, Backpacking Oregon, Backpacking Washington, Backpacking Wyoming, One Best Hike: Mount Rainier's Wonderland Trail, One Night Wilderness: Portland,* and *Top Trails: Olympic National Park & Vicinity.* Lorain is a photographer and recipient of the National Outdoor Book Award. His photos have appeared in numerous magazines, calendars, and books.